THE L[illegible] SMALLPOX

TRAGEDY IN BIRMINGHAM

ISBN: 9781980455226

Cover image shows the centrifugal rash of smallpox on a female.
Image source: https://pixabay.com/en/female-woman-figure-standing-lady-24482/ CC0 Creative commons

If you believe you can add value to subsequent editions of this book or want to share information and insights on the 1978 smallpox incident, please visit: fb.me/lastdaysofsmallpox

ABOUT THE AUTHOR

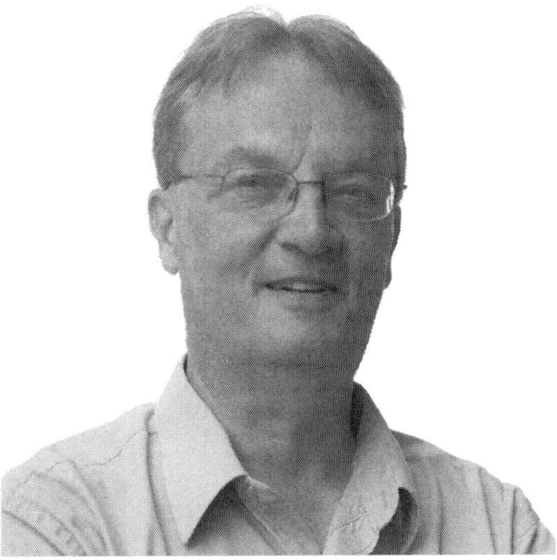

Mark Pallen is a Research Leader at the Quadram institute in Norwich and Professor of Microbial Genomics at the University of East Anglia. He completed his undergraduate medical education in Cambridge and London and his specialist training in microbiology at St Bartholomew's Hospital. While working on a PhD at Imperial College in the mid-1990s, Mark led a team to victory in the TV quiz show University Challenge. Shortly afterwards, he gained his first professorship at Queen's University Belfast, before taking up a chair at the University of Birmingham in 2001. During his twelve years in Birmingham, Mark developed a keen interest in the 1978 smallpox incident.

Mark's academic interests include microbial genomics, bioinformatics, ancient DNA, public understanding of science (particularly evolution) and the life and legacy of Charles Darwin. He is the author of the Rough Guide to Evolution. Mark is married with four children and two dogs and divides his time between Worcestershire and East Anglia.

THE LAST DAYS OF SMALLPOX

TRAGEDY IN BIRMINGHAM

MARK PALLEN

Dedicated to the memory of Janet Parker
And to all victims of smallpox

Dedicated to the memory of Henry Bedson
And to all who fought to end
The horror that was smallpox

Most world-historic events—great military battles, political revolutions—are self-consciously historic to the participants living through them. They act knowing that their decisions will be chronicled and dissected for decades or centuries to come. But epidemics create a kind of history from below: they can be world-changing, but their participants are almost invariably ordinary folk, following their established routines, not thinking for a second about how their actions will be recorded for posterity. And of course, if they do recognize that they are living through a historical crisis, it's often too late—because, like it or not, the primary way that ordinary people create this distinct genre of history is by dying.
Steven Johnson (2006) *The Ghost Map*

There is not the least reason in the world why we should not be very proud of the fact that these Britons have been in the forefront of this research, have been in the forefront of eradicating smallpox from the world, and men like Professor Bedson and his three colleagues are the men who were there, as it has been described in this case, pushing back the frontiers of scientific and medical knowledge to bring about these wonderful things, following in a fine tradition that this country can be proud of.
Brian Escott-Cox QC, summing up in *Cook v. University of Birmingham*, 1979

CONTENTS

Part One

Origins

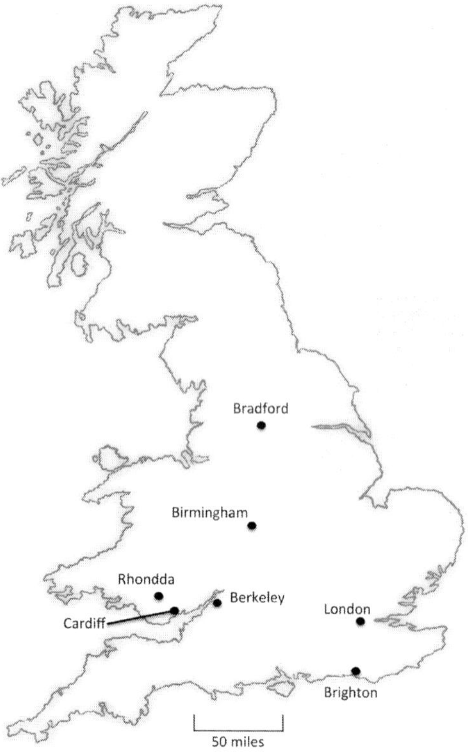

SMALLPOX IN GREAT BRITAIN
Showing Jenner's village of Berkeley
and the sites of selected twentieth-century outbreaks.

1

FROM BERKELEY TO BIRMINGHAM

You have erased from the calendar of human afflictions one of its greatest. Yours is the comfortable reflection that mankind can never forget that you have lived. Future nations will know by history only that the loathsome smallpox has existed and by you has been extirpated.
Thomas Jefferson (1806), writing to Edward Jenner[1]

ENGLAND'S M5 MOTORWAY is not particularly notable. It was not the country's first motorway to be built, nor is it the longest. But it has a hidden importance, as it links the Gloucestershire village of Berkeley to Britain's second largest city, Birmingham: the beginning-of-the-end and the end-of-the-end of smallpox. Historically, a full one hundred and eighty-two years separate Berkeley from Birmingham, but by a curious twist of fate, geographically they are less than sixty-six miles apart—a short drive of just an hour and twenty-three minutes, most of it along the M5.

The beginning-of-the-end of smallpox came on 14 May 1796, when, at his home in Berkeley[2], the English scientist Edward Jenner inoculated James Phipps, the eight-year-old son of his gardener, with material from cowpox blisters on the hand of a cowgirl, Sarah Nelmes.[3] A short while later, he challenged the boy with material from a smallpox patient and found that the boy was protected against the deadly infection. In so doing, he invented the practice of *vaccination* and initiated a chain of events that led to the eradication of smallpox.[4] Just ten years later, Thomas Jefferson, founding father of the American Republic, wrote in his prophetic letter to Jenner 'Future generations will know by history only that the loathsome smallpox existed.'

However, Jefferson was being presumptuous. Smallpox killed millions between Berkeley and Birmingham. It took a worldwide effort to chase it from the dry uplands of Ethiopia, from the swampy marshlands of Bangladesh, from the scenic coastline of Somalia. It cost billions of dollars. Millions of people played their part.

Triumph came, when the last naturally occurring case of smallpox was diagnosed in the hospital cook, Ali Maow Maalin, in the picturesque seaport of Merca, Somalia, on 26 October 1977.

IN AUGUST 1978, the smallpox virus crept like a thief in the night from a laboratory in Birmingham to re-inhabit human flesh and blood. What happened next has all the hallmarks of a Greek drama or Shakespearean tragedy, with the shocking, mysterious appearance of a dreaded disease in the heart of England; a frantic effort to save a university, a city and the world from disaster; a tragic heroine, who suffered a terrifying fate; and a persecuted protagonist, driven to mortifying despair, treated as a scapegoat during an official inquiry, but later exonerated in a court of law.

In this book, the reader will learn what happened when smallpox struck Birmingham in that fateful summer of 1978. However, to understand what happened in Birmingham—and what might have happened—we first need some context.

In Part One, we explore the origins and history of smallpox. In Part Two, we learn what happened when this viral trickster repeatedly struck the people of Britain during the twentieth century. In Part Three, we tell the heady story of smallpox eradication—a towering achievement put at risk by the events in Birmingham. Part Four provides a detailed account of the 1978 outbreak, drawn from records of the time and reminiscences of those who lived through it. Part Five describes the official investigation into the outbreak. Part Six documents the court case that largely discredited the official account. Finally, in Part Seven, we end with a look at what has happened to smallpox since 1978 and the many resonances between then and now.

Let us start in Birmingham, forty years before that tragic last summer of smallpox.

2

A CHILD IS BORN

The smallpox was always present, filling the churchyards with corpses, tormenting with constant fears all whom it had stricken, leaving on those whose lives it spared the hideous traces of its power, turning the babe into a changeling at which the mother shuddered, and making the eyes and cheeks of the bighearted maiden objects of horror to the lover.
T.B. Macaulay (1848) *The History of England from the Accession of James the Second.*

WE ARE IN BIRMINGHAM, England, early in 1938. The world is on the brink of a World War. A baby girl, called Janet, is born to Hilda Witcomb and her husband Frederick.[1] Smallpox still looms large on the world stage, menacing every continent and almost every country.[2] In a broad swathe of territories bounding the Tropics, from Brazil via sub-Saharan Africa and the Indian subcontinent to Indo-China, the most severe form of smallpox, *variola major*, is still a clear and present danger, killing 15–30% of those it infects. Those not killed are often left blind or horribly scarred for life. Curiously, in the early twentieth century, a milder form of the disease, *variola minor* or *alastrim*, with a death rate of less than 1%, has taken root in the West.

For generation after generation, smallpox has been a recurrent threat—an acute contagious disease, characterised by a fever and a rash (the *pocks*).[3] Only humans catch smallpox, usually through direct contact with another human. In its classical presentation, smallpox tracks a reliable course, with an incubation period of around twelve days, during which patients are not infectious and feel and look fine. This is followed, for a few days, by a prostrating flu-like illness, with a high fever, headache, backache and vomiting. Then, a rash appears, starting in the mouth, but within a day or so severely affecting the face, spreading lightly across the trunk and limbs to engulf the hands and feet. This concentration on peripheral sites makes it a *centrifugal* rash, in contrast to the *centripetal* rash of chickenpox, which is most dense on the trunk.

The spots progress through a predictable series of changes: starting out as flat and red *macules* that by day two become raised solid circumscribed bumps known as *papules,* which may have a dent in the centre. By day three or four, the papules fill with clear fluid to become *vesicles*. Within a couple more days, the spots fill up with cloudy fluid to become round, firm *pustules*, which sit like pearls embedded deep within the skin. In the severest cases, the pustules fuse together to produce *confluent smallpox*. If the patient survives, within a fortnight after the rash appears, the pustules empty and crust over to form scabs, which flake off, leaving permanent pitted scars—the *pockmarks*.

Sometimes smallpox takes a nastier more lethal course: as *malignant smallpox*, characterised by a low velvety rash and toxic shock, or *haemorrhagic smallpox*, where patients bleed out from the mouth, bowels, bladder or vagina.

IN THE YEAR of Janet's birth, globally, there are still tens of millions of cases and millions of deaths from smallpox. With smallpox packed into humans of every creed and colour, the planet carries a viral load of variola that tops three thousand million million virus particles—there are ten thousand times more smallpox virus particles on Earth than there are stars in our home galaxy, the Milky Way.[4]

But within the lifetime of that baby girl, every viral star in the variola firmament will be extinguished. And Janet and her birthplace, Birmingham, will play their own tragic part in this story.

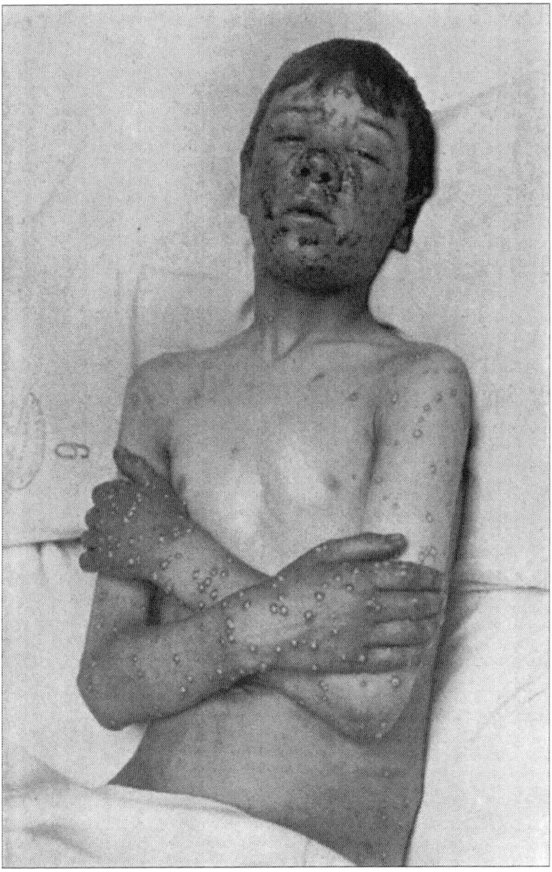

SMALLPOX RASH ON AN ADOLESCENT MALE
Note how the trunk is spared and the tense pearly appearance of the pustules.
{Source: Ricketts (1908)}

3

PERSONAL INTERLUDE

END OF THE STEADY STATE

The summer of 1978 marks a major transition in my life: the end of school. As a thirteen-years habit suddenly ends, a school friend sums it up with the phrase 'end of the steady state'. I am going to start studying medical sciences at Fitzwilliam College, University of Cambridge in October, but that leaves a long hiatus, which I fill with work at a local geriatric hospital—my experience of medicine starts quite literally at the bottom, cleaning the backsides of elderly folk.

I have no personal memory of the Birmingham smallpox incident that summer. However, I do have a clear recollection of explaining to someone how impressed I was that the World Health Organization had eradicated smallpox and how this had informed my choice of career.

At university, I decorated the wall of my student room with a picture of a bifurcated needle cut out of a magazine to celebrate the triumph of eradication. A few years later, I remember one of my former class mates boasting that he was so nerdy that he had even bought a copy of the Shooter Report into the 1978 smallpox incident.

Smallpox then slipped out of my consciousness for a couple of decades. However, looking back, it is clear that, even as a young man, I counted the eradication of smallpox as one of the crowning triumphs of the human intellect and of human endeavour—and I still do!

4

VIRUS WORLD

LOUIS PASTEUR IS BURIED in a neo-Byzantine chapel in the heart of Paris.[1] This august setting is amply justified, as this French scientist ushered in one of the greatest advances in human thought—*the germ theory of infection*: the notion that invisible microscopic organisms cause disease in humans, plants and animals.[2] The walls of Pasteur's crypt are lined with exquisite marble, above which sit mosaics illustrating vignettes from his productive life. The final mosaic highlights Pasteur's work on vaccination against rabies, with a vivid representation of the shepherd Jean-Baptiste Jupille struggling against a rabid dog.[3]

Pasteur saved Jupille's life, but the scientist remained puzzled by rabies. He could grow the causative agents of most of the infectious diseases on which he worked and use a microscope to visualise them—these agents we now call bacteria. However, the cause of rabies eluded him—and for good reason, as we now know it was caused by a virus rather than a bacterium.[4]

Pasteur's associate, Charles Chamberland, invented a filter, made from porcelain, that could be used to remove microbes from a liquid suspension. Initially, it was thought that such filters could retain all infectious agents. However, in 1892, Dmitri Ivanowski, working in St Petersburg, used a filter on an extract of plants with tobacco mosaic disease and showed that, even after filtration, the extract remained infectious. Six years later, the Dutch scientist Martinus Beijerinck, after similar experiments, proposed the idea of a new kind of infectious agent, which he termed *filterable virus*, that was much smaller than bacteria and would grow only in the presence of living cells. The adjective was soon dropped and modern usage of the term *virus* became widespread. In 1906, the Italian pathologist, Adelchi Negri, showed that Jenner's vaccine was a filterable virus and in 1925, British microbiologist Mervyn Gordon wrote an authoritative report on the viral nature of the germ causing smallpox.[5]

However, what, aside from size, makes viruses different from bacteria?

VIRUSES ARE LIKE ZOMBIES—they are not quite dead, not quite alive, and to keep going, they have to feed on living flesh.[6] It is tempting to dismiss viruses as 'infectious chemicals', rather than as 'properly living things'—because properly living things are made of cells, membrane-bound bags of lively chemical reactions. Properly living things are like engines, turning over energy. They have a metabolism. Properly living things eat and excrete. Viruses don't do that. Instead, viruses feed off living cells: they are energy parasites.

It is worse than that. Cells make their own proteins in complex specialised molecular factories called ribosomes. Every cell makes its own ribosomes and is heir to an unbroken lineage of ribosomal genes, passed from mother to daughter cell stretching back more than three billion years to the very dawn of cellular life. Viruses have no ribosomes of their own—instead, they are freeloaders, hijacking the protein factories of the host cells to get their own proteins made.

The most destructive viruses live a nomadic lifestyle. Of no fixed abode, they take over cells, trash them and move on. Each infected cell falls victim to a viral flash mob, as the orderly molecular society of the cell is press-ganged into the creation and provision of virus factories, spewing out fresh virus particles.

Not all viruses are quite so riotous. Some domesticate their host cell, causing it to create new virus particles, without trashing it. Some turn into sleepers, lying dormant for decades; others integrate themselves so deeply into their host cell that they effectively become part of it. A large portion of the human genome is formed from the remnants of such *endogenous viruses*, which have acted as a crucible of evolution, for example, in driving the evolution of the mammalian placenta.[7]

When one thinks of the magnificence of life on Earth, viruses do not spring to mind. How can something seen only with a powerful microscope compare to the grandeur of a blue whale or a soaring majesty of a giant redwood, the rich vibrancy of the Amazonian rain forest or the kaleidoscopic glory of a coral reef? Yet, when it comes to sheer numbers, viruses are the dominant biological entity on our planet. In environment after environment, viruses have turned out to be far more abundant than the cells that they prey upon. Each millilitre of ocean water contains several million virus particles[8]—a global total of 10 followed by 30 noughts!

While we can argue about whether we should call viruses 'minimal life forms' or 'infectious chemicals', one thing is clear: they contain genes, the units of genetic information encoded in the molecule DNA or its close cousin RNA. Some viruses carry only a handful of genes: the Ebola virus can kill a man with only eight genes. By contrast, the variola virus that causes smallpox is a whopper, with around two hundred genes.[9]

Where did viruses come from? There is no evidence that all viruses have a common ancestor, so the viral lifestyle may have arisen more than once.[10] There are currently three potential explanations for their origins. According to the *degeneracy hypothesis*, viruses evolved from small cells that parasitised larger cells and then lost genes that enabled them to survive outside a cell. In support of this, there are many kinds of bacteria that live inside other cells and depend on them for their survival: for example *Chlamydia,* which causes sexually transmitted infection. However, when you look closely, such cellular parasites do not really resemble viruses.

An alternative explanation comes from the *escape hypothesis*, which posits that viruses evolved from genes that escaped from the genome of a larger organism to became autonomous and infectious. In the case of the smallpox virus and its relatives, there are dozens of genes involved in subverting the host's immune system that appear to have been stolen from their vertebrate hosts.[11] However, this hypothesis does not account for the origins of the specifically viral genes that have no counterparts in cellular life.

That brings us on to a third explanation: *the virus-first hypothesis*, which claims that viruses hail from a time before cells first appeared on the Earth. This line of thinking gained impetus with the discovery of a giant virus called mimivirus in an unlikely setting—living inside amoebae inside a cooling tower in the English city of Bradford.[12] Mimivirus is remarkable not just for the hefty size of its viral particles and of its genome—in which it matches bacteria—but also because it carries genes for protein synthesis and metabolism. In the light of these findings, a provocative new theory has emerged, in which the smallpox virus is now seen as a diminutive giant virus, a remnant of a primordial viral world that pre-dated the world of cells.[13]

So, with a deep ancestry blended with a recently acquired toolkit for subverting the immune system, the smallpox virus represents a well-honed blend of ancient and modern—a miniscule machine perfectly adapted to infect humans. But how, when and where did this virus first spillover into our species?

5

OUT OF AFRICA

And on the pedestal these words appear:
'My name is Ozymandias, king of kings:
Look on my works, ye Mighty, and despair!'
Percy Bysshe Shelley (1818) *Ozymandias*

Semper aliquid novi Africam adferre
(Africa always brings something new).
Pliny the Elder (c. 76 CE) *Historia Naturalis Book 8, Section 42*

THERE IS NOT MUCH notable about the reign of Ramesses V.[1] It lasted barely four years: from 1149 to 1145 BCE. He was certainly no match for his great ancestor, Ramesses II, the Ozymandias of poetic fame, who died six decades earlier. Nor was he one of the pharaohs that made it into the Bible. His was a time of instability in Egypt, threatened by Libyan raiders. Perhaps the only notable event during his time in charge was an extensive census recorded on what is now called the Wilbour Papyrus.

However, Ramesses V made it into the history books—not from the course of his life, but from the nature of his death. His mummy was re-discovered in 1898. Soon afterwards, in 1911, the pioneering Anglo-German palaeopathologist Marc Armand Ruffer published a research note on the mummy, suggesting the 'probable existence of smallpox as evidenced by as characteristic an eruption as the conditions of preservation of such ancient material permits.'[2]

Later authorities agreed with this conclusion, reporting 1–5 mm pustules on the pharaoh's lower face, neck, shoulders, arms, lower abdomen and scrotum, with an absence of rash on the chest and upper abdomen.[3] In 1979, veteran of the eradication campaign, Donald Hopkins, subjected some tiny pieces of the mummy's skin to electron microscopy. Although Hopkins failed to see any poxvirus particles, after seeing the rash first hand, he was convinced it was smallpox.

Ramesses V marks the first tangible evidence of smallpox in humans—but where did he get smallpox from? In fact, where does anyone get smallpox from? The textbook answer is that you catch smallpox from someone else who has smallpox. More precisely: you usually catch it when you have had face-to-face contact with someone with smallpox. That was the assumption during the eradication campaign—and it was an assumption that, by and large, worked.

How far back can you push this assumption? Some of the pathogens and parasites that bother humans—including head and body lice and the herpes virus that causes cold sores—go back in an unbroken chain of transmission to the birth of our species and beyond.[4] However, smallpox isn't one of them. There is no equivalent of smallpox in our closest relatives, the great apes.

Numerous viruses circulate among wild animals and repeatedly spill over into humans—examples include Ebola, influenza and sudden acute respiratory syndrome (SARS).[5] Most of the time these immigrant viruses meet a dead end, unable to move from one human to another effectively enough to be maintained within our species. Yet, sometimes they do adapt, slot into a new lifestyle and even colonise the globe, benefitting from the way humans crowd together in cities and move across long distances. The most notorious example is HIV—human immunodeficiency virus, the cause of AIDS—which spilt over into humans from our primate cousins and, in little more than a half century, has spread from Africa across the whole planet.[6]

Given its absence from great apes—sometime, somehow, somewhere—smallpox must have jumped into humans from another species. In the run up to the eradication campaign, how this happened was not just an academic question—if spillover of smallpox from animals to humans happened once, what's to stop it happening again and thereby undermining all our efforts at extinguishing this fearsome disease?

MINDFUL OF THE THREAT of killer viruses lurking in the wild, researchers began systematic examinations of wild animals.[7] In 1962, scientists at the Institut Pasteur in Dakar, Senegal, started to work their way through the insect-eating bats that inhabited the region. A couple of years later, a more extensive programme of viral surveillance of small mammals began at the Virus Research Laboratory in Ibadan, Nigeria, in collaboration with two American partner organisations, the Smithsonian Institute in Washington DC and the Yale Arbovirus Research Unit.

Between 1964 and 1971, the researchers in Africa sampled nearly seven and a half thousand wild animals, representing over a hundred species encompassing rodents, hyraxes and hares, insectivores, carnivores and anteaters, primates and bats. Collecting took place at three-dozen sites in Nigeria, Dahomey and Togo, spanning five ecological zones, from the dank coastal lowlands to the airy heights of the Jos plateau. Their efforts yielded sixteen different types of virus, from the well known (bluetongue or West Nile virus) to the exotic (a virus with the unlikely name of Arumowot).

One of the most commonly sampled animals was Kemp's gerbil (also called the naked sole gerbil), a small rodent found all over west and central Africa, from Guinea to Ethiopia. At seven inches long, Kemp's gerbil is the largest of the West African gerbils, midway in size between a mouse and a rat. It is nocturnal, lives in burrows and eats the roots of savannah grasses and crop plants. In April 1968, the team captured nearly a hundred naked sole gerbils from the area around the town of Kouandé in the dry mountainous northwest of Dahomey (the country now called Benin). One of these rodents, captured on 23 April, carried something unexpected.[8]

The liver and spleen of the gerbil were removed aseptically and shipped in liquid nitrogen to Ibadan, where the specimens were ground up and centrifuged. Fluids from the centrifuge tubes were injected into the brains of six suckling mice. Some of the mice got sick, so their brain tissue was extracted, freeze-dried and sent to Yale.

When scientists at Yale injected the brain tissue into a fresh crop of suckling mice, they found infectivity blocked by antibodies against vaccinia virus (the smallpox vaccine). This suggested that the samples contained a poxvirus closely related to smallpox. They needed expert advice, so the Yale team sent four frozen suckling mice to poxvirus experts at the Centers for Disease Control (CDC) in Atlanta, Georgia. The CDC's virologists performed a standard procedure for poxviruses—they inoculated a suspension of material from the mouse brains into twelve-day-old fertilised hens' eggs.

UNTIL THE LATTER HALF of the twentieth century it was not easy to diagnose smallpox in the laboratory, even though the virus particles can just about be seen under the light microscope. The Scottish physician John Brown Buist first spotted the virus this way at the University of Edinburgh in 1886, using a stain developed by the pioneering microbiologist Robert Koch.[9] German scientist Enrique Paschen made similar observations in 1906.[10]

By the mid-1940s, visualisation of the minute egg-shaped *Paschen-Buist* bodies under the light microscope had become a standard method for detecting the smallpox virus in clinical samples. However, the technique became redundant just a few years later, when the far more powerful electron microscope yielded detailed images of the smallpox, chickenpox and vaccinia viruses.[11] In these images, the poxviruses are seen as brick-shaped particles, clearly different in appearance from the virus that causes chickenpox. However, even with electron microscopy, it can be impossible to distinguish between different kinds of poxvirus.

In the early decades of the twentieth century, virologists became better and better at growing the vaccinia and variola viruses in tissue culture.[12] Initially, they started with mashed up organs from laboratory animals, but eventually they managed to coax single types of cells to grow in the lab and maintain the virus. However, even today, cell culture remains a cumbersome approach, with exacting requirements.

In 1932, American virologists Alice Woodruff and Ernest Goodpasture, working in Tennessee, made a breakthrough, when they showed that vaccinia virus could be grown in fertilised hen's eggs.[13] A few years later, John Nelson followed suit at the Rockefeller Institute in New Jersey by growing the smallpox virus in eggs.[14]

When propagated on eggs, the virus preparation is inoculated on to the chorioallantoic membrane, an air-breathing film, permeated by a dense network of blood vessels, that plays a role similar to the placenta in mammals. When suitable dilutions of variola are applied, the virus produces large opaque white pocks on the membrane within forty-eight hours, which are distinctive enough in size and density to allow a differentiation between variola and vaccinia. The chickenpox virus does not grow on egg culture. Eggs provide a ready way of growing up sufficient quantities of the virus to create stock cultures, suitable for archiving, distributing to other labs or performing additional rounds of tests.

AT THE CDC, THE GERBIL VIRUS grew well on the chorioallantoic membrane, producing dense white pocks. Worryingly, most of the pocks were similar in size to those produced by variola virus and were markedly larger than those caused by the related mousepox (ectromelia) virus, a common problem in laboratory mice. With some related poxviruses, such as cowpox, rabbitpox, or monkeypox, there is bleeding into the pocks on the membrane, but the CDC scientists found no evidence of that here. With vaccinia virus, there is often a dying away of cells at the heart of the pocks (*central necrosis* in the jargon)—but there was no evidence of that here. Instead, on egg culture, the gerbil virus looked more like smallpox than any other virus.

The virus grew readily on a wide variety of mammalian cells in cell culture. On cultured lawns of cells, different viruses produce different cell-damaging effects (known as *cytopathic effect* or CPE). The gerbil virus, now dubbed gerbilpox or taterapox (after the Latin name for the gerbil), produced a CPE similar to that of variola virus and distinct from that of the mousepox, monkeypox, rabbitpox, cowpox, or vaccinia viruses. In immunological tests, it also clearly fell into a subgroup of poxviruses, which includes variola virus.

Isolated just after the peak of a local epidemic of human smallpox, this virus was as close to the smallpox virus as you could get without actually being variola. For the scientists studying it, explaining away this virus presented a considerable challenge. Did it represent a chance infection of a gerbil from a human—a one-in-a-million event that was never likely to recur? Or did humans originally acquire smallpox from a gerbil?

KEMP'S GERBIL IS NOT the only contender for the initial source of smallpox in humans. Two years after the gerbil gave up its poxviral cargo in Africa, a pair of Iranian scientists isolated poxviruses from camels in Iran. In Liverpool, the British virologist Derrick Baxby evaluated the camelpox viruses using the same battery of laboratory tests that had been deployed on the taterapox virus.[15] Just as with gerbilpox, in every test the camelpox viruses were indistinguishable from some strains of variola virus. In a subsequent study, Baxby even showed that smallpox virus could be used to vaccinate camels against camelpox.[16]

It is now clear that camelpox affects camels across the globe.[17] With over twenty million camels scattered across the world and a history of domestication stretching back over five thousand years, the camel provides an attractive explanation for the origins of human smallpox, even though there is no evidence from modern times that camels can give humans smallpox or vice versa.[18]

In recent years, advances in DNA sequencing have shed light on the relationships between smallpox, taterapox and camelpox.[19] Just a few thousand changes in the 180,000 characters in the poxvirus genome separate the three viruses. However, the DNA sequences show that the two animal viruses are more closely related to each other than either is to smallpox—so we still cannot say whether the primordial smallpox germ first spilt over into humans from a camel or from a gerbil.

It also remains unclear how long ago this happened. Early dating estimates based on DNA sequences placed the origins of smallpox tens of thousands of years ago[20]; but more recent estimates place the divergence of smallpox from taterapox and camelpox just a few thousand years ago—in fact, not long before Ramesses V fell ill.[21]

Russian poxvirus experts Igor Babkin and Irina Babkina suggest that smallpox originated when all three hosts—camels, humans and gerbils—first came together 3500-4500 years ago, when humans introduced camels to the Horn of Africa.[22] Ironically, in a pleasing circularity, this part of the world is also where the last natural case of smallpox occurred. However, as we shall see, between spillover and eradication, this virus brought untold misery to its new host species, particularly as it spread from the Old World to the New.

6

FROM THE OLD WORLD TO THE NEW

AFTER RAMESSES V, there is nothing much to say about smallpox in the historical or archaeological record for more than two thousand years. Some claim that smallpox may have been behind the plague of Athens or some other outbreak of disease from ancient or early medieval sources. However, this is all speculative or inconclusive. You look in vain for smallpox in the Bible or in Hippocrates.

The earliest credible description of smallpox hails from the golden age of Islamic scholarship: from the pen of Muhammad ibn Zakariya al-Razi (Latinised as Rhazis) in his treatise *On Smallpox and Measles*, written in the early tenth century CE.[1] Although smallpox probably rose in prevalence in Europe and Asia during the Middle Ages, as a mass killer it seems to have played second fiddle to *Yersinia pestis,* which brought the Black Death to Europe in the fourteenth century CE, killing up to a third of the population.[2]

However, as Europeans 'discovered' and colonised the New World in the fifteenth and sixteenth centuries, smallpox took on a fearsome new role as the destroyer of nations. In his 1997 book, *Guns, Germs, and Steel,* Jared Diamond attempts to explain why European populations succeeded in colonising so much of the world.[3] In this tightly argued classic of interdisciplinary reasoning, Diamond argues that the dominance of Eurasian civilisation is not the product of any supposedly innate superiority of the people involved. Instead, he argues, it was made possible by a set of historical, social and geographical preconditions limited to the Eurasian landmass, priming the development of advanced technologies such as guns and steel. He also suggests a key role for *germs* such as the smallpox virus, which, during the process of colonisation, decimated the populations of the New World.

Why should these diseases prove so much more devastating to the inhabitants of the New World than to the colonising Europeans? Diamond's explanation is that diseases like smallpox arose when humans first came into close contact with domesticated animals and starting living at high population densities. These prerequisites had been in place in Europe and Asia for many thousands of years, where the inhabitants had long been exposed to a rich collection of dangerous pathogens and so had acquired immunity through the process of natural selection. The inhabitants of the New World, having no experience of such pathogens, remained exquisitely vulnerable.

The earliest eyewitness account of smallpox in the Americas comes from the missionary monk Motolinía in his *History of the Indians of New Spain*, written in the first half of the sixteenth century.[4] Motolinía wrote of ten plagues that afflicted the people of the Americas, foremost among them being smallpox. He claims that an African slave brought the disease to Mexico in April 1520. Subsequently, in most provinces smallpox killed half of the Native American population, who, according to Motolinía, 'died in heaps like bedbugs' with survivors left 'covered with pockmarks'.

Over the centuries that followed, with epidemic after epidemic, smallpox decimated Native American populations[5]—and in so doing helped create the modern white-dominated Americas. In some cases, whites even considered using the deliberate spread of smallpox to native populations as an instrument of genocide. The best attested example comes from the correspondence between Sir Jeffrey Amherst, Commander-in-Chief of the British forces in North America, and Colonel Henry Bouquet, who together conspired to use smallpox to wipe out a coalition of Native American tribes during Pontiac's War.[6]

However, the Old World also supplied the New with a remedy against smallpox—as Jefferson's correspondence with Jenner shows, vaccination found ready acceptance in the Americas. Jenner himself contributed to such efforts. After the death of an Iroquois chief from smallpox, Jenner sent a book explaining vaccination to the Council of the Five Nations. In response, the Five Nations presented Jenner with the gift of a belt and a string of wampum beads, while proclaiming, 'We shall not fail to teach our children to speak the name of Jenner and to thank the Great Spirit for bestowing upon him so much wisdom and so much benevolence.'[7]

There is so much more to say about the role of smallpox in world history. However, this is not the place to give a full account of the horrors of smallpox in the eighteenth and nineteenth centuries, nor how Jenner's vaccination slowly started to triumph—this has been covered amply elsewhere.[8] Instead, we must move quickly on to the twentieth century—but before we do, let's pause just briefly in Pennsylvania in 1863.

7

GETTYSBURG 1863

We believe, that we but echo the feeling of the whole country without distinction of party, in sincerely hoping that the president will soon be restored to full health and strength. Men of his habit of body are not usually long lived, and the small-pox to a man of his age, even when the health is usually good, is a very serious matter. His death at this time would be a real calamity to the country, and would tend to prolong the war.
Editorial in the *New York World* newspaper, 5 January 1864

IN NOVEMBER 1863, at the age of 54, Abraham Lincoln, the sixteenth president of the United States—who has steered the Union through its bloodiest war and greatest political crisis—comes face to face with two life-threatening adversaries.

On 8 November, as the President sits for what is to become the iconic photograph of his life, no one is aware that he has just picked up a dangerous infection.[1] The following day, watching John Wilkes Booth play the villain in a play at Ford's Theatre in Washington, the President and his sister-in-law get the feeling that the actor's most menacing lines are directed at Lincoln himself—their intuition is spot on, because eighteen months later Booth assassinates Lincoln in that very same theatre.[2]

On 18 November, the President sets off from the nation's capital by train for a small town in Pennsylvania to dedicate a battlefield cemetery.[3] On the journey, Lincoln tells his secretary John Hay that he is feeling weak. The next morning, he complains of dizziness. Nonetheless, the nation's leader completes a carriage tour of the battlefield and cemetery, before travelling by horse to the site of the dedication, where he sits patiently through a two-hour oration from the Massachusetts politician Edward Everett.

Then, with the smallpox virus coursing through his veins, Lincoln takes to his feet and gives one of the greatest speeches of all time. Yet, during that Gettysburg address, Hay notes Lincoln's face has a ghastly colour and the President appears 'sad, mournful, almost haggard'.

After the speech, Lincoln boards the 6:30pm train back to

Washington, feeling feverish, headachy and weak. Back at the White House, the high fever, headache, backache, weakness and malaise continue.

On the fourth day of the illness, a rash appears and the following day Lincoln's doctors conclude that he has smallpox. The President responds with characteristic good humour, suggesting that, with a waiting room full of visitors, 'For once in my life as President, I find myself in a position to give everybody something!' It takes nearly a month for the President to recover and return to his usual activities.

Lincoln's physicians tell him that he has a mild version of smallpox—'a touch of the varioloid'. However, in a tightly argued piece published in 2007, two professors from Texas make it clear that Lincoln suffered from the more severe form of smallpox, variola major, which had a mortality rate of 30%. Lincoln probably caught the infection from his ten-year-old son Tad and he probably passed it on, with lethal consequence, to his African American servant William H. Johnson, who nursed Lincoln through his illness.[4]

Smallpox at Gettysburg prompts a great *what if*—what if Lincoln's immune system had not prevailed and he had succumbed to smallpox in 1863?[5] Would his successor, Vice-President Hannibal Hamlin, have been more or less successful in bringing the Civil War to a close than Lincoln? Would the ardent abolitionist Hamlin have done a better or worse job than Lincoln's real-world successor, Andrew Johnson, in achieving reconciliation between North and South or between former slaves and former slave-owners in the reconstructed Union?

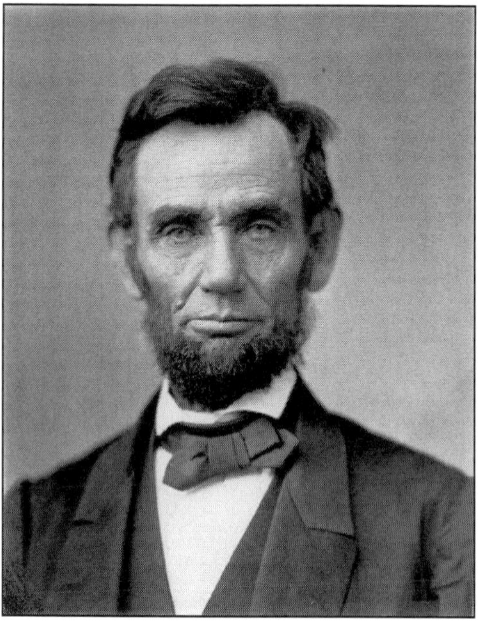

ICONIC PORTRAIT OF ABRAHAM LINCOLN
Taken by Alexander Gardner shortly after
Lincoln became infected with smallpox.
{Source: commons.wikimedia.org/wiki/
File:Abraham_Lincoln_O-77_matte_collodion_print.jpg}

Part Two

The Trickster

8

INTO THE TWENTIETH CENTURY

BY THE EARLY TWENTIETH CENTURY, smallpox had become marginalised as a cause of death in Europe and North America, thanks to two developments: the widespread adoption of vaccination and the spread of a milder form of the disease, known as variola minor or alastrim.[1]

Alastrim had the same incubation period and symptomatology as classical smallpox, but was associated with a death rate of less than 1%, compared to up to 30% for variola major. Providing cross-protection against its more severe sibling, alastrim slowly elbowed variola major out of many temperate countries. Nonetheless, every few years, there were importations into the US, UK and continental Europe from countries where smallpox remained endemic. As a result, outbreaks of smallpox flared up in Western society with frightening frequency, typically sputtering on through several rounds of infection, before being brought under control by case finding, quarantine and vaccination.[2]

When you look back at the textbook descriptions of smallpox, there is a temptation to make it look like an infection that was easy to recognise and control—after all, it produced a characteristic rash and had a predictable incubation period.

However, hindsight is deceptive.

MOST MYTHOLOGICAL TRADITIONS feature one or more *tricksters*—characters that don't play by the rules, shape shifters that hide and deceive by appearing to be what they are not.[3] The Norse had Loki, the Bible has Satan as a serpent, while in West Africa and the Caribbean, you will find Anansi the shape-shifting spider—and in outbreak after outbreak, smallpox played the role of a twentieth century trickster, popping up unexpectedly and unrecognised, spreading through routes unseen and unknown, until someone somehow connected the facts.

Smallpox was all too often mistaken for chickenpox—this happened in outbreaks in Gloucester in 1923, in London in 1927, in Edinburgh in 1942, in Middlesex in 1944, in Birkenhead in 1946, in Bilston in 1947 and in Glasgow in 1950.[4] In the first of three outbreaks that struck Scotland in 1942, a ship's engineer's smallpox was misdiagnosed as measles.[5] In Tottenham in 1957, smallpox masqueraded as leukaemia.[6]

Sometimes fleeting encounters were enough to spread the infection—walking past an open window or popping one's head through a doorway.[7] In 1913, a single individual infected nearly a hundred people during a journey by train from Kent to Manchester.[8] Sometimes, the viral trickster lurked in the laundry or popped up in a cotton mill.[9] In a 1967 South London outbreak, the authorities even worried about whether a phone box could be infectious.[10]

Often it was hard to find a direct face-to-face link between consecutive cases or outbreaks—for example, in 1942, smallpox somehow jumped from Glasgow in the west of the Scottish Lowlands to Fife in the east and then on to the capital Edinburgh, but no one was able to work out how.[11] Sometimes smallpox hitched a ride into the country even when the carrier had been vaccinated. This happened in 1944 when a 23-year-old soldier brought a particularly virulent strain of variola virus to Middlesex that caused three deaths from devastating haemorrhagic smallpox, even though the serviceman had been vaccinated in infancy and revaccinated a couple of years earlier.[12]

Sometimes the most notable aspect of an outbreak was not the disease itself, but the response to it—an importation of smallpox into New York City in 1947 led to an intensive month-long campaign to vaccinate millions of New Yorkers.[13] However, in some outbreaks—including in Edinburgh in 1942—as many died from the side effects of vaccination as from smallpox itself.[14]

The public did not always comply with medical advice. In 1946, smallpox was carried from town to town in the north of England by what were styled *freedom-loving tramps*—itinerant vagrants, who jumped quarantine.[15] The last outbreak on US soil, in Texas in 1949, included scenes reminiscent of a horror movie, as a patient delirious with smallpox twice escaped from hospital to wander the streets, sporting an infectious mass of pus and crusts.[16]

In the post-war period, there were dozens of smallpox outbreaks in industrialised countries, with more importations of smallpox into the United Kingdom than into any other comparable country.[17] If we are to reach Birmingham in 1978 in a timely fashion, we cannot hope to review all of these outbreaks—but to place the last days of smallpox into context, we should at least survey some of them. Let's start in Brighton.

9

BRIGHTON 1950

Though smallpox, once it develops, usually behaves in an extremely orderly way, there is... considerable caprice in the way in which infection may or may not be spread.
Gerald Breen (1956)[1]

IT'S CHRISTMAS EVE, which this year falls on a Sunday. It's cold: across the British Isles, it has been the coldest December since 1890, with frequent fog and snow.[2] We are in Brighton, a Georgian seaside resort on England's south coast, home to just over 150,000 souls. Two men—one in his twenties, the other in his fifties—are about to enter a pub.[3]

The younger man is an RAF serviceman, Flight Lieutenant Hunter, who has been looking forward to spending Christmas with his 26-year-old fiancée, Elsie Bath, who works as a telephonist in the Brighton Telephone Exchange. The older man is Elsie's father, Harold Bath, a 53-year-old taxi driver, who lives with his daughter in an unassuming terraced house close to the main railway station.[4]

However, preparations for the holidays haven't been going to plan. For nearly a fortnight Elsie has been suffering from a flu-like illness and, after developing a rash, has been admitted to the nearby Bevendean Hospital for Infectious Diseases. Harold also feels unwell and has spent the last day or so in bed.

One can imagine the conversation between the airman and his prospective father-in-law that night before Christmas. The old man felt bloody awful and the young one was getting over what he thought was malaria. Nonetheless, with the lady of the house away in hospital and the festive season about to start, the two of them agreed that they could not just stay at home and fester. Surely after a few beers, poor old Harold wouldn't feel so bad?

So they set off. They did not stop at just one pub. Instead, despite the inclement weather, the two of them undertook a pub-crawl through the alehouses of Brighton and nearby Hove. Several pints down, they crash out at a friend's place for the night, with the older man sleeping on the couch, the younger man sharing a bed with their impromptu host.

Tired and hung-over, the two men somehow make it through Christmas Day. But, on Boxing Day, Harold's condition deteriorates and he is forced to join his daughter as a patient in the Bevendean Hospital for Infectious Diseases.

With two members of the same family holed up in the same hospital with similar symptoms at the same time, the doctor at Bevendean calls for help from colleagues who specialise in public health. A short while later, after examining Harold and Elise and interviewing Hunter, the Medical Officer of Health for Brighton, Dr Rutherford Cramb, and his deputy, Dr William Parker, deliver their verdict: all three of them are suffering from smallpox.

WHEN POOR HAROLD BATH dies of haemorrhagic smallpox two days later, local undertakers and a crematorium refuse to handle his body. To control the outbreak, Cramb and Parker are joined by Dr Gerald Breen[5], a consultant in infectious diseases at the South Middlesex Hospital, and Dr Liselotte Lennhoff[6], a local infectious disease physician and a refugee from Nazi Germany. Harold's taxi is tracked down and disinfected and a nationwide search begins for everyone who has ridden in it, chasing up leads as far away as Devon, Scotland and Northern Ireland.[7] Subsequent investigations reveal that Harold and Elsie acquired the infection from Hunter, who brought it with him—perhaps in a rug—when he flew in from Pakistan at the end of November.

By now, smallpox has been in Brighton for a month—spreading unsuspected and unseen. During a visit to the hairdresser, Hunter directly or indirectly infects a 27-year-old housewife, who infects her son and her brother. The infection jumps from Elsie to a fellow telephonist and then on to another colleague in the telephone exchange.

The wily virus hitches a ride on infected clothing from the Bath family to a local laundry,[8] where more than sixty staff serve over a thousand customers. On 27 December, a sorter at a receiving depot for the laundry falls ill with smallpox. She survives. A few days later, a second sorter at the same branch, a 28-year-old woman who has never been vaccinated, comes out in a rash and is dead within a fortnight. Four more cases crop up among laundry staff over the next week and a half—tragically, one of them, a 53-year-old woman, spreads the infection to her Sunday school class before dying from haemorrhagic smallpox. The laundry premises and vans are fumigated twice, before being forced to close.

Bevendean Hospital is placed under quarantine, with staff and patients locked in and allowed to communicate with relatives only via postcards that are sterilised on the way out. Supplies and food are left in a garage outside the gates and, with local help, flowers, chocolates, cigarettes and beer are smuggled into the hospital. At least one captive scales the wall and pops out for an illicit pint.

However, these preventative measures come too late to prevent smallpox from ripping through the hospital, striking down nine nurses (three of whom die), two domestics, a one-year-old patient with measles and a hospital gardener, who had the simple misfortune to assist with the Christmas decorations on an infected ward. One of the Bevendean nurses infects an assistant in a greengrocer's shop[9]—who dies from semi-confluent smallpox—as well as a nine-year-old schoolboy, who survives.

Yet, as Gerald Breen notes, this is a capricious virus that doesn't play by the rules—sometimes it fails to strike when intuition says it should. After all, before the diagnosis, Hunter travels back and forth by train to Scotland, visits a cinema, a theatre and an ice-rink, and goes on a pub crawl with his prospective father-in-law in Brighton—but subsequent investigations find no evidence of infection in any rail passengers, passers-by or fellow drinkers.

As the outbreak rages through that harsh winter, 14,000 contacts are traced and followed up and sanitary inspectors make 65,352 surveillance visits. Two contacts have attended weddings and so bride, groom and guests have to be tracked down. Over 120,000 are vaccinated, including all of Brighton's district nurses, midwives, welfare officers, refuse collectors, rent collectors, police and public transport staff and the entire crew of a ship from a submarine depot in Scotland.

Local conferences and sporting events are cancelled. The cast of the pantomime *Mother Goose* at Brighton's Theatre Royal, including the actress Beryl Reid, are quarantined and forced to queue for vaccination. A café owner in Chichester puts up a sign saying 'Visitors from Brighton not welcome' and staff on the Brighton train from Victoria cry 'All aboard the Plague Special'! Public anxiety is fuelled by a film noir, *Panic in the Streets*, showing at the cinemas, centring on a search in New Orleans for someone spreading pneumonic plague.

No new cases are found after 22 January. By the time the all clear is sounded on 6 February, a total of thirty-five people have contracted smallpox in Brighton, of whom ten are dead. A civic thanksgiving service is held in the parish church of St Peter on 11 February.

10

BRADFORD 1962

IT'S 11 JANUARY and it's a Thursday afternoon in Bradford, a northern-English city in the foothills of the Pennines.[1] Dr Derrick Tovey is puzzled by two blood samples that have just arrived at his path lab. As he looks down the microscope at blood films from the samples, he can see that they are almost identical. However, they are both highly unusual—both show florid signs of damage to blood cells. Why have two such similar but unusual samples turned up at the same time? Tovey, with a colleague, consults the textbooks. They chance upon an old haematology book and are surprised to find that the changes they are seeing can occur in smallpox.

The first of the samples has come from Hettie Whetlock, a 49-year-old native of Bradford who works as a cook at Bradford Children's Hospital. She was admitted the day before to the Leeds Road Fever Hospital with a rash and fever of unknown origin. Tovey phones a specialist at the fever hospital and informs him that Whetlock has blood changes indicating an overwhelming viral infection. Almost apologetically, Tovey adds that similar changes have been described in smallpox. After a pregnant pause at the other end of the phone, the infectious disease consultant responds with 'You may well be right'.

Tovey then tells him about the other sample—from a 40-year-old abattoir worker called Jack Crossley, who was admitted two days ago to St Luke's Hospital with a bleeding disorder thought to be a complication of meningitis. He died shortly after the blood sample was taken and is now lying in the hospital mortuary. The infectious disease specialist rushes to the mortuary and finds a tell-tale pinprick rash on Crossley's arm. The two men realise that they are now facing a potentially catastrophic outbreak of smallpox.

With the weekend looming, rather than wait for a definitive diagnosis from the laboratory, they immediately convene a 'council of war', consisting of Tovey, three medical officers and the regional infectious diseases consultant. They soon establish that Crossley and Whitlock both visited Bradford Children's Hospital over the Christmas period and that four children at the hospital have now developed rashes, along with a toddler convalescing at another hospital nearby. All five children are quickly transferred to the Oakwell Smallpox Hospital, around eight miles away in Birstall, where two of them die.

The next day the investigators make the link to a 9-year-old Pakistani girl, who, a few weeks before, had flown in from Karachi, fallen ill with a fever and rash and spent the Christmas period in the Children's Hospital. They discover that the poor girl died on 30 December and a local pathologist, Norman Ainley, performed a post-mortem.

As soon as he makes the link to the Pakistani girl, Tovey informs fellow pathologist Ainley. Panic strikes as Ainley realises he has had intimate contact with a victim of smallpox, but he himself has never been vaccinated. Despite frantic attempts at vaccination, Ainley falls ill that very evening. The next day he is admitted to the local Smallpox Hospital, where he dies a few days later. Ainley's widow Margaret is released from quarantine just in time to join five hundred people at a memorial service for her husband in Bradford Cathedral.[2]

By mid-January, ten second-generation cases of variola major have come to light in Bradford, five of them fatal. Every hospital in the city is closed to non-urgent admissions while the situation is brought under control. In a heroic effort, over 1,400 contacts are traced and 285,000 people are vaccinated (practically the city's entire population) within just five days, drawing on vaccine supplies shipped in from Canada. The Medical Officer of Health holds exhausting daily press conferences. Local football matches are postponed.

Luckily, there are only three third-generation cases—two old men and an 11-year-old boy—who all survive their smallpox. However, the vaccination campaign brings its own victims, with six vaccinees suffering side effects severe enough to require hospitalisation. Three infants die from swelling of the brain caused by the vaccine—tragically, one of them, an eighteen-month-old boy, has not actually been vaccinated, but has become infected with the vaccinia virus after sharing a bath with his recently immunised sister.[3]

THE BRADFORD SMALLPOX OUTBREAK would have been little different from other post-war outbreaks in the UK had it not collided with the politics of immigration.[4] By the weekend, the outbreak is front-page news. *The People* sports a caption: *Smallpox Storm. "Keep out Pakistanis" call by MPs as thousands of Britons queue at clinics. The Yorkshire Post* runs with headlines *Pakistanis blamed in*

Smallpox City and *Anger in Bradford*. Racist Tory MP Sir Cyril Osborne writes in to the *Daily Express*, exclaiming 'this weekend's smallpox deaths should lie heavily upon the Labour Party's conscience'. A few days later, *The Guardian* prints a troubling report of a 'hooligan fringe' responsible for breaking windows and daubing Pakistani premises with racist insults, while children are calling the disease *Paki-pox* and asking Pakistani bus conductors for a 'two-shilling smallpox fare'. [5]

The English sense of fair play is also in evidence. A reader writes in the local paper: '...smallpox is the enemy of mankind as a whole. Those who irrationally feel they must have a human culprit should remember that in Bradford they must start with an innocent little girl, who suffered and died unwillingly. She happened to be brown...'[6]

After a window is smashed in a Pakistani butcher's shop, a local man walks in and proclaims, 'We're not all like that. I like Pakistanis. Take no notice of this sort of thing. Here you are, for the window'—and thrusts a ten-shilling note into the shopkeeper's wife's hand.[7]

Minister for Health, Enoch Powell, is forced to respond to a question in parliament from fellow MP Kenneth Robinson: 'Will you join us in deploring the exploitation of this outbreak in the interests of racial prejudice and in an attempt to justify the Government's immigration bill'. Powell responds evasively that he is unaware of any such efforts to exploit the outbreak.[8]

The final word on what happens when smallpox hits Bradford goes to Margaret Croft[9], writing in *The Guardian* on 24 January:

'Sir, Your reporters have given a fair enough picture of the feeling in Bradford about the outbreak of smallpox, although it is impossible for anyone to know what the unvocal majority are thinking. May I add a few points? The big stores in the city centre have also had a big drop in customers, yet none of them has coloured assistants. Our local paper *The Telegraph and Argus* has published admirably sane editorials and a lot of readers' letters: 37 between 17 and 20 January. Of these, 14 show some degree of racial prejudice, nine simply criticised the Government for lax immigration health regulations, seven pleaded for racial tolerance, four praised the splendid work of Bradford doctors and nurses, two commented on the cancellation of football matches, and one criticised a Shipley clinic, which temporarily ran out of vaccine. I work in Bradford and have not yet seen any signs of hooliganism. Some of us have gone out of our way to show the Pakistanis that we do not hate them, although not so far as handing out ten-shilling notes. The affair has made us more conscious of the Pakistanis' presence but people are calming down—not that there was ever a panic. We have all got sore arms—white, brown and black alike—and are talking about our scabs.'

11

SOUTH WALES 1962

IT'S 8 FEBRUARY and we are in the Rhondda—a Welsh valley famed for mining, Methodism and male voice choirs.[1] Our story begins in a modest semi-detached house in Maerdy, a village at the head of the smaller of the two valleys in the Rhondda. A local 23-year-old married woman, Margaret Mansfield, née Evans, is nearing the end of her second pregnancy and has moved back in with her mum to prepare for a home birth. But, these last few days, Margaret has not been feeling at all well—she has been drowsy and has come out in a rash. One of her eyes is badly bloodshot.

The midwife does her best to see the poor woman through labour, but Margaret starts to bleed heavily from her womb and gives birth to a dead macerated baby. She is rushed to East Glamorgan Hospital, where she receives a blood transfusion and a retained placenta is removed. Margaret dies in the anaesthetic room. A post-mortem is performed, attended by local obstetrician Mr Robert Hodkinson. The pathologist records the cause of death as heart failure as a result of acute liver failure caused by pre-eclampsia and loss of clotting factors.[2]

The bodies of Margaret Mansfield and her stillborn child are put on display in an open coffin at her home in the neighbouring village of Ferndale for a few days, while family and friends pay their last respects. Then, they are both buried.

A WEEK LATER, Marion Jones—a 24-year-old neighbour of Margaret's mum—falls ill. By 20 February, Marion has developed a rash. Marion's GP suspects smallpox, but has to wait a few days for a local smallpox expert, Dr Morley-Davies, to confirm the diagnosis. On 25 February, Mrs Jones is sent to Penrhys Smallpox Hospital, which sits on a windswept hill above the Rhondda.

That same day, a local infectious disease expert, Dr John Pathy, is called to East Glamorgan Hospital to examine Robert Hodkinson, who has been admitted suffering from severe back pain and a rash. Pathy quickly makes a clinical diagnosis of smallpox and Mr Hodkinson, who has never been vaccinated, joins Mrs Jones at the Penrhys Smallpox Hospital—where he dies on 6 March.

Investigations reveal that three family contacts of Margaret Mansfield have fallen ill with what has been diagnosed as chickenpox: her one-year-old son Terence, her married sister—28-year-old Mrs Patricia Pugh[3], who dies from smallpox—and Margaret's brother, Brian, who passes on the infection to his one-year-old son. From Patricia Pugh, the infection spreads to ten more cases. Smallpox jumps from Marion Jones to infect her husband Malcolm and five members of her family in the lower Rhondda.

A local four-year-old boy, Stephen Howells—treated in the same anaesthetic room as Margaret Mansfield[4]—falls ill on 14 February, and is at first misdiagnosed as having chickenpox. Infection spreads from the boy to his mother and a 9-month-old contact in hospital—both die from smallpox—and, probably, from Stephen to another hospital contact, 50-year-old Albert Cook.[5]

Smallpox mysteriously strikes two more patients in the village of Tonyrefail, just south of the Rhondda: a 49-year-old council worker, Trefor Thomas, who dies from haemorrhagic smallpox on 13 March, and his 81-year-old aunt, Edith Lewis, who survives. The link between these two patients and those in the Rhondda remains obscure.[6]

SMALLPOX'S FORAY into Wales did not begin with Margaret Mansfield. On 12 January, a Pakistani man, Shuka Mia, arrived in the UK from Karachi and travelled by bus, train and taxi to the Welsh capital, where he lodged above a local curry house.[7] On 15 January, Mia was admitted to Lansdowne Isolation Hospital with an undiagnosed fever. The next day, when a rash appeared, John Pathy made a diagnosis of smallpox and Mia was transferred to Penrhys Smallpox Hospital, where he stayed until 6 March.

Earnest efforts were made to trace Shuka Mia's contacts on the train and in Cardiff, but remarkably no new cases turn up in Cardiff or England. However, somehow, smallpox jumped from Cardiff to the Rhondda. Interestingly, the gap between Mia's arrival in Cardiff (13 January) and Mansfield falling ill (5 February) comes out as double the usual generation time for smallpox, so the most likely route is a missing case: someone who came into contact with both Shuka Mia and Mrs Mansfield. Suspicion falls on an unidentified fifteen-year-old girl, who came into contact with Mia and lived in the village of Tonteg, halfway between Cardiff and the Rhondda.[8]

However, there is a more unsettling explanation: that smallpox was passed on after Shuka Mia entered Penrhys Smallpox Hospital on 16 January travelling by air or through contaminated items. After all, Margaret Mansfield's home in Ferndale is only half a mile downhill from the hospital and this is not the first time that suspicions have fallen on a smallpox hospital as a source of infection in the local population.[9]

At the start of April, the local newspaper sounds the all clear in the Rhondda. The tally of smallpox cases in the Rhondda has come to twenty-four, with six deaths. All seems well—for a while.

GLANRHYD HOSPITAL IN BRIDGEND, eighteen miles west of Cardiff, is part of a vast national infrastructure of 'lunatic asylums' that have grown up in the UK, functioning as a set of self-contained communities for the long-term mentally ill. Sophia Evans is a 75-year-old inpatient on Glanrhyd's Langland Ward, one of forty-five confused and/or bed-ridden middle-aged or elderly female patients on the ward.[10] On 17 March, Sophia collapses with suspected pneumonia and is treated with penicillin. She develops a rash, which is dismissed as an allergic reaction to the antibiotic. Subsequent symptoms include a sore throat, conjunctivitis and ulcers on the tongue. The rash spreads to cover her body. On 25 March, she dies. No post-mortem is performed.

On 6 April, the local Medical Officer of Health Dr Evans and a local smallpox expert Dr Waddington visit Langland Ward. The two of them conclude that eight patients are suffering from smallpox—six of the eight go on to die from the infection. A fresh generation of smallpox cases starts at Glanrhyd Hospital on 18 April, when all surviving patients are moved a few miles north to Blackmill Isolation Hospital.

By the end of the Glanrhyd outbreak, nearly half of the forty-five patients on Langland Ward have developed smallpox and thirteen are dead—a vicious mortality rate of over 60%. When the final all clear is sounded on 21 May, over four months have passed since Shuka Mia brought smallpox to Cardiff and around 900,000 people in South Wales have been vaccinated.

Forty years after the outbreak, in a newspaper interview,[11] Marion Jones and her husband Malcolm describe how people crossed the road when they saw them after their brush with smallpox: 'Some people were marvellous, but some were frightened. If you saw us you would have been afraid. We had no hair and we had a face full of scars.'

12

PERSONAL INTERLUDE

BLUE LIGHT

Being a doctor is a strange job, in that you are supposed to care about your patients—but not too much. Your patients expect you to appreciate their problems, but also to maintain a professional distance. No one wants a doctor who feels their pain enough to cry with them.

As a medical student in the early eighties, I received no training in how to cope with the emotional demands of the job and just once I let the guard slip.

It was during a brief stint with the obstetrics flying squad. For the one and only time in my medical training, I had the chance to ride in an ambulance, with blue lights flashing as we sped through the streets of London's East End. We arrived to find a young woman giving birth to a stillborn child on her sofa in a council flat. A short while before, she would have been full of the anxious optimism of impending motherhood. But now she was suffering the agony of labour without the ecstasy of a live birth.

I maintained my cool at the scene, but when a fellow student and I got back to the London Hospital in Whitechapel, I broke down in tears. He chastised me for my momentary emotional incontinence and I soon recovered my composure. A few years later, by the time I had become a house officer, I had developed a thick skin—I remember feeling completely numb after seeing a four-year-old child die from asthma or a middle-aged mother die from a stroke while I was on duty.

But all these years later, when I read about what happened to Margaret Mansfield, forced to give birth at home to a macerated child—mother and baby murdered by smallpox—my eyes again fill with tears and my blood boils with anger at this cruel virus.

13

STAFFORDSHIRE 1966

The Region consists of a continuous succession of industrial towns.... Little countryside is seen; smoke from several hundred factory chimneys generally overlies much of the area. Residents of the area jokingly comment that "In the Midlands the birds wake up coughing, not singing!"
CDC report on the 1966 Staffordshire smallpox outbreak[1]

A MAN WALKS INTO A PUB with his father and his girlfriend one Sunday lunchtime in late February 1966. The pub is the White Cock Inn at Blythe Bridge, in Staffordshire in the English Midlands.[2] The young man is 23-year-old Tony McLennan[3], who lives with his parents in the nearby town of Stone. When the barman spies Tony's face, he mutters: 'that's the worst case of acne I have ever seen'.

Tony is just getting over a nasty flu-like illness, having spent several days in bed at his fiancée's flat in nearby Willenhall, laid low with a fever, headache, backache and vomiting. He also has developed a rash—clearly still in evidence—but it has been dismissed by a GP as a sweat rash or drug reaction.

On the previous Friday night, as Tony starts to feel up to socialising, he attends a folk dance and banquet. Over the weekend, Tony borrows his dad's razor and slices through one of the pustules on his face. Eight or nine days later, Mr McLennan Senior develops a papule on his face and both parents subsequently fall ill with a flu-like illness followed by a rash.

The McLennans are suffering from variola minor—the less serious form of smallpox. In addition to his mum and dad, Tony has managed to infect three other people: a 16-year-old girl from the nearby town of Willenhall, who works in a chemist's shop with Tony's girlfriend; a 25-year-old schoolteacher, who sits opposite Tony at the dinner-dance; and a 72-year-old man who just happened to be drinking in the White Cock Inn when Tony pops in.

Smallpox smoulders on for several weeks in Willenhall, hiding in plain sight before anyone recognises it. The girl in the chemist shop infects her sister and her boyfriend, who infects his sister and two brothers. Infection spreads via a local youth club. When a 16-year-old girl from the club is seen in hospital, smallpox is at last recognised for what it is and subsequently confirmed in the lab as variola minor. However, by then the teenager in question has already infected her mother and brother and, while in hospital, infects a five-year-old boy recovering from measles. The old man from the White Cock Inn has infected his fourteen-year-old grandson and a six-year-old granddaughter, who in turn have infected their cousins. The cousins infect their family and a playmate in nearby Cheadle.

On Good Friday, 8 April, White Cock man's grandson joins an excursion by bus to the seaside resort of Blackpool just as he develops a rash. During the trip, the teenager infects two of his friends plus—through a chance encounter at a motorway service station—a hitchhiker on his way up to the Lake District, who goes on to infect his mother as soon as he gets home.

In early June, a fresh outbreak surfaces in a primary school in the Welsh town of Pontypool, involving eight children, some of whom are admitted to Penrhys Hospital in the Rhondda. A couple of family outbreaks crop up in July—one in the West Midlands, the other in Greater Manchester. A look-back reveals that smallpox has been grumbling on for several weeks in both locations, ricocheting between generations in each family. No links are ever established between these three outbreaks and the initial outbreak in Staffordshire.

Overall, there are over seventy cases of variola minor in England and Wales that year. The question of how and where Tony McLennan acquired smallpox remains unanswered—an active social life involving frequent contact with immigrants at parties and in pubs seemed explanation enough at the time. No one made much of the fact that, working as a photographer at the Medical School in Birmingham, McLennan had shared a building with a smallpox lab. Luckily, smallpox did not kill anyone[4] when variola minor struck England and Wales in 1966. When history repeats itself twelve years later, the story has a more tragic ending.

14

BIRMINGHAM 1967

IN THE SIXTEENTH CENTURY, the English burnt witches and were afraid of ghosts—in the Twentieth Century, they burnt hospitals and feared viruses.

It's early 1967—and the schizophrenic sixties, liberal, but violent, are in full swing. In January, American forces step up the war in Vietnam[1], while in March, the UK authorities are forced to take drastic action to control an oil spill off the Cornish coast from a tanker, the Torrey Canyon—by dropping 150 tons of napalm.[2] On 2 May, Harold Wilson announces that the UK is going to apply for membership of the European Economic Community.[3]

The next day, a 33-year-old Scotsman, Alasdair Geddes, arrives in the heart of England to look around the East Birmingham Hospital, weighing up whether to press ahead with an application to become a Consultant in Infectious Diseases.[4]

ALASDAIR GEDDES was born and raised in Fortrose, a village in the Scottish Highlands, not far from Inverness. The local school, Fortrose Academy, provided him with a sound education and the young Alasdair enjoyed an idyllic childhood climbing cliffs, fishing, sailing, working on a farm and watching soldiers prepare for D-Day.

As a young man, Geddes studied medicine in Edinburgh, where he developed an interest in antibiotics. He completed his first medical jobs in Edinburgh and Perth and spent two years in the Royal Army Medical Corps, reaching the rank of captain.

Following a chance conversation in a pub, he is offered an infectious diseases position and gains experience in his chosen discipline in Edinburgh and Aberdeen. He starts to do research on antibiotics, with early publications in *The Lancet* and *British Medical Journal*. In 1965, Alasdair tours the east coast of the US and attends a conference in Washington DC. By 1967, he is ready to take up a consultant job.

When he arrives at the East Birmingham Hospital on the morning of 3 May, Alasdair has little idea what the hospital or the city has to offer. As a result, he is keen to meet the hospital's only other Consultant in Infectious Disease, Dr Ron Fothergill. However,

Dr Geddes wonders what on Earth he is letting himself in for, when he is told that he will have to wait till the afternoon to see his potential new colleague—because Dr Fothergill had been called away to supervise the burning down of a local smallpox hospital!

IN BRITAIN AT THAT time, first-line hospital provision for smallpox consists of a network of small hospitals, used exclusively for the care of patients suffering from proven or suspected smallpox.[5] The aim is that patients needing admission to such hospitals should not have to travel for more than two hours by ambulance. Between cases and outbreaks, smallpox hospitals are left empty, but kept in good order by resident caretakers.

Birmingham City Council built Witton Isolation Hospital in 1894 in a semi-rural location.[6] But by the 1930s it has been encircled by the suburb of Kingstanding, six miles north of the city centre. Nonetheless, even in the sixties, the hospital grounds present a green oasis in the urban sprawl—with mature trees, ample lawns and neat rows of daffodils. Up until the early 1960s, Witton Hospital serves as the chief smallpox hospital for Birmingham—and is called into action during the outbreaks that strike in 1962 and 1966. Remarkably, during the 1966 outbreak, a thief risks catching smallpox by stealing theatre shoes and a pair of wellington boots from the hospital, just as a new suspected case is being admitted.[7]

Once the final patient is discharged on 4 May 1966, a terminal fumigation is carried out. The hospital's days are numbered, as the central heating system is no longer reliable—besides, it seems unwise to maintain an isolation hospital in such a built-up area, particularly when there is another smallpox hospital not far away in rural Warwickshire.

The resident caretaker moves out in December 1966, leaving the hospital derelict and empty.[8] In April 1967, a passer-by sees intruders in the hospital from the top of a passing bus and reports the problem to a journalist at the Birmingham Mail. As a result, Birmingham's Medical Officer of Health, Dr. Ernest Millar, and the Ministry of Health soon settle on what we might call the 'Torrey Canyon solution'—destruction of the hospital by fire.

So, just as Alasdair Geddes arrives in Birmingham, firemen enter the derelict hospital, throw open the windows and set the buildings alight. Dramatic news bulletins vividly document the thick billowing smoke, the hungry fire devouring buildings and the flaming timbers crashing down.[9] The ensuing conflagration sterilises the site.[10]

A short while later, when the MP for nearby Selly Oak, Harold Gurden, discusses the burning of Witton Hospital in parliament, he drags in the question of immigration. In response, Julian Snow from the Ministry of Health exclaims 'I fear that immigration in Birmingham, like smallpox, tends to be an emotive word.'[11]

Despite this unusual set of circumstances, Alasdair Geddes takes up the consultant job in the East Birmingham Hospital and settles in nearby Solihull.

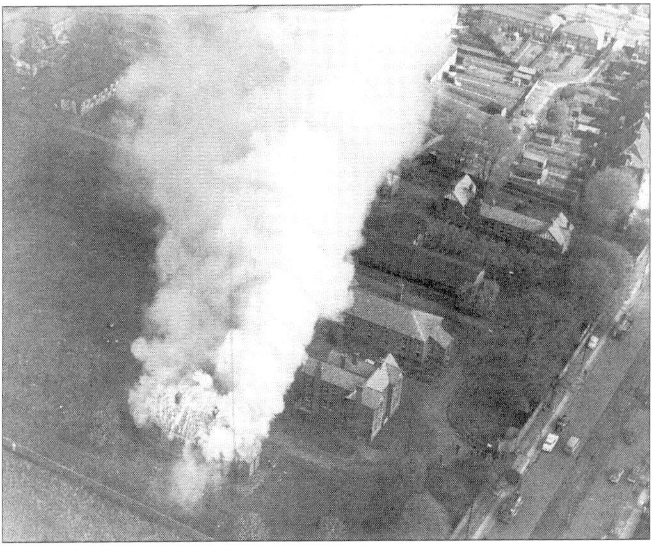

WITTON HOSPITAL

Smoke billowing from the smallpox hospital after it has been deliberately set alight.

{Source: Birmingham Mail}

15

WEST GERMANY 1970

MESCHEDE IS A SMALL town nestled in northern Germany's Ruhr valley, where the river flows through the heavily wooded Sauerland hills. The town dates back to medieval times, while the sandstone and shale on which it sits date from the Devonian period.[1]

On New Year's Eve 1969, Bernd Klein, a twenty-year-old backpacker, flies home to West Germany from Pakistan. Over the past five months, Klein and five friends have travelled overland in a Volkswagen camper van through Yugoslavia, Turkey, Iraq, Iran and Afghanistan. The group split up in Pakistan, leaving Klein to fend for himself in Karachi, where he stayed in a dingy hotel in a run-down part of town and was treated for hepatitis in hospital.

Klein is met by his father and his brother at Düsseldorf airport and makes the two-to-three-hour train journey due east to Meschede. The town is carpeted in snow.

On Saturday 10 January 1970, Bernd Klein develops a fever and the following day is admitted with suspected typhoid fever to an isolation unit at St. Walberga Hospital. He is confined to a single room, Room 151, on the ground floor of the three-storey building. Once he has settled in, Klein does not feel too bad and keeps himself amused with sketching and painting. He manages to clean himself using the sink in his room, but has to suffer the indignity of filling a bedpan, to be emptied by a pair of nuns/nurses.

By Wednesday, Bernd Klein is suffering from a rash. Smallpox is suspected on clinical grounds and confirmed two days later by electron microscopy. He develops a nasty cough. On 16 January, he is transferred to a new purpose-built smallpox hospital in nearby Wimbern, where he makes an uneventful recovery.

The St. Walberga Hospital has already been closed because of an ongoing community outbreak of influenza, but smallpox means that it stays closed. All staff and patients are immunised. Most receive the usual live vaccinia virus vaccine; the frailer patients are given a dead inactivated vaccine or an anti-variola antibody preparation. Most patients have been immunised in the past, but not for several decades. Direct contacts are put into isolation in Wimbern, while all the others are confined to the hospital building in Meschede during the quarantine period.

Despite these precautions, smallpox jumps from Bernd Klein to infect seventeen other people who were in the hospital buildings from 13 to 16 January. These include three nurses, thirteen patients and a transitory visitor who was in the building for just 15 minutes. Two die from their infection: 79-year-old Anton Hömberg, and a previously well, but unvaccinated 17-year-old trainee nurse, Barbara Berndt.

In a second round of cases, two more patients are infected, one of whom dies. Fear of smallpox leads to vaccination of 100,000 in the Ruhr valley and to death threats, which mean the Klein family are forced to flee their family home. The cold war at its height, East German border guards set up a vaccination station on the highway linking West Germany with West Berlin.

THE MESCHEDE OUTBREAK WAS unusual in that smallpox spread across three floors to patients who appeared to have had no direct contact with Klein at all. This flies in the face of the accepted wisdom that smallpox patients can infect only direct contacts within a two-metre radius—and, like Dr Who's daleks, smallpox was not supposed to be able to climb stairs.

WHO investigators entertained several explanations for what happened. Direct face-to-face transmission could be ruled out as all the hospital staff agreed that Bernd Klein did not leave his room during his stay at the St. Walberga Hospital. In addition, during his transfer out of the hospital, he was encased in an airtight plastic isolation device aimed at preventing transmission. Indirect transmission via an infected member of staff could be excluded because there simply wasn't enough time between Klein's arrival and the onset of symptoms in the subsequent round of cases, with an epidemic curve centred around a fortnight later.

A second potential explanation was transmission via inanimate objects. However, this did not fit, as Klein's linen was disinfected before cleaning and supplies for food and linen were shared with the adjacent large general hospital, yet there were no cases there. A priest who offered communion to patients was considered as a vector, but ruled out as his movements did not fit and Bernd refused to see him.

The investigators were forced to accept an unorthodox explanation—airborne spread across a wide area—which best accounted for the distribution of cases across three floors, the uniform attack rate across all floors, plus the infection of the transient visitor and of a patient on the second floor who had not left her room at all in January. A smoke test confirmed that the flow of smoke particles mapped neatly on to the distribution of patients, and Klein had a nasty cough, which may have forced variola virus particles from the throat out into the hospital air.

Not everyone was convinced: even some smallpox experts remained sceptical of airborne spread as an explanation, preferring to focus instead on potential spread via a night nurse or duty doctor or via the patient himself. However, as we shall see, Meschede made airborne spread of smallpox a talking point eight years later in Birmingham.

16

LONDON 1973

'As this report will reveal, smallpox is no respecter of persons or reputations and one of its chief characteristics seems to be that it strikes at the most inconvenient times in the most inconvenient places...'
Cox, McCarthy & Millar (1974)[1]

IT'S SATURDAY 17 MARCH, we are in London and it is St. Patrick's Day—a day celebrated by Irish people the world over. However, it is not easy being Irish in London right now, as the IRA has just launched their mainland bombing campaign and many English people are blaming *all* their Irish neighbours for the actions of *a few* militant republicans.

By a curious coincidence, two Irish women have been thrown together in adjacent beds in the same hospital. The two women hail from different parts of Ireland and belong to different generations: 23-year-old Ann Algeo comes from Northern Ireland, while 66-year-old Nora Hurley is from south of the border. Mrs Hurley, a spritely Irish widow, has been on the ward since the previous Wednesday, under treatment for an arthritic back. To celebrate their shared Irishness that special day, Nora Hurley gives her young compatriot a sprig of shamrock and lends her a copy of *Ireland's Own*, a weekly magazine offering undemanding Irish tittle tattle.

Later that day, Nora's 34-year-old son Thomas and his 29-year-old wife Margaret come to visit. During the course of the evening, Ann Algeo hands back the copy of *Ireland's Own* to Thomas or Margaret—she also shares something altogether less wholesome.

ANN ALGEO GREW UP as a Catholic in Northern Ireland, reaching her teens during the early years of the Troubles.[2] Just before violence peaked in the province[3], she moved south to gain a BA in Zoology from Trinity College Dublin. After graduating in the summer of 1972, she went travelling and worked in South Africa for a while.

On New Year's Day 1973, aged twenty-three, Ann Algeo began a new job at the London School of Hygiene and Tropical Medicine, working in the Mycology Reference Laboratory. Despite the London

School's solid reputation and impressive exterior, the labs inside are cramped, dirty and dingy.

Ann works in a lab dedicated to research on farmer's lung: an allergic reaction to inhaled fungal spores. However, in the course of her research, she requires almost daily use of equipment across the corridor in the pox lab, where she makes friends with a young research technician, Mr P. J. Bruno. On Wednesday 28 February, Ann watches Mr Bruno harvest eggs infected with a strain of variola major.

Ann falls ill on 11 March with a fever, a headache, backache and vomiting. A couple of days later, Ann visits a local GP who prescribes a painkiller and an antibiotic and advises her to stay off work. She takes to her bed for a couple of days. By Friday 16 March, she is covered in small itchy spots and the GP arranges for admission to hospital. The closest hospital, St Mary's at Paddington, is full, so Ann ends up in a satellite hospital, St Mary's Harrow Road, just over a mile away.

Ann's fading rash is labelled a drug reaction and her illness as a fever-of-unknown-origin. She is admitted to Ward 4, a medical ward for female patients. She starts off in the open part of the ward, but a day later she and Mrs Hurley are moved into a five-bedded unit set aside from the main ward.

That fateful Saturday, a house officer notices six pustules on Ann Algeo's chest and back. A short while later, the doctor on duty over the weekend notices a pustule on Ann's right hand, as well as smaller pustules on the chest and scalp. Curiously, with the appearance of the pustules, Ann Algeo has started to feel a lot better—well enough to nag the doctors to let her go home.

DR DONALD MACKENZIE is director of the lab that employs Ann. Perhaps as a result of his own experience of working in Northern Ireland,[4] he takes a special interest in the lively young Irish woman.[5] He arranges collection of skin scrapings, which test negative for fungal infection. MacKenzie pays Ann a visit on the Wednesday afternoon and remains puzzled by her illness, particularly the pustule on her right hand. He phones his colleague Charles Rondle, who runs the pox lab. Rondle thinks it highly unlikely that Ann is suffering from a poxvirus infection, but suggests that, if MacKenzie is still worried, he should get some skin scrapings looked at under the electron microscope.

MacKenzie presses his deputy, Miss Philpott, into obtaining some more skin scrapings when she visits Ann Algeo the next day. Miss Philpott takes the scrapings to the London School and watches as they are processed by the electron microscopist, Dr Ellis. A first attempt to visualise any viruses fails. However, second time around, Ellis turns up twelve brick-shaped particles, which, he explains, are clearly poxvirus particles, although he cannot tell whether they represent smallpox or monkeypox. Curiously, Miss Philpott leaves it until nine o'clock the next morning before passing on the news to her boss.

At ten o'clock that morning, MacKenzie discusses the findings by phone with Dr Kelly, the medical house officer looking after Ann Algeo. Kelly summarises their discussion in Ann Algeo's medical notes: *skins scrapings show poxvirus particles, poxviruses are used in the lab. Probably not smallpox but may be monkeypox. She has been vaccinated.*

MacKenzie passes the information on to the head of department, Professor Geoffrey Edsall, who summons Rondle to work.[6] On reviewing the evidence, Rondle concludes that Ann Algeo is suffering from a pox infection and is sufficiently worried to phone smallpox expert Professor Keith Dumbell. Later that afternoon, Rondle is shocked to hear from Mr Bruno that Ann Algeo has watched the technician harvest smallpox-infected eggs.

A DIAGNOSIS OF SMALLPOX now in the frame, one might have hoped that a well-oiled infection control apparatus would swing into action—sadly, that is not what happened. Instead, efforts were slow, grudging and poorly organised.

Ward 4 is closed and all the patients are asked to remain there in isolation, although they are not told why. One patient refuses and leaves the ward. Local medical officer Dr Marjory Dawson and the ward sister vaccinate patients, hospital staff and Ann Algeo's two flat mates, who are visiting her on the ward. Ann Algeo is sent off to Long Reach Smallpox Isolation Hospital in Dartford, arriving shortly before midnight.

Attempts to identify contacts falter over the weekend and only pick up steam the following Monday, 26 March, when Nora Hurley is added to the list. However, two days are wasted, due to a mix-up over Hurley's address, before a health inspector arrives at her top-floor council flat at 3pm on the Wednesday—a full five days after the smallpox alarm was first raised. Nora Hurley is vaccinated, but no one mentions smallpox, examines her or asks her who visited her in hospital. She assumes the vaccination is done to help her arthritis.

THOMAS AND MARGARET HURLEY live with their two sons, Nigel

aged nine and Anthony aged eleven, in a two-bedroomed terraced house in the North London suburb of Harrow. Thomas Hurley works as foreman to a gang of electricians. That last week in March, his work has taken Thomas as far afield as Aylesbury, Hemel Hempstead and Basildon. Thomas enjoys a drink in his local pub, *The Red Lion* in Harrow's High Road.

On Thursday 29 March, Thomas Hurley notices that a sausage he is eating tastes a bit off. The next day, Thomas returns home before midday and takes to his bed. He blames the sausage, but Margaret has also fallen ill with nausea, fever and headache. Their condition worsens over the weekend and they both develop a rash. On Monday evening, 2 April, they are admitted to the West Hendon Hospital with a diagnosis of viral gastroenteritis.

Their condition goes from bad to worse. Margaret starts bleeding into her urine and from injection sites. Doctors are puzzled. This looks like some kind of severe viral infection, but they simply do not consider smallpox to be a serious contender for two Irish people living in the middle of Harrow.

The news of Ann Algeo's smallpox breaks in the newspapers, but the mystery of the Hurleys' illness is solved only after a chance encounter between Thomas's mum Nora and a woman called Jessie MacKenzie, who works at the Camden Old People's Welfare Association. At first, they discuss Nora's pension book. Then, Nora reveals how worried she is about her son and daughter-in-law, so ill in hospital. She also expresses bewilderment as to why a doctor did something to her arm a few days before. Jessie connects what she is hearing to the newspaper reports and promptly phones the West Hendon Hospital, informing them of the links between the Hurley family and a case of smallpox.

Staff and contacts in the hospital are promptly vaccinated and quarantined. Margaret and Thomas join Ann Algeo in Long Reach Hospital. Margaret Hurley dies from haemorrhagic smallpox on 6 April. She is cremated.

Thomas Hurley dies from confluent smallpox on 15 April. His body is immersed in disinfectant-soaked sawdust within a coffin rendered airtight with putty. On 20 April, his last remains are transported through the Dartford Tunnel and through London's East End to his final resting place in Camden Cemetery. The coffin is wrapped in plastic and buried six feet under in a part of the cemetery put out of use for the next six months. Gravediggers and undertakers are vaccinated and kept under surveillance for sixteen days.

DURING THE OUTBREAK, the World Health Organization (the WHO) declares London a smallpox-infected area, disrupting business and holiday travel. To bring smallpox under control, hundreds of contacts are traced and up to four million people are vaccinated. Twelve people are admitted to Long Reach Smallpox Isolation Hospital. Contaminated homes and wards are disinfected with formaldehyde. The entire stock of the Red Cross library at St Mary's Hospital Harrow Road, amounting to about 4000 books, is fumigated in batches of 175 volumes.

In the wake of the outbreak, Sir Keith Joseph, Secretary of State for Social Services, sets up a committee of inquiry chaired by war-hero-turned-QC Philip Cox.[7] The resulting report reads like a tragic novel and ends with a *cri-de-coeur*: 'In financial terms alone the cost of this outbreak, bearing in mind, for example, the cost of medical supplies, administration of the vaccination programme and time lost from work, particularly from reactions to vaccination, might be reckoned in millions of pounds. But it is to the immeasurable cost in terms of human suffering and loss of life that we should look for the motivation to take any action now which will secure our people from any such tragedy in the future.'[8]

17

LOOK BACK IN ANGER

What a book a devil's chaplain might write on the clumsy, wasteful, blundering low and horridly cruel works of nature!
Charles Darwin (1856)[1]

Smallpox virus is a terrific virus. It does its job magnificently well. That doesn't mean that it's a good thing. It doesn't mean that I don't want to see it stamped out.
Richard Dawkins (1995)[2]

IT IS EASY, WHEN LOOKING BACK over outbreaks of smallpox from the twentieth century, to treat these narratives as exercises in detection fiction—intellectual games that engage the reader's curiosity—or as tales of horror, enjoyed from the safety of the armchair.

However, smallpox was no fictional creation of Agatha Christie or Edgar Allen Poe, H. P. Lovecraft or Stephen King. This was a real-life adversary, an endless source of human misery, a vicious virus that stole children from their parents, parents from their children, killed doctors and nurses, broke hearts and sundered lovers. Smallpox fed off the very life ties that make us human: killing a woman who had just given birth, ruining the lives of an affianced couple, capitalising on the act of caring for the sick, jumping from the dead to the living. In its wake, smallpox brought suspicion and shame, hatred and blame.

But where lies the blame? We casually say 'Case 1 infected Case 2 with smallpox'. Yet, in all those twentieth-century outbreaks, no one with smallpox can be held morally responsible for infecting anyone else with the disease, through deliberate action or inaction. You cannot blame a young girl for bringing smallpox to Bradford or a young woman in labour for infection in the Rhondda.

So, who or what is to blame?

CHARLES DARWIN STRUGGLED with use of language in formulating his theory of evolution. He identified a process that explained why living things often appear so perfectly adapted to their environment and he decided to call that process *natural selection*. However, in doing so, Darwin was breathing agency into an inanimate process—after all *selection* implies a *selector*.[3]

Darwin also realised that the cruelty of nature was hard to square with the idea of a benevolent creator. In particular, he was appalled by the amoral behaviour of the ichneumonid wasp, writing, 'I cannot persuade myself that a beneficent and omnipotent God would have designedly created the Ichneumonidae with the express intention of their feeding within the living bodies of Caterpillars.'[4] The same arguments apply to the variola virus, as it feeds on human flesh—in response to the Genesis creation narrative, one is driven to ask: on what day did God create smallpox?

Over a century later, Richard Dawkins infused agency into genes in his best-selling book, *The Selfish Gene*: 'The argument of this book is that we, and all other animals, are machines created by our genes'.[5] These attempts by Darwin and Dawkins to add agency to natural processes apply with added vigour to the variola virus.

For this selfish replicator, the disease smallpox is merely a means to an end—humans are just the virus's way of making more virus. Natural selection has honed the virus to an abhorrent perfection, deftly hijacking human tissues while avoiding the immune response. Sometimes from a viral perspective, it makes sense to crash and burn as a lethal case of haemorrhagic or confluent smallpox; sometimes, it is more favourable to evolve into something less virulent, like alastrim, leaving victims infectious for longer. Yet, in all cases, the virus cares nothing for its human hosts—and nothing for their wants, their hopes, their loves, their lives.

Arguments may rage as to whether it is misguided to ascribe agency, motive or even blame to something that is mindless. But emotional responses are not driven by pure reason. Had a human killed, maimed and scarred as smallpox did, calls for justice would ring loud. So, when considering the death and destruction caused by smallpox, there can be only one appropriate emotion—and that is *anger*!

But as the phrase 'don't get mad, get even' suggests, anger without action is not enough. In the latter half of the twentieth century, anger at a virus, twinned with compassion for our fellow humans, combined to drive this vicious killer off the face of the earth.

Part Three

Eradication

18

THE EXPANDING CIRCLE

As man advances in civilisation, and small tribes are united into larger communities, the simplest reason would tell each individual that he ought to extend his social instincts and sympathies to all the members of the same nation, though personally unknown to him. This point being once reached, there is only an artificial barrier to prevent his sympathies extending to the men of all nations and races.
Charles Darwin (1871)[1]

THE CENTURY THAT CONNECTS the 1870s to the 1970s provides scant evidence for Darwin's expanding circle of sympathy—with an unending litany of manmade megadeaths: *manifest destiny* as a pretext for the massacre and displacement of Native Americans; imperialist wars across the globe, from China to Africa; two World Wars and a Cold War that brings Stalin's Gulag, Mao's Great Leap Forward and vicious wars in Korea and Vietnam.[2]

Yet, if the world were run solely on realism, it would be a grey and miserable place. Repeatedly over the centuries, idealists have set new targets, which realists would initially judge unrealistic, or even undesirable. In the 1770s, Thomas Paine ignited the American Revolution with an idealistic pamphlet.[3] In France, the nineteenth century opens to the cry of *liberté, egalité, fraternité*, while Britain in the decades that follow sees the abolition of slavery and the emancipation of Catholics. Later that century, Americans fight a brutal Civil War to defend the ideal that all men are created equal. During the late nineteenth and early twentieth century, a wave of political idealism takes hold in the Anglo-Saxon world, with UK Prime Minister Gladstone and, later, US President Woodrow Wilson articulating foreign policies that reflect the internal ideals of their societies.[4]

Such idealism is soon subsumed into ideology—particularly in the brutal middle decades of the twentieth century. However, even at the height of the Cold War, the West and the Soviets both subscribe, however imperfectly, to shared ideals—of feeding the hungry, educating the ignorant and healing the sick. In the wake of the Second World War, this sense of common humanity leads to the formation of the United Nations and its subsidiary agencies, crucially, including the World Health Organization or WHO.[5]

THE WHO WAS LAUNCHED IN 1948 under the stewardship of Dr Brock Chisholm, a maverick Canadian psychiatrist, whose conviction politics earned him the title of 'Canada's most famously articulate angry man'.[6] It is Chisholm's idealism that leads to the title *World Health Organization*, with a global—rather than merely international—reach. In harmony with its grand ambitions, the new organisation takes up home in the imposing Palace of Nations, overlooking Lake Geneva, with a clear view of the Alps.[7]

The new organisation's goals and policies are set by an annual World Health Assembly (WHA), which, to start with, meets in Geneva. Repeatedly during its first decade, the WHA discusses the global problem of smallpox. Chisholm himself proposes a smallpox eradication programme, but the assembly dismisses the very idea as unrealistic.[8]

The decisive call for change has to wait until May 1958, when delegates from over eighty member states convene for three weeks at the Eleventh WHA in the American city of Minneapolis. The city and the country are playing host, thanks to the efforts of local Senator Hubert Humphrey—an idealist internationalist, keen to highlight American support for the organisation.[9]

During the WHO's early years, the Soviet Bloc boycotts the organisation, protesting at what it sees as a poor allocation of resources to Eastern Europe. However, the WHO stubbornly ignores Soviet absenteeism, arguing that its constitution contains no provision for withdrawal, so all these countries still count as members, leaving a route open to Soviet re-engagement. In 1958, in line with Soviet leader Khrushchev's new policy of peaceful coexistence with the West, for the first time the Soviet Union sends a delegation to the WHA, headed by their Deputy Health Minister, Viktor Zhdanov.

And so it comes to pass that in Minneapolis in the American Midwest, thanks to the hospitality of an American idealist and the intervention of a clear-sighted Soviet clinician, the WHO finally grasps the thorny rose of idealism with the firm hand of realism to set in motion a train of events that culminates in one of humanity's greatest achievements: the eradication of smallpox.

19

ZHDANOV

Considering it opportune to raise the problem of the world-wide eradication of smallpox in the near future, requests the Director-General to study and report to the Executive Board at its twenty-third session on the financial, administrative and technical implications of a programme having as its objective the eradication of smallpox.
Viktor Zhdanov (1958) Resolution WHA11.54

JEREMY BENTHAM SET OUT the principles of utilitarianism in the late eighteenth century.[1] Chief among these was the felicific calculus, an attempt to calculate the utility of an act in terms of the ability of the act and its consequences to maximise pleasure and minimise pain for sentient beings.[2] In the early twenty-first century, the effective altruism movement took on the mantle of utilitarianism with renewed enthusiasm, using evidence and reason to weigh up the most effective ways to improve the world. Early in his 2015 book, *Doing Good Better*, Scottish philosopher William MacAskill applies the felicific calculus to the question of who in human history had done the most good for humanity. He overlooks Socrates or the Buddha, Jesus or Muhammad, Lincoln or Martin Luther King, Mahatma Gandhi or Nelson Mandela. Instead, the answer he comes up with was a forgotten Soviet doctor: Viktor Zhdanov.[3]

VIKTOR MIKHAILOVICH ZHDANOV[4] was born in 1914 into the family of a rural doctor in the village of Shtepin, tucked away in the south-eastern corner of Ukraine in what is now the Donetsk region, close to the Aral Sea. As a hint of the greatness that was to come, while at school, the young Zhdanov wrote a physics textbook for his classmates. On leaving school, to fund his medical studies and to gain preferential treatment during the admissions process, he worked on a farm for several months, where his natural leadership skills soon led to him being elected foreman.

Zhdanov then moved a few hundred miles north to the Ukraine's second city, Kharkov, to start his medical training. While studying at the Kharkov Medical Institute, the lively medical student enjoyed a full programme of extra-curricular activities, including playing the piano as an accompaniment to silent movies and writing and directing an opera. He graduated from the Institute at the age of twenty-two, then spent ten years working his way up the ranks as an army doctor in Siberia and Turkmenistan, eventually becoming a Major General. During this time, Zhdanov learnt how to deal with bureaucrats and gained a mastery of epidemiology out in the field. Crucially, he was involved in efforts to eliminate malaria and dysentery, in the development and implementation of quarantine measures and in the containment of imported infections, all of which laid the foundations for his later thinking.

In 1946, at the age of thirty-two, Zhdanov defended a doctoral thesis entitled *Infectious hepatitis (Botkin's disease): Etiology and Epidemiology* and throughout his life he maintained the critical mind-set of a research scientist. That same year, following his release from the army, he became Chief of the Epidemiology Department in the Metchnikoff Institute of Epidemiology and Microbiology in Kharkov. Within two years, he had become Director of the Institute. Within four years, he was a professor and had been elected a corresponding member of the USSR's Academy of Medical Sciences.

A good listener, hard-working, well organised, sharp-witted, knowledgeable, with an extraordinary thirst for life, Viktor Zhdanov had all the makings of an inspiring and effective leader. In 1951, he became Chief of the Department of Sanitary and Epidemiological Services, with responsibility for communicable disease control across the whole of the Soviet Union. Fuelled by Soviet idealism and Soviet successes in controlling smallpox and Guinea worm, he was increasingly drawn to the idea of disease eradication. In 1952, with fellow microbiologist Timakov, Zhdanov published a report outlining the prospects for eliminating selected infectious diseases, stressing that increased investment in the short term was sure to deliver decisive savings in the long term.

In 1955, Zhdanov became Deputy Minister of Health and Chief Medical Officer, serving under the Soviet Minister of Health, the neurologist Dr. Maria Kovrigina. In this role, he formulated a strategy for tackling health problems that combined scientific analysis, wide-ranging discussion and decisive action. Such an approach was to serve him—and the world—well, when he turned his mind to the eradication of smallpox, not just from the Soviet Union, but from the entire globe.

AND SO IN 1958, as spring was turning into summer in

Minneapolis, Zhdanov presented a report to the eleventh WHA. According to the official history of smallpox eradication, the report was rather long and couched in overly formal language, but few other declarations have had such power to change the course of history. As a sophisticated orator, Zhdanov tailored his rhetoric to the local audience, opening his address with an uplifting exhortation from US founding father Thomas Jefferson, in his 1806 letter to Edward Jenner: 'future nations will know by history only that the loathsome small-pox has existed.'

Zhdanov's report rammed home the point that no nation was free of the risk of smallpox until all were free of the disease, highlighting the recurrent costs of vaccination and revaccination across the globe and stressing that there were good grounds for believing that eradication was theoretically and practically possible. Zhdanov recommended that a system used in England to manage the disease, the so-called Leicester system, be adopted widely: this system encompassed prompt identification and isolation of new cases together with quarantine and surveillance of contacts. His report concluded with a bold claim: 'As regards its complete eradication throughout the world, we think that this can be achieved within the next ten years.'

Zhdanov did not instantaneously win over his audience in 1958. The delegates did, however, ask the Director-General of the WHO to give fuller consideration to the prospect of smallpox eradication. The Soviet Union, and its ally Cuba, quickly followed up Zhdanov's suggestion with practical help by supplying the WHO with 25 million and two million vials of vaccine, respectively. At the subsequent World Health Assembly in 1959, agreement was reached to launch a global eradication campaign for smallpox.

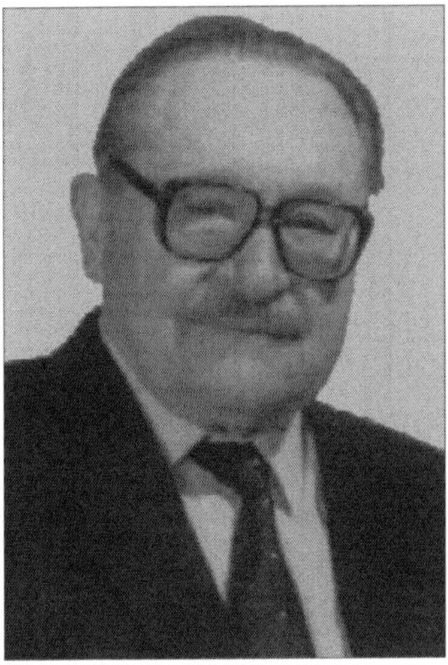

VIKTOR ZHDANOV 1914-1987
Soviet virologist who convinced the World Health Assembly to adopt a programme to eradicate smallpox
{Source: ru.wikipedia.org/wiki/Файл:Zhdanov_VM.jpg}

20

D. A.

It is not the critic who counts; not the man who points out how the strong man stumbles, or where the doer of deeds could have done them better. The credit belongs to the man who is actually in the arena, whose face is marred by dust and sweat and blood; who strives valiantly... who spends himself in a worthy cause; who at the best knows in the end the triumph of high achievement.
Theodore Roosevelt (1910)[1]

ALTHOUGH THE SPEECH that launched the eradication campaign had been given in America, the USA was initially slow to follow the Soviet Union's lead. However, in 1964—which, as International Cooperation Year, marked the twentieth anniversary of the United Nations—President Lyndon B. Johnson pledged his country's commitment to this bold effort. Shortly afterwards, in a nice symmetry with initiation of efforts by the Soviet Union's Zhdanov, an American, Donald 'D.A.' Henderson, was propelled into leadership of the smallpox eradication campaign.[2]

Donald Ainslie Henderson was born in 1928 in Northwood, Ohio, an emerging suburb of Cleveland on the southern shore of Lake Erie. His father was an engineer, his mother a nurse. He was a nerdy child—classmates nicknamed him 'Doc Henderson' or 'Biology Boy'. Henderson gained a chemistry degree from Oberlin College, a liberal arts college thirty miles southwest of the family home. Inspired by a Canadian uncle, D.A. entered the medical profession, gaining his MD in 1954 from the University of Rochester Medical Center in upstate New York.

During his residency, interactions with polio patients prompted an interest in infectious disease. Faced with the prospect of a rather dull two years of military service, the young Dr Henderson signed up with the US Epidemic Intelligence Service—a mobile hands-on outbreak investigation corps at CDC (which at that time stood for the *Center for Communicable Diseases*) based in Atlanta, Georgia. He clearly had an aptitude for the work, as by 1961 he had become chief of the surveillance section at the CDC. The following year, D.A. established a smallpox surveillance unit, marking the beginning of an obsession with this infection that would dominate his life.

In 1966, the World Health Assembly narrowly voted in favour of a ten-year intensified global eradication campaign for smallpox. Impressed by Henderson's efforts on smallpox control in Africa, the WHO's Secretary-General, the Brazilian malariologist Marcolino Gomes Candau, approached Henderson to ask if he would accept the role of Director of the WHO Smallpox Eradication Office.

Fearful that he was being set up to fail, the 38-year-old Henderson was initially reluctant. After all, global efforts to end hookworm, malaria and yellow fever had run into the sand and nearly half the delegates in the World Health Assembly—and even Candau himself—were doubtful that the campaign would succeed. And Henderson was just a year into the smallpox and measles eradication campaign he had set up in Africa. On top of that, the paltry $2.4m annual budget set aside for global eradication (just 5% of the WHO's budget) was not even enough to cover the costs of the smallpox vaccine, let alone all the other running costs. Plus, there was a political angle: with East versus West, North versus South, Henderson could see that they wanted an American to blame when things went wrong.

Nonetheless, casting his doubts aside, Henderson accepted the challenge and moved with his family to Geneva to work at the WHO headquarters, now in a new modernist building set back between the lake and airport. On 1 January 1967, the Global Intensified Smallpox Eradication Programme began, with smallpox still circulating in over thirty countries. Over the next decade, from his cramped accommodation in Geneva, Henderson led the eradication campaign, channelling efforts through WHO Regional Offices to over 150,000 field workers.

Never, before or since, in the history of disease control has so much been achieved with so little in terms of financial investment. A forceful individual, Henderson led from the front—the epitome of Roosevelt's man-in-the-arena—repeatedly spending time 'in the trenches', as he put it, filing progress reports from country after country. He also made sure that his colleagues, however senior in the campaign, got out of their offices to see what things were like on the front line.

Henderson and his co-workers at first struggled with the problem of poor quality vaccine stocks. D.A. led the way in establishing adequate procedures and facilities for vaccine production. He persuaded laboratories in Canada and the Netherlands to act as quality control centres, testing vaccine samples for the programme. Initially relying on donations from the

Soviet Union, the campaign eventually moved vaccine manufacture into resource-poor countries. It is estimated that 2.4 billion vaccine doses were administered during the eradication campaign.

Vaccination traditionally relied on scarification, scratching the vaccine into the skin, but this was a low-throughput technique. Hydraulic-powered jet injectors that could deliver a thousand vaccinations an hour were used in the early phase of the eradication campaign, but these proved costly high-maintenance devices that required skilled operators. Instead, smallpox was driven off the planet with a beautifully simple device: a modified sewing needle.

Designed in the early 1960s by Benjamin Rubin and Gus Chakros of Wyeth laboratories, the *bifurcated needle* consisted of a five-centimetre-long narrow steel rod, equipped with two prongs at one end.[3] The gap between the prongs held a single dose of reconstituted freeze-dried vaccine, which was driven into the skin of the upper arm by fifteen rapid jabs. Afterwards, the needle was sterilised and used again. The bifurcated needle was so easy to use, it took just an hour to train someone, who could then vaccinate up to 1,500 people in a single day. The bifurcated needle brought the added bonus of needing only a quarter of the vaccine that the jet injector used to produce immunity. Hundreds of millions of people were vaccinated using this simple piece of metalwork.

At inception, the eradication campaign adopted the principle of mass vaccination, aiming to create sufficient *herd immunity* to snuff out transmission of the smallpox virus. The idea behind herd immunity was that, even if a small proportion of the population remains unvaccinated, by vaccinating most of the population chains of transmission of infection could no longer be maintained.

However, mass vaccination soon proved inefficient and ineffective, as the virus was still capable of sustained transmission even in a solidly immunised population, with over 80% vaccine coverage. The focus switched to *ring vaccination*—a policy developed by the American medical missionary Dr William Foege in Nigeria. The policy capitalised on the slow spread of the infection (12 days per generation) and relatively low transmission rate (typically just 3-4 new cases arising from each infected individual). This meant that, once a case had been identified, there was sufficient time to create a protective ring by quarantining and immunising all those who had been exposed to the infected individual.

Foege was not the first to come up with the idea of isolating contacts to wall off smallpox—as Zhdanov noted, a similar approach had been developed in Leicester in England in the late nineteenth century. However, in showing that surveillance twinned with targeted quarantine and vaccination worked so well in the field, Foege changed the way people thought. This strategy was given added strength when Dr A Ramachandra Rao showed that the approach brought transmission to a halt in the Indian state of Tamil Nadu within just six months. As a result, from 1969 onwards, the smallpox eradication campaign relied on the principle that 'knowledge is power', focusing on active, intensive surveillance and vigorous containment of outbreaks, rather than onerous and wasteful mass vaccination.

Henderson played the diplomat, working with the Soviet Union at the height of the cold war. He built a relationship with Haile Selassie's private doctor and used it to break through Ethiopian bureaucracy. He visited Yugoslavia during Europe's last outbreak and led the fight in India during the crucial phase of the final most intense campaign, *Operation Smallpox Zero*.

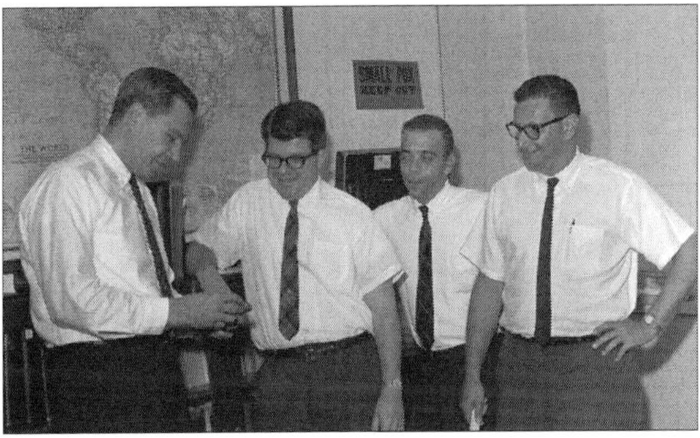

D. A. HENDERSON (1928-2016)
Far left, with the smallpox eradication team in 1966
{Source: commons.wikimedia.org/wiki/
File:Smallpox_eradication_team.jpg}

THIS IS NOT THE PLACE to document the details of how smallpox was squeezed out of every corner of the globe. For those keen to pay supreme respect to this remarkable achievement, there is a holy book, a weighty tome of over a thousand pages, to be held with care and read with reverence—the mammoth WHO publication, *Smallpox and its Eradication*, often dubbed 'the Big Red Book'. Or there is Henderson's own personal account of the campaign: *Smallpox—Death of a Disease*.[4]

Suffice it to say that the campaign overcame numerous hurdles—physical (mountains, rivers, floods) and social (ignorance, political wrangling, vested interests, national pride, fraudulent under-reporting of cases, famine, war, displacement of people). Every conceivable form of transport was used to deliver vaccine to its targets: jeeps, motorcycles, pushbikes, mules, boats, even elephants! Doctors swam across rivers, bearing vaccine and vaccination equipment on their heads and emerged with leeches clinging to their bodies. In Ethiopia, health workers were shot dead by suspicious tribesmen. In India, devotees of the smallpox goddess Shitala Mata were followed home to uncover new cases of the disease, while the mighty Tata Industries lent staff to the campaign.

One by one the regional goliaths of endemic smallpox fell to the slingshot of vaccine delivered by bifurcated needle—Brazil and Indonesia, West Africa, India. A 1970 incursion into Yugoslavia was snuffed out. By 1975, smallpox was confined to two localities and only in one of them did the serious form, variola major, still inhabit human flesh and blood.

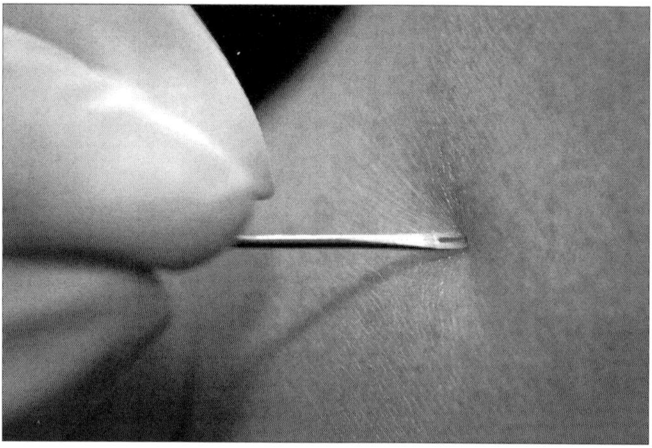

A BIFURCATED NEEDLE

Used during the eradication campaign to deliver smallpox vaccine

{Source: pixnio.com}

21

PERSONAL INTERLUDE

WMD

One of the advantages of working your way up through a profession is that you get to meet the heroes of your youth—the people that inspired you when you were just starting out, when they seemed as unreachable as the gods. I had the opportunity to meet D. A. Henderson just the once—and I made a hash of it!

It was on Monday 7 April 2003, in Edinburgh, at a meeting of the Society for General Microbiology. The Iraq war had started barely three weeks before and that week the news feed was full of pictures of Saddam Hussein's statue being toppled in Baghdad. In the wake of 9/11, D.A. had been appointed as Director of the newly created Office of Public Health Preparedness to coordinate the US national response to public health emergencies, which included bioterrorism and biowarfare. He had been invited to give a keynote address at the conference on smallpox vaccines. He explained that, with the threat of variola virus as a biological weapon, efforts were underway to procure supplies of vaccinia virus, develop newer versions of the vaccine and vaccinate those in the front line should a deliberate release of smallpox occur.

A little before 4pm, during the Q and A session at the end of D.A.'s talk, I stuck my hand up, opened my mouth and challenged my hero: 'So given recent events in Iraq, where are these weapons of mass destruction then?' D.A. responded without hesitation: 'We don't know. We haven't found them yet, but we are sure they are out there somewhere.'

D.A. turned out to be right on smallpox and its eradication, but wrong on WMDs in Iraq. But I still feel embarrassed for challenging him on this. Nonetheless, in his role in homeland protection, D.A. was able to apply his influence to good effect. Armed with a copy of a report into a 1942 Edinburgh outbreak[1], given to him by Alasdair Geddes—which highlighted ten deaths from vaccination—D.A. reined in the Bush administration's impulse to vaccinate the entire US population in response to a purely hypothetical risk. In so doing, he saved thousands more lives, on top of the millions already saved by smallpox eradication, and so he remains a hero to me!

22

WHITEPOX

The smallpox eradication campaign would not have been undertaken, had there not been good epidemiological evidence that there was no non-human reservoir of the virus. Some doubt has arisen in recent years, because six viruses reported as having been isolated from animal tissues have all the laboratory properties associated with variola viruses.[1]
Dumbell and Kapsenberg, 1982

A MAJOR CONCERN DURING the eradication campaign were the risks that smallpox could hide in non-human animal hosts or that another poxvirus might jump into the niche vacated by the vanquished variola virus. In particular, attention focused on two viral spectres: monkeypox and whitepox.

Monkeypox first surfaced in the late 1950s as a disease of captive monkeys. The first human case was recognised in August 1970 in a 9-month-old boy in the northern part of what is now the Democratic Republic of Congo. Over the next five years, twenty cases were recognised in central and west Africa.[2] Although the infection in humans was indistinguishable clinically from smallpox, it showed a limited propensity to spread from human to human and the monkeypox virus was easily distinguishable from variola virus in the laboratory.

The whitepox story begins in the autumn of 1964, when scientists working at the Rijks Instituut voor de Volksgezondheid in Bilthoven in the Netherlands recover two cultures of poxviruses from monkey kidney cells.[3] The cells had come from two apparently healthy wild-caught crab-eating macaques, imported from Malaysia and housed in a monkey colony free of any pox-like disease.

On laboratory testing, the two new viruses, termed 64/7255 and 64/7275, could be easily distinguished from other animal poxviruses, but, like gerbilpox and camelpox, they showed an uncannily close resemblance to the smallpox virus. Like variola, they produced white pocks on the chorioallantoic membrane of hen's eggs, so they quickly earned the name *whitepox*. They appeared to differ from variola viruses only by their tendency to cause patching bleeding and tissue damage when injected into the skin of rabbits.

In the seventies, the hunt for an animal reservoir of monkeypox began in earnest. Hundreds of monkeys, rodents and miscellaneous other mammals were tested from across tropical Africa, the Americas and Asia. Almost all failed to yield anything interesting.[4]

However, from 1970 to 1974, the Russian virologist Svetlana Marennikova at the Research Institute for Viral Preparations in Moscow reported isolating four new poxviruses from tissues from four species of mammal captured at various sites in the Equateur Province of Zaire, an area of dense tropical rain forest, which had been free of smallpox for several years.[5] All the new viruses closely resembled variola in producing white pocks on the chorioallantoic membranes of eggs and so were added to the list of whitepox viruses. The diversity of sites and sources was a major concern: a chimpanzee captured near the town of Basankusu, an unidentified species of monkey captured near the Ubangi river and two African rodents captured near the inland port of Bumba.

FOR THOSE TRYING TO eradicate smallpox, there were a number of worrying questions. Could whitepox viruses act as a source of smallpox, once the disease had been eradicated from all of humanity? Could the disease re-emerge from an animal source? How would we be able to tell the difference between deadly transmissible smallpox and other less worrying but closely related poxviruses?[6]

A major step forward in distinguishing between the various kinds of mammalian poxviruses in the laboratory came in 1961 with a study reported by two British microbiologists working in Liverpool: Dr Henry Bedson and Dr Keith Dumbell. In the study, published in the *Journal of Hygiene*, the 31-year-old Bedson and his colleague Dumbell systematically examined the effect of temperature on pock formation by poxviruses on the chorioallantoic membrane, and established that there was a characteristic 'ceiling temperature' for each virus, beyond which the virus would not grow.[7]

For the first time, the 'Bedson ceiling test' provided a simple method to distinguish variola major viruses, which will grow up to 38.5°C, from the less hazardous variola minor viruses, which will not grow above 37.5°C. Crucially, this paper set Bedson on the path to becoming a leading expert on the differentiation between smallpox and other poxviruses.

23

BEDSON

HENRY SAMUEL BEDSON was born on 29 September 1929.[1] As the son and grandson of academics, his path was laid down early in life. Three years before he was born, Henry's father Sam took up a newly created Freedom Fellowship in virology at The London Hospital in Whitechapel. The year Henry was born, Sam discovered the causative agent of a form of pneumonia caught from birds called psittacosis. The microbe was, at least at first, named *Bedsonia* in his honour.[2] In later life, these achievements earned Bedson Senior a knighthood and Fellowship of the Royal Society.

Henry grew up a grammar school boy in Brighton and Hove. He was the middle of three sons, but Henry alone followed his father into medicine: the elder brother became a civil engineer and the younger, a vet. Once a year, Bedson Senior took his three sons off on a fly-fishing holiday in the north of England, which endowed the young Henry with a lifelong passion for the art of dry-fly fishing—dubbed by Izaak Walton the contemplative man's recreation. The young Henry was also an accomplished cricketer, particularly behind the wicket and as a cover-point fielder.

Henry spent his time as a medical student at The London Hospital Medical College[3] in the London's East End. He qualified in 1952, the same year his father retired from a chair at the very same college. After his house officer jobs, Henry followed the family line into the speciality of pathology (the UK term for what elsewhere is called 'laboratory medicine'). He joined the Royal Army Medical Corps and served for a couple of years in a small military hospital in Hong Kong. After a short stint back at The London Hospital, he took up a research fellowship at the University of Liverpool, working under Allan Downie, the country's leading poxvirus expert. In 1959, Bedson became assistant lecturer, and a year later was appointed a full lecturer.

Bedson arrived in Liverpool as a bachelor. A year or two later, his boss, Allan Downie, was laid low with a prolapsed disc. The older man was a little surprised at the number of visits he received from his young apprentice while convalescing in the Liverpool Royal Infirmary. The real reason for the repeated visits became clear when

Bedson announced his engagement to a staff nurse on the ward—a plain-speaking Yorkshire woman, Ann Patricia (known as 'Pat') Ducker, who hailed from Bramhope, just north of Leeds. Henry and Pat were married in 1961—the same year he invented the 'Bedson ceiling test'.

While at Liverpool, Henry worked alongside—and became close friends with—three other early-career poxvirus enthusiasts: Kevin McCarthy, Charles Rondle and, in particular, Keith Dumbell. Bedson and Dumbell become godparents to each other's children and their wives complained that the two men were so similar that they could finish off each other's sentences.

Each Friday lunchtime, the four young virologists ran an informal wine-tasting session, drawing samples from a bottle smuggled into the departmental lunch in a brown paper bag. One weekend, Henry provided practical help to his friend Keith, helping to repair some old guttering. On another occasion, the usually modest Henry tried to show off in front of his friends at a restaurant in Liverpool's China Town by ordering from the menu using the Cantonese he had picked up in Hong Kong—but was brought down to size when the waiter failed to understand a word he was saying!

In 1964, at the height of Beatlemania, the Bedsons left the coastal city of Liverpool to move a hundred miles inland, so that Henry could take up a position as Senior Lecturer at the University of Birmingham. By then, Henry looked every inch the archetypal English boffin: short and slight of stature, balding, quietly spoken with a reserved, intense manner, but optimistic in outlook and well liked by colleagues. He maintained a stiff upper lip, stoically keeping his feelings to himself, even if inside he was feeling upset.

In the years that followed, Pat gave birth to a boy, Peter, in December 1964 and two girls: Catherine Ruth (known as Ruth) in March 1966 and Sarah Elizabeth in December 1967. Henry embraced family life, sharing music with his children and spending time with family and friends at his holiday home in Llangynog in North Wales.[4]

By 1969, Henry had been promoted to Reader in Virology—by 1976, he was Professor and Head of a newly formed Department of Medical Microbiology at the University. As he rose up the career ladder, Henry's interests focused on the enigmatic whitepox viruses and some apparent hybrid viruses, that appeared to be part-vaccinia, part-variola. He embraced techniques from the emerging field of molecular biology. During the final stage of the eradication campaign, the WHO valued Henry's opinion and sent him to

Pakistan and Afghanistan to assess the progress of the eradication efforts there.

AND SO IT CAME TO PASS that Professor Henry Bedson, blessed with an aptitude for technical innovation and faced with the challenge of sorting a lethal highly spreadable virus from its less harmful cousins, came to be working on live, virulent variola virus, right in the heart of England.

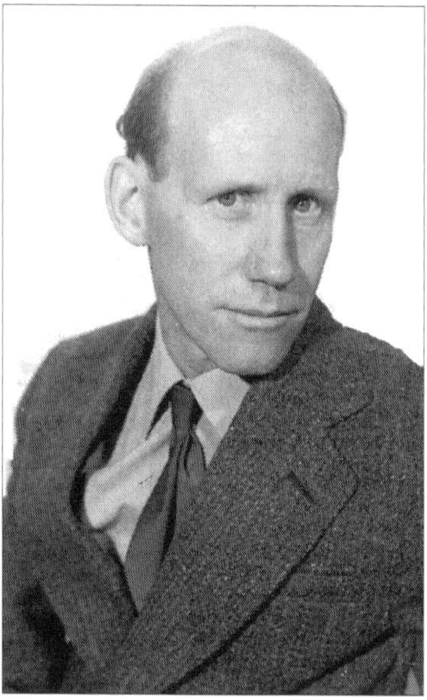

PROFESSOR HENRY BEDSON

Poxvirus expert and head of the smallpox lab
at the Birmingham Medical School

{Source: Birmingham Mail}

24

BANGLADESH 1973

BANGLADESH WAS TWICE BORN IN BLOODSHED: once in 1947, when, during the partition of British India, Muslim-majority East Bengal was sundered from Hindu-dominated West Bengal; and then again in 1971, when, after a vicious civil war, East Pakistan became the newly independent 'Country of Bengal'.

Despite the handicaps of a high population density and a flat, swampy, flood-prone terrain, by 1970 this corner of the planet had shaken off the scourge of smallpox—beating its larger neighbours India or West Pakistan to local eradication.[1] However, the civil war led to massive displacement of people, with nearly one in seven inhabitants fleeing temporarily to India. There in refugee camps, some of the temporary exiles acquired smallpox and, when the war finished, they went home and reintroduced the disease to their newly independent motherland. Aided by social upheaval, floods and famine, smallpox flourished in Bangladesh, with 90,000 cases by the end of 1971.

Victory over smallpox in Bangladesh took nearly four more years and a heroic effort from more than 24,000 workers, including 200 international workers—among them a Scottish doctor we have already met: Alasdair Geddes.[2]

He was there in 1973, because the UK Department of Health wanted some of the country's younger infectious diseases doctors to gain experience of smallpox before it disappeared. Not yet forty and not yet married, Geddes was selected to represent his country in the WHO smallpox eradication effort in Bangladesh. The challenges were immense: a population of 80 million, a flood-prone landscape and a host of inaccessible villages.[3]

GEDDES ARRIVED IN BANGLADESH with a problem. Despite being sent by the British government and the WHO, no one had told him that he needed a visa to enter the country. Without the necessary paperwork, as soon as he arrived at Dacca airport, Geddes was detained by the immigration authorities, who threatened to send him back to London on the very same plane that had just delivered him. Suddenly, a tall white man jumped over the barrier at the airport and handed what was probably a bank note to the Immigration Officer and Geddes was through! The white guy turned out to be a graduate of Birmingham Medical School called Nick Ward, who headed up the Smallpox Eradication team in Bangladesh.

Once in Dacca, Geddes noticed a couple of blue Land Rovers being readied for deployment in the field, one stuffed full of food and drink (mainly Coca-Cola), the other left bare. To his horror, he soon discovered that the full vehicle was for an American team, while his own team were to be dispatched in the empty vehicle—because Nick Ward believed that eating local food with the natives was more likely to elicit a co-operative response. This view was vindicated on their first evening in rural Bangladesh, when the owner of a village café treated them like royalty, feeding them chickens the size of blackbirds, while the locals were forced to watch the team feasting through a glassless window. However, the negative side of dining with the locals soon became clear, when Geddes fell ill with amoebic dysentery.

Under Nick's leadership, Geddes and the team crisscrossed the country by Land Rover, boat, bike and foot, seeing hundreds of cases of smallpox and vaccinating everyone they encountered. By day, as they entered remote villages, local young women fled into the bush, only be to hunted down and dragged back by the Bangladeshi members of the smallpox team, before grudgingly consenting to vaccination. In the evenings, the team visited markets with photographs of smallpox patients, asking whether anyone had seen a case. Reports of positive sightings evoked a rapid response as members of the team were dispatched to investigate.

Geddes spent seven weeks in Bangladesh, before the oil crisis in October 1973 meant he was summoned home. He had done his bit to wipe this evil virus off the face of the Earth. Having seen plenty of smallpox in the tropical landscape of Bengal, he never expected to encounter this viral adversary again in the temperate urban backdrop of the English Midlands—but he did.

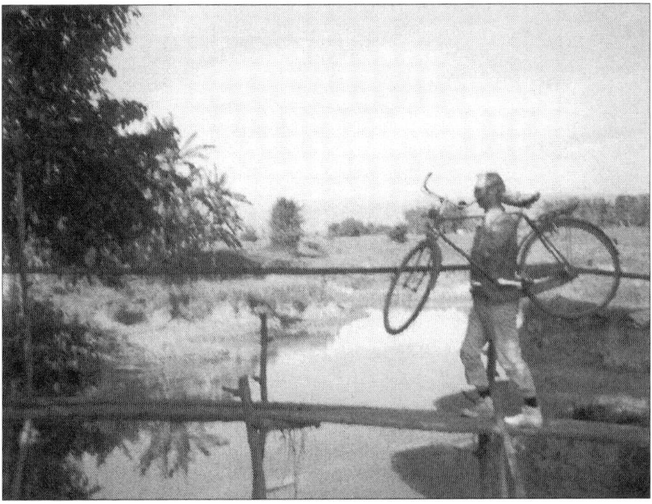

ALASDAIR GEDDES IN BANGLADESH
Carrying a bicycle across a narrow footbridge in 1973.
{Source: A. Geddes}

25

BANGLADESH 1975

The rule of the Final Inch! The realm of the Final Inch! In the Language of Maximum Clarity it is immediately clear what that is. The work has been almost completed, the goal almost attained, everything seems completely right and the difficulties overcome. But the quality of the thing is not quite right...

Solzhenitsyn (1968) *The First Circle*, quoted in a progress report to smallpox staff, 27 October 1975[1]

IT IS 16 October 1975 and we are in the Bangladeshi village of Kuralia on Bhola Island, situated at the mouth of the Meghna River in the mighty Ganges Delta. Today marks the culmination of a global eradication campaign stretching back nearly two centuries to Jenner. A young girl has just developed a rash—signalling the onset of the last naturally acquired case of variola major, the life-threatening form of smallpox.[2]

The WHO launched *Operation Smallpox Zero* in 1975. The last case of the disease in India was reported on 17 May that year in Bihar. By early November 1975, the eradicators thought they had closed in on the last case of variola major: a boy in Chittagong in Bangladesh, on the eastern side of the Bay of Bengal. Stan Foster, the American in charge of the eradication campaign in Bangladesh, started to receive congratulatory telegrams. Then comes a telegram announcing a new case on Bhola Island.

Bhola Island (also called Dakhin Shahbazpur) is the largest island in Bangladesh, with a surface area of nearly 1,500 km^2. A sandy mudflat, where rice, bananas and palm trees grow in profusion, but which repeatedly suffers appalling devastation whenever a cyclone strikes the Bay of Bengal. In 1975, it was home to nearly a million people.

The last case of variola major came to the world's attention thanks to the detective work of an eight-year-old girl called Bilkisunnessa who lived in Kuralia. In November 1975, she reported a cluster of smallpox cases to a local care worker, including a ten-year-old boy called Haris, who had infected his two-and-a-half-year old niece, Rahima Banu Begum. For her sleuthing, Bilkisunnessa received a reward from the WHO of 250 Bangladeshi taka (around $60)—equivalent to nearly a month's wages for the average Bangladeshi.[3]

It took Stan Foster twenty-four hours to reach the village from Dhaka by a combination of speedboat, steamer, jeep, motorcycle and foot. Once the diagnosis was confirmed, Rahima was put into quarantine, with guards at her home and food and money supplied to the family. Foster and another eradicator, Daniel Tarantola, assembled a large team of field workers, who vaccinated everyone within a mile and half—about 18,000 people—and searched every house within five miles for additional cases.

They found none: and so Rahima Begum has gone down in the history books as the end of a long lineage of human-to-human transmission of variola major that stretched back for centuries, maybe even millennia. Rahima made a complete recovery and, despite the stigma of suffering from smallpox, went on to marry at the age of eighteen and played mother to four children.[4] Rahima's smallpox scabs were saved and transported to a secure facility in the USA to serve as last relics of a global killer. Nearly twenty years later, they yielded a genome sequence from the last naturally acquired strain of variola major.[5]

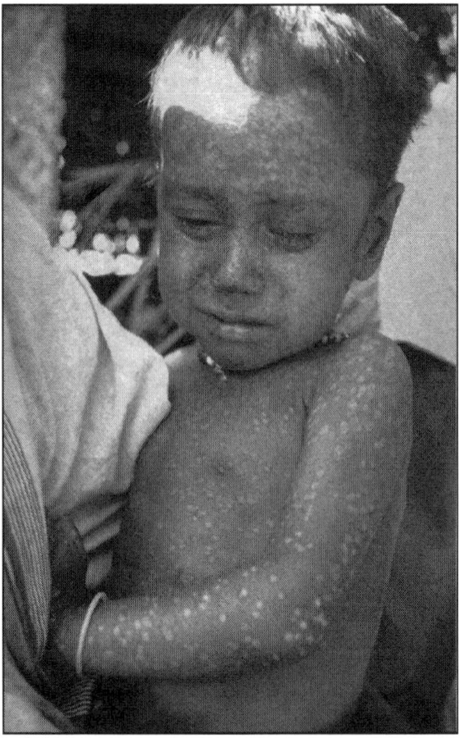

RAHIMA BANU IN 1975

Last case of naturally-acquired variola major.

{Source: commons.wikimedia.org/wiki/File:Rahima_Banu.jpg}

26

SOMALIA 1977

SMALLPOX, IN THE WEAKENED form of variola minor or alastrim, sputtered on for more than two years in the Horn of Africa.[1] Wrestling it to extinction in the face of social and political opposition, civil war and an inhospitable terrain took a form of heroism that is the stuff of legend. As Haile Selassie lost hold on the far-flung provinces of Ethiopia, helicopter teams taking vaccine supplies to remote areas were shot at and, on occasion, kidnapped or lost. Vaccination teams sometimes had to travel overland on mule or by foot for ten days to reach a destination.

The fall of Selassie and a new Ethiopian government in 1974 delivered fresh impetus to the campaign, so that over the next two years smallpox was swept out of the country's central highlands and Ogaden desert. The viral trickster made its last stand in neighbouring Somalia, where social, political and geographical obstacles were even more taxing than in Ethiopia. Three thousand staff struggled with an epidemic that reached its peak in April 1977 and encompassed over a thousand cases.

The last ever case of variola minor occurred in October 1977: Ali Maow Maalin, a 23-year-old hospital cook and part-time vaccinator (but himself unvaccinated) from the busy port of Merca. Maalin had acquired the infection during a 15-minute ride with two infected children from a camp of nomads. In response to his infection, 54,777 people were vaccinated within two weeks. Then transmission ceased—smallpox hit zero!

THE SMALLPOX ERADICATION CAMPAIGN cost around 300 million US dollars.[2] That sounds a lot, but it amounts to only 1-2% of the cost of the Apollo programme that put just twelve men on the surface of the moon.[3] For less than a dime per person, five years after the last man walked on the moon, smallpox had been wiped from our planet. The audacious hopes of Jenner, Franklin, Chisholm, Zhdanov and Henderson had come to fruition—but Maalin was not to be the last case of smallpox. Smallpox the infection had been extinguished, but the virus that caused it lived on in labs around the world.

27

PERSONAL INTERLUDE

COMING TO BIRMINGHAM

During the summer of 2001, I was excited to be leaving Queen's University Belfast for a new Chair in Microbial Genomics at the University of Birmingham. During my nearly two years in Northern Ireland, I had managed to accumulate a considerable strain collection that included lots of pathogenic strains of E. coli and Salmonella—and I wanted to move them to Birmingham with me, along with my VW Golf.

Back then it was not uncommon for scientists to transport strains, appropriately and safely packaged, in their own cars. However, the Irish Sea presented a problem, as the rules did not allow such strains to be transported on the fast ferry service from Belfast to England. I was sorely tempted just to load the strains into the boot of my car and take them with me, particularly as security measures had been relaxed considerably in the wake of the Good Friday Agreement.

As I started the journey home, the newspapers reported that Imperial College had been prosecuted for constructing a hybrid virus with genes from the Hepatitis C and Dengue viruses, without agreed safeguards in place. An article in the Guardian pointed out parallels with the 1978 smallpox incident in Birmingham. As I arrived at the ferry terminal in Belfast, I imagined a future headline: 'Maverick new professor sacked for bringing dangerous pathogens to smallpox university'.

Just as I approached the ramp leading on to the ferry, my Golf and I were pulled over for a security check. I was asked to open the boot, which I did, revealing it to be entirely empty. In a parallel universe, an alternative me was led away in handcuffs.

Luckily, in the real universe, the chief technician at Queen's had already arranged for my strains to be transported through an official route. On 1 July 2001, I took up my new job and moved into laboratory and office accommodation on the lower ground floor of the East Wing of the Medical School at the University of Birmingham, just downstairs from what used to be the smallpox lab. A few weeks later, I met Alasdair Geddes, whose vivid recollections of the remarkable events of the summer of 1978 provided the impetus for the book in front of you.

PART FOUR

ONE AUGUST EVENT

Alien they seemed to be;
No mortal eye could see
The intimate welding of their later history,
Or sign that they were bent
By paths coincident
On being anon twin halves of one august event,
Till the Spinner of the Years
Said 'Now!' And each one hears,
And consummation comes, and jars two hemispheres.
Thomas Hardy (1912) *Convergence of the Twain*

28

PAKISTAN 1970

Lives of great men all remind us we can make our lives sublime
And departing leave behind us footprints on the sands of time.
Henry Wadsworth Longfellow (1838) *A Psalm of Life*[1]

WE ARE IN A LAND between East and West, where Eurasian and Indian plates collide, embracing the Indus valley, flanked to the west by the Baluchistan plateau and to the north by the foothills of the Himalayas. Historians may argue whether great men really do shape history or merely ride its currents.[2] Yet, several great men have clearly left footprints on this landscape.

Sometime before 400 BCE, Siddhartha Gautama established a new religion, Buddhism, which rapidly permeated the region. In the third century BCE, the Macedonian general, Alexander the Great, swept in from the West, ushering in a new era of Indo-Greek civilisation. The resulting fusion of Greek sculpture with Buddhist religious art culminated in the familiar statues of the Buddha scattered across Asia. Buddhism lasted a thousand years in Pakistan before, in the eighth century of the Common Era, the region fell under the influence of another protagonist who left his footprints on the sands of time, Muhammad, and of another religion, Islam.

IN 1970, THE SMALLPOX eradication campaign was in full swing, but there were still thousands of cases every year in Pakistan. The variola major virus, the cause of the more lethal form of smallpox, was proving surprisingly tenacious. Surviving for century after century here, this virus had become a microcosm of Buddhism, caught up in an endless cycle of reincarnation, jumping every couple of weeks from one human body to the next.

But the virus evolved. Every infection represented a lineage that had completed the cycle of reincarnation thousands of times—transmitted endlessly from Buddhist to Buddhist, from Buddhist to Muslim and then from Muslim to Muslim. In recent years, a new lineage had emerged, producing a slightly different profile of proteins and behaving slightly differently when grown in the laboratory. It might even have been a little more virulent. In the years that followed, it was to spread as far south as Vellore in India and was to track through the Middle East before jumping into Yugoslavia, deep within Europe.

In February 1970, two samples of the new lineage are taken from patients in Pakistan, one from a three-year-old boy called Abid, the other from an eighteen-year-old man called Taj.[3] Each sample is packed full of a million or more particles of the variola virus.

Freighted by air, these representatives of what we might call the Abid Dynasty ascend high into the stratosphere. The viral pilgrims migrate northward from Pakistan into the heart of the Soviet Union. There, they join an elite set of reference strains, sent to research centres around the world.

Within a few years, the Abid lineage has taken up residence in laboratories in three continents, including the laboratory of Professor Keith Dumbell at St. Mary's Hospital Medical School in London. On 26 May 1978, Dumbell hands some vials of smallpox virus over to his friend and fellow smallpox expert Henry Bedson and the Abid lineage makes the one-hundred-mile journey from London to Birmingham.

FREED FROM THE ENDLESS cycles of host-to-host transmission—from the samsara of entry, infection and escape from human tissues—the Abid Dynasty has achieved viral enlightenment, nirvana in the laboratory. Whether propagated endlessly in a paradise of laboratory culture or left to sleep frozen or freeze-dried, the virus has become immortal, tamed, otherworldly.

But within twelve weeks of its arrival in Birmingham, there will come a convergence of the twain—virus and victim—as variola escapes back into the wild world of humankind and brings tragedy to Britain's second city.

29

THE PHONEY WAR

FOR OVER TEN MONTHS, humanity's viral load of variola has stood at zero. But now, the Abid Dynasty is reincarnated in a new human avatar. Sometime in late July or early August 1978, virus meets woman.[1] A few variola virus particles, perhaps even a single particle, enter a cell in her throat, lungs or skin, commandeering the cell into creating virus factories.

The virus declares war on its new victim, but, to begin with, it is a phoney war. The initial infection produces no symptoms or identifiable damage. A recent study by a team from Stanford has documented in exquisite molecular detail how cells respond to poxvirus infection.[2] The Stanford microbiologists expected to see massive changes in the way genes were switched on or off, as the cell sensed the virus setting up to devour it from within. Instead, even in obviously damaged cells, they encountered what they described as 'stunned silence'.

The smallpox virus, like all poxviruses, carries an arsenal of deadly silencers that cloak it from the cell's usual defences, jamming up the signalling pathways that would otherwise scream 'Danger!' Instead of assault and battery, it deploys stealth—or even seduction.[3]

After setting up base camp in peripheral cells, the virus spills into the new victim's blood. It is then taken up by macrophages, a type of warrior-cell-cum-waste-disposal-unit at the heart of the body's immune system.[4] The macrophages carry the virus to the lymph nodes and similar collections of immune cells throughout the body. Within these cellular fortresses, cycle after cycle of viral replication occurs. Virus Abid is re-arming, preparing for the tipping point, for the viral offensive. After silent infiltration of enemy territory, the offensive will begin.

30

BIRMINGHAM 1978

AT FIRST GLANCE, BIRMINGHAM is an improbable place.[1] By population, it is the UK's second city, after London. Four hundred and sixty feet above sea level, this midlands metropolis sits high on its own uplands, the Birmingham plateau, bounded to the north and south by the valleys of the Trent and the Avon, to the west by the Stour and Severn and to the east by the Blythe. Even today, trains struggle to climb the Lickey Incline on the southern approach to the city—the steepest such incline in the country. Forty-five miles to the north of the city, the Peak District shades into the southern end of the Pennines, the series of hills dubbed 'the backbone of England'.

Yet, there is nothing obvious in the landscape to justify Birmingham's existence. There is no port or harbour here; the city lies a hundred miles from the nearest coast. Although it sits on a small river, the River Rea, this hardly seems enough to act as a nucleation point for a sprawling metropolis. Instead, this is a city whose existence is better explained by history and industry, rather than mere geography.

THE ROMANS BUILT A FORT a few miles south of the current city centre, at a crossroads on Icknield Street. Later, the Anglo-Saxons settled here to create *Beormingahām* or the homestead of Boerm's people. In the twelfth century, the local Lord of the Manor, Peter de Birmingham, acquired a royal charter, allowing him to hold a weekly market in what was to become the Bull Ring, jumpstarting Birmingham's life as a trading centre.

Several centuries later, seditious Birmingham sided with Parliament and the Puritans in the English Civil War. Around the same time, Birmingham experienced its first population explosion, fuelled by a booming manufacturing industry dominated by metal goods. By 1700, Birmingham had become the fifth-largest town in England and Wales; far enough from London to avoid the strangling influence of the guilds, yet close enough to the capital and the country's ports to engage in trade. The town's smithies exploited twin resources of the surrounding landscape: iron and coal.

By the early eighteenth century, Birmingham had also become a centre of religious dissent, home to Quakers, Unitarians and

Presbyterians. This local tradition of free thought primed an unprecedented coupling of intellectual enlightenment and industrial innovation in the city and its environs. In 1709, less than forty miles to the north west of the city, Quaker Abraham Darby I established the first blast furnace to smelt iron with coke rather than charcoal. In 1741, the world's first cotton mill opened in the city.

By the second half of the eighteenth century, as science and industry went hand in hand, the modern world was born here in Birmingham. The city played host to the Lunar Society of Birmingham[2], a dining and discussion club, which included many of the country's leading thinkers-and-doers: Joseph Priestley, Matthew Boulton, Josiah Wedgwood, James Watt, William Withering and Erasmus Darwin.

Together, Boulton and Watt developed the steam engine, freeing humanity of an age-old reliance on muscle power, while Boulton's Soho Manufactory and Wedgwood's pottery firm signalled the birth of the factory system. Priestley largely established chemistry, Withering founded pharmacology, while polymath Erasmus Darwin captured the spirit of the age in overblown epic poetry.[3]

By the nineteenth century, Birmingham had earned a reputation as *the city of a thousand trades*, plugged into the rest of the world, first by an extensive canal network and then by the railways. With industrialisation and urban growth came squalor. In response, in the late nineteenth century, under the leadership of local mayor Joseph Chamberlain, Birmingham's slums and its city centre underwent a series of ambitious improvements, reshaping it into a modern world-class city.

As the twentieth century dawned, with help from Chamberlain, the city also gained its own University. Snug in the city's leafy southern suburbs, the new University of Birmingham sported an understated grandeur, built of warm but imposing red brick, clad with friezes depicting the fruits of industry, capped with domes reminiscent of Byzantium and centred around a looming clock tower worthy of the Venetian skyline.

ON BALANCE, UNTIL ITS final quarter, the twentieth century was good to Birmingham. In 1906, Herbert Austin acquired a site for his car-making factory in Longbridge, a few miles south of the University. Aside from making cars, the site was to play a decisive role in both World Wars, turning out munitions and parts for tanks and aircraft.

Birmingham suffered badly during the Blitz, which destroyed many of the city's fine buildings. However, the post-war years brought a new affluence to the city and the region. By the late 1960s, Longbridge was the largest car plant in the world, with a 25,000-strong workforce and a range of best-selling products, including the iconic original two-door Mini.

In the decades after the Second World War, Birmingham underwent a transformation—physical and demographic—that left it a modern metropolis or a concrete jungle, depending on one's point of view. The city's skyline expanded heavenward. Road transport through the city now flowed freely through a series of expressways and tunnels, but pedestrians were wary of being mugged in urine-soaked underpasses.

Birmingham was now connected to the rest of the country by a network of motorways, which fed right into the city centre via the notorious Spaghetti Junction and seven-lane Aston Expressway. Birmingham was connected to the wider world by its own international airport. In a short movie, American actor Telly Sevalas (TV detective *Kojak*) lauded the city's mix of old and new as 'his kind of town.'[4]

IN THE LATE SEVENTIES, 'Brum' was not just the second largest city in the UK, with a population of just over a million people, but also the beating heart of the West Midlands conurbation, which encompassed over two million inhabitants. To the west, sprawled an urban landscape known as the Black Country, whose inhabitants dismissed the neighbouring city as 'Brummagen'. The Black Country merged westwards into Wolverhampton. To the east of Birmingham was the well-to-do metropolitan borough of Solihull and, beyond that, Coventry. To the north sat suburban Sutton Coldfield and, a bit further north, Staffordshire and the Potteries. As a mark of the importance of the West Midlands on the national stage, in 1976, the National Exhibition Centre was established at a point where Solihull meets Birmingham.

In the 1960s and 1970s, the West Midlands played a pivotal role in the birth of the indigenous musical genre of Heavy Metal, spawning legendary bands such as Black Sabbath, Led Zeppelin and Judas Priest. In the post-war years, immigration made the region more cosmopolitan. Irish labourers helped construct the region's roads and urban environment. Pakistanis started running restaurants and cafés, culminating in the creation of the 'Birmingham balti', a distinctive local curry served in a metal bowl with a massive naan bread. In 1975, the Birmingham Central

Mosque joined the city's skyline as the largest mosque in Western Europe.

However, the indigenous population was not always welcoming to the newcomers. In 1964, Tory MP for Smethwick, Peter Griffiths, ran, and won, an election campaign with an anti-immigration stance bolstered by posters featuring the slogan: 'If you want a nigger for a neighbour, vote Labour.'[5] In 1968, local MP and racist rhetorician Enoch Powell gave his infamous 'rivers of blood' speech in Birmingham, prophesying inter-racial violence.[6]

After the Provisional IRA bombed the city's pubs in November 1974, killing 21 people and injuring 182, there was a backlash against the Irish community and the 'Birmingham Six'—all Irishmen who had lived in the city since the 1960s—were beaten by police and prison officers, framed and imprisoned for the crime.[7]

In July 1975, Rastafarian reggae artists Bob Marley and Third World played the Birmingham Odeon.[8] In their wake, many young black Brummies, fed up of discrimination in the work place and harassment by the police, began to reject the ideal of integration and instead started seeing Africa as their home and the city and country they lived in as 'Babylon'.[9]

Just over a year later, on 5 August 1976, English Rock legend Eric Clapton let rip a racist rant while drunk at a concert in Birmingham, dropping the line 'I used to be into dope, now I'm into racism'. Despite having worked with Bob Marley, Clapton went on to use the Birmingham gig to voice his support of Enoch Powell, parroting a National Front slogan 'Keep Britain white!' and peppering his speech with offensive talk of 'wogs' and 'coons'.[10]

By 1978, Birmingham reggae band Steel Pulse had released their landmark album *Handsworth Revolution*, complete with album cover showing Rastas thriving in a post-apocalyptic urban jungle. In the south of the city, members of what was to become multiracial reggae band UB40 started rehearsing that summer in a local basement.[11] UB40 took their name from an official government form used to sign on for unemployment benefit. In so doing, they captured the local zeitgeist of a city sliding into economic decline.

Fordism—Henry Ford's take on Matthew Boulton's production line economy—delivered wealth to the city throughout the post-war years. However, in the 1970s, Birmingham and the West Midlands went from being the country's wealthiest region outside the Southeast to its most deprived. As hundreds of thousands of local jobs were lost, this sudden crash in prosperity stoked the fires of discord between classes and between communities.

By the mid-1970s, British Leyland, then-owner of the

Longbridge plant, was facing collapse. The government provided a £2.4 billion bailout, but this was not enough to ensure industrial harmony or quality production. Instead, union convenor at Longbridge, Derek 'Red Robbo' Robinson, stirred up over 500 disputes in just two years.[12] With the precipitous decline in manufacturing, the West Midlands fell into a serious financial and industrial malaise.

IN THE LATTER HALF OF 1978, the United Kingdom as a whole could hardly be described as a nation at peace with itself or the world. Two years of punk rock had driven a wedge between the generations. We were still at war with the Provisional IRA over Northern Ireland. Our nuclear weapons were still targeted on Moscow. Although notionally a parliamentary democracy, the trade unions jostled with Jim Callaghan's Labour government as to who ran our country.

The newspapers that year devoted many column inches to strikes and other industrial action, threatened or already underway, as the Callaghan government tried to enforce a 5% pay deal in the public sector. The press, although free, was not always rational or responsible. It fanned the flames of a scare over whooping cough vaccine[13] and, the year before, newspaper vied with newspaper as to how much sensationalist coverage they could devote to a sex-in-chains scandal involving a Mormon missionary.[14]

Margaret Thatcher, already known as the Iron Lady, was Leader of the Opposition and that year the Tories took the unprecedented step of hiring an advertising firm, Saatchi & Saatchi, to revamp their image and get their message across ahead of an anticipated general election.[15] In the months that followed, Callaghan considered calling an autumn election, but made the worst mistake of his career in deciding not to—the Winter of Discontent that followed would prepare the way for a Thatcher government.[16] Abba provided a catchy but vacuous backdrop to the closing years of a dreary decade.

YET, DESPITE ALL this local, national and global discord, Birmingham felt safe. Far from the coast, it was safe from flooding. In the heart of England's green and pleasant land, there were no poisonous spiders and snakes, no predatory human-eating carnivores and no malaria or cholera—and, in this post-eradication world, Birmingham seemed to be safe from smallpox.

On its leafy campus, nestled in the sedate southern suburbs, the University of Birmingham must have felt safe too. For three quarters of a century it had flourished as Britain's first 'redbrick' university, a safe and solid choice for an education outside of the golden triangle of London, Oxford and Cambridge.[17] In his 1975 novel *Changing Places*, local English-professor-turned-novelist David Lodge had satirised it as the University of Rummidge, gently mocking the safe conventional conformity of British academic life.[18]

In May 1978, the University gained its own railway station, opened by then Secretary of State for Transport Bill Rodgers MP (later to gain notoriety as one of the 'gang of four' who founded the SDP).[19] The railway line and adjacent Birmingham and Worcester canal bisected the campus, with the bulk of the University to the south and the Medical School and Queen Elizabeth Hospital to the north. With a workforce of several thousand, the Edgbaston campus was one of Birmingham's largest employers. During term-time, the University thronged with thousands of students. In retrospect, with hundreds of thousands within an hour's walk and millions within an hour's drive, it was an odd place in which to locate a smallpox laboratory.

SO WHAT WAS BIRMINGHAM in the summer of 1978: Rummidge or Babylon? Safe city or metropolis on the brink? It all depends on your perspective. But something was about to happen. Into this troubled tinderbox of a million souls, of economic decline and political discord, of racial tension and class struggle, of truculent trade unions and tasteless tabloids, the spark of smallpox was about to settle. And no one could know how far the viral flame and accompanying fumes of fear were going to spread.

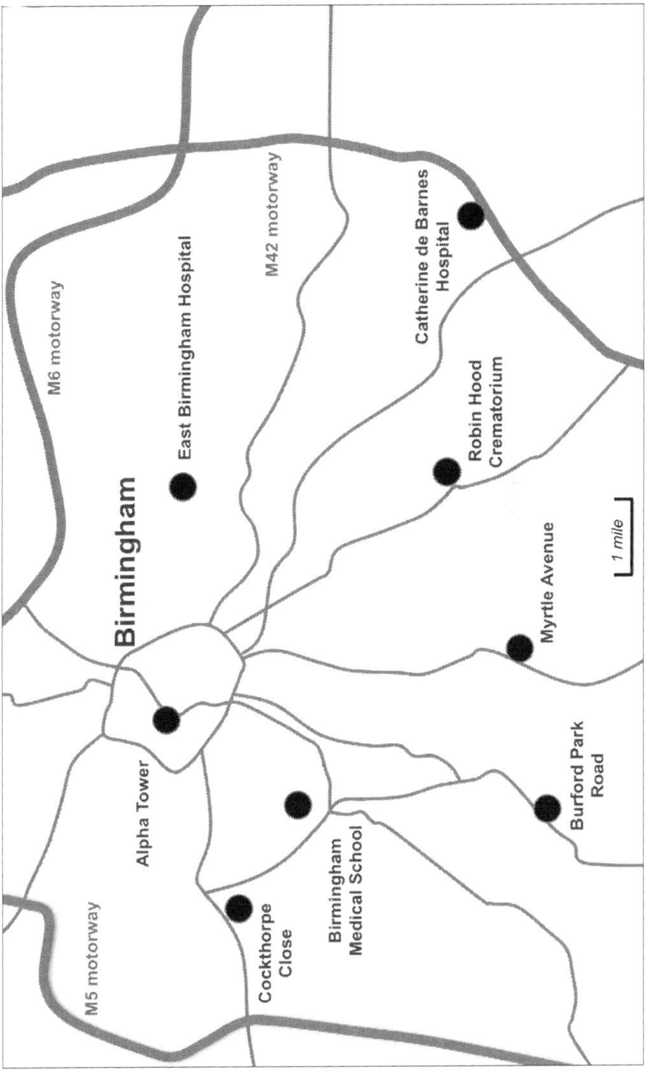
Birmingham
M6 motorway
East Birmingham Hospital
M42 motorway
Catherine de Barnes Hospital
Robin Hood Crematorium
Myrtle Avenue
1 mile
Burford Park Road
Alpha Tower
Birmingham Medical School
Cockthorpe Close
M5 motorway

31

THE FLUEY PHOTOGRAPHER

'FLU'—WE HAVE ALL had it. Or at least we all say we have had it. Along with an upset tummy, feeling 'fluey' is the commonest excuse to avoid coming into work. The term has even been co-opted in the battle of the sexes in the phrase *man-flu*, for flu that isn't really flu at all. But real flu isn't something you can argue with. It forces you to bed; it forces you to snatch a restless haunted sleep.

Janet Parker felt fluey. It was odd to catch flu in August. Yet Janet had all the right symptoms: a skull-cracking headache and world-weary muscles that ached and ached. It was a Friday—Friday 11 August 1978. The constitutionally calm, 'no-panic Janet' did not want to make a fuss; one day to go till the weekend. She had work to do, so she soldiered on. She went into work.[1]

THERE WAS NOTHING REMARKABLE about Janet. Nothing to suggest that she would end up in the history books or to justify the tragic fate that befell her. Born just before the War, she lived through the thrifty fifties and the swinging sixties—hers was the first generation to call themselves 'teenagers'. In a picture taken at her wedding, she appears fresh-faced, sporting a bob cut and fringe, with bright eyes and a vibrant, almost cheeky half-smile: a sunny young woman, with her whole life ahead of her.

In a subsequent pair of photos, taken a decade or more later, Janet looks rather more solid and sensible. In a holiday photo, she sports a white polo-neck sweater, a sensible smart jacket and trousers and a light-coloured cap—with just the hint of a smile. In what appears to be a passport photo, she is no longer smiling. Her lower face carries a wide full-lipped mouth and her broad jaw line now looks more angular, rugged, almost masculine. Her darkish wavy hair, now fringeless and parted on the left, is just long enough to touch her collar. Her sensible blouse and dowdy cardigan suggest a sound, even-tempered, reliable mind-set.

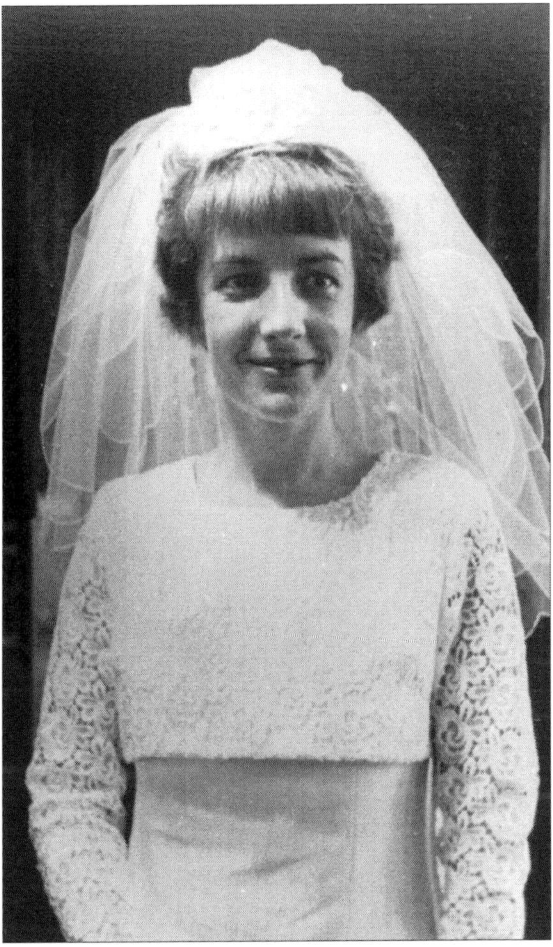

JANET PARKER AS A YOUNG WOMAN
Aged twenty-seven at her wedding in 1965.
{Source: *Birmingham Mail*}

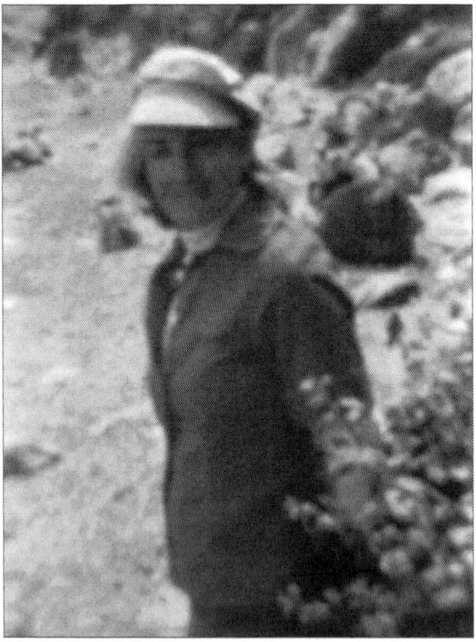

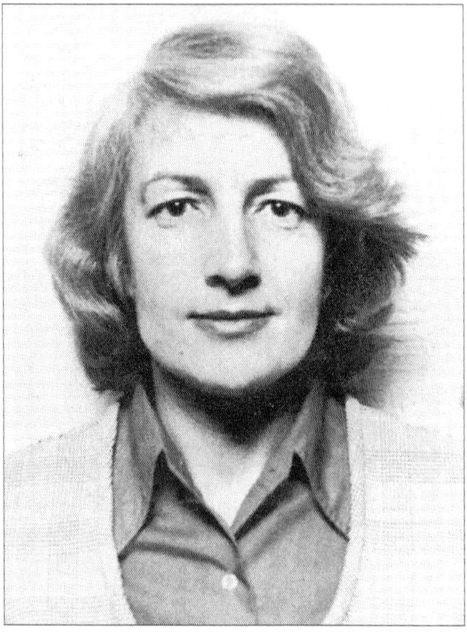

JANET PARKER IN LATER LIFE
{Source: *Birmingham Mail*}

Janet was educated at Kings Norton Grammar School for Girls. As a grammar-school girl, she must have been bright enough to pass the selective eleven-plus entrance examination, which would have allowed her to benefit from a selective but free education paid for by Birmingham City Council. She spent a couple of years in the Department of Metallurgy at the University of Birmingham, before embarking on a career in photography in her early twenties. She spent fifteen years working as a photographer with the West Midlands Police Force. During this time, through the court appearances necessitated by her work, she made a strong impression on the lawyers she encountered—local barrister Brian Escott-Cox later described her as 'an attractive young woman, with a bright aura, who clearly knew what she was doing.'

In 1965, at the age of twenty-seven, she met the man of her life, Joseph Parker, while he was visiting Birmingham Police HQ to repair a faulty switchboard and they married in the September of that year.[2] Twelve years her senior, Joseph confessed that he was a bit of a loner before he met Janet. He worked as a Post Office engineer at a time when, in Britain, the Post Office still looked after telecommunications.[3] Typically for industrial relations in the UK in the late 1970s, at the time our story begins, Joseph and his fellow Post Office engineers were in dispute with their employer over the length of their working week.[4]

Early in 1978, Janet celebrated the big 'four-O': her fortieth birthday. She entered middle age enjoying the settled domesticity of married life. Janet lived with Joseph in an unremarkable suburb, Kings Norton, in the southern reaches of Birmingham's urban sprawl.[5] A medieval village, complete with village green, Kings Norton had expanded considerably after the Industrial Revolution, linked to the outside world first by the Redditch Road, then by a canal and then by a railway. In the late 1970s, Kings Norton's chief claim to fame was that, with neighbouring Selly Oak, it formed half of the fictitious Kings Oak, home to the Crossroads Motel, focus of a low-budget but well-loved British soap opera, where improbable things happened in suburban Birmingham.[6]

Unlike the large Georgian house that became the Crossroads Motel, the Parker residence in Burford Park Road was a modern, modest, affordable home, a detached bungalow benefitting from off-street parking and a convenient location, less than fifteen minutes by car from the city centre and from the Medical School, where Janet worked.

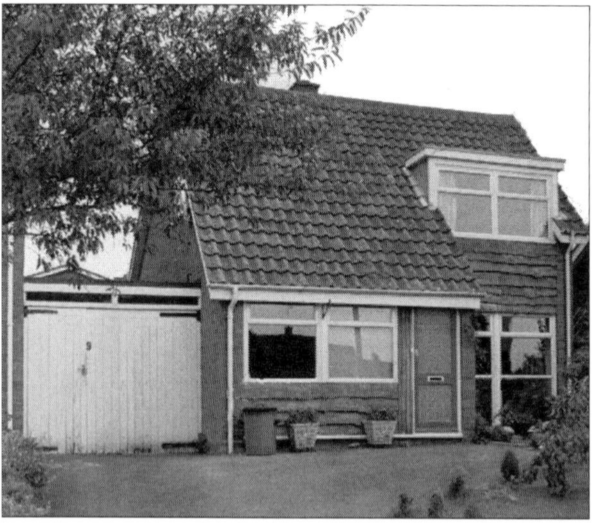

9 BURFORD PARK ROAD

Janet Parker's home in the Birmingham suburb of Kings Norton

{Source: Birmingham Mail}

Janet and Joseph loved their cars and they bought British: she had a Triumph Spitfire, a nifty little sports car, while he had a more solid and sensible Triumph 2500, both manufactured at the Canley works in nearby Coventry.[7] Janet and Joseph had no children, but they had dogs. Plus Janet's parents were near at hand: Fred and Hilda Witcomb lived just ten minutes' drive away in Myrtle Avenue, a quiet cul-de-sac in the suburb of Kings Heath. From here, Janet's father travelled by bus to work at J. W. Barrett, a jewellery firm in Birmingham's Jewellery Quarter.[8]

Three years earlier, in 1975, Janet had decided she had had enough of the erratic hours associated with police work, so she had taken up a new, predictable, nine-to-five job as Medical Photographer in the Anatomy Department at the Birmingham Medical School, in leafy Edgbaston. Her work chiefly involved using a microscope to photograph tissue sections on slides, but occasionally she was called on to photograph primates in the University's animal house. She sometimes undertook private photographic work, mainly taking passport photographs for staff in the Medical School. She was responsible for placing orders for all the photographic materials that she used, which meant a lot of time spent on the telephone. Janet had developed what was described as 'spinal trouble', which restricted her movements somewhat. This meant she tended to stick to the Photography Department, with occasional forays into the Educational Services Unit.

In her new work place, Janet had rapidly developed a small circle of loyal friends—half a dozen of them got together to form a coffee club. She took her lunch and tea with them in the technician's common room. Her workmates described her as kindly, mature, level-headed, possessing a quiet sense of humour and easy to work with. In her spare time, she was trying to better herself by taking a distance-learning course with the Open University and had planned to use her annual leave to attend an Open University event. Like many other technical staff at the University, Janet joined the union, the Association of Scientific, Technical and Managerial Staffs (ASTMS), Britain's largest union for white-collar staff. At least once she joined a picket line at the Medical School.[9]

THAT FRIDAY, 11 AUGUST 1978, although feeling fluey, Janet travelled to and from work with Joseph by car. The next day, when the weekend started, she felt better and grabbed some fresh air on a brief walk in Kings Norton. By Sunday, she was feeling rough again. That day, two neighbours, Millicent Rowley and her husband, from 11 Burford Park Road, called in to see Janet.

The fog of 'flu' thickened over the next few days. By Monday 13 August, Janet had developed red spots on her trunk, limbs and face. She had been looking forward to attending a weeklong Open University course at Nottingham University, but the rash was enough to change her mind. Had she gone, she would have been exposed to around three thousand people and would almost certainly have triggered a massive nationwide outbreak of smallpox.

Janet's General Practitioner, Dr Lewis Arundel, saw Janet on a home visit on Tuesday 14 August and made a tentative diagnosis of chickenpox. As Janet had just started experiencing symptoms of cystitis (painful and frequent passing of urine), he prescribed an antibiotic, oxytetracycline. She also started taking a painkiller-pick-me-up called Hypon (a mixture of aspirin, codeine and caffeine). Janet's mother was sceptical of the diagnosis, as she had nursed Janet through chickenpox as a child.

Two days later, Arundel's partner, Dr George Horry, visited Janet. He noticed the worsening rash and, mindful of the fact that oxytetracycline could cause a rash, made a diagnosis of drug reaction and stopped the medication. He prescribed two other antibiotics instead: cotrimoxazole, for the presumed urinary tract infection, and erythromycin, to cover the possibility of a respiratory tract infection.

On Monday 21 August, Fred Witcomb drove his ailing daughter to the parental home in Myrtle Avenue. As the second week of her illness progressed, even under the care of Mum and Dad, Janet was getting worse, as additional spots sprung up on her face, limbs and trunk. She had one more visitor: an aunt, Mrs Allen. She started taking a sedative, sodium amytal, to calm her nerves and help her sleep.

32

THE VIRAL OFFENSIVE

IN 1968, THE VIET CONG LAUNCHED the Tet offensive, suddenly everywhere, striking at more than a hundred towns and cities across the length and breadth of South Vietnam.[1] A poorly equipped but determined army was taking on a superpower, the most sophisticated and well armed in the world. It faced tactical defeat, but gained a strategic victory.

By mid-August 1978, variola virus is suddenly everywhere across the length and breadth of Janet Parker's body. A virus armed with just a couple of hundred proteins is taking on a multicellular superpower: an organism of a hundred trillion cells, protected by a highly sophisticated immune system.[2]

The storm has been brewing silently for nearly two weeks. Now, the virus sweeps through her bloodstream in a massive virus shower, a so-called *secondary viraemia*, which triggers the onset of symptoms. It has made her feel fluey. Her back aches. Her head aches. Her belly aches. Her temperature soars. The virus invades the linings of her mouth, tongue and throat to produce internal spots. As it bursts out into her breath, she reaches the peak of infectivity, becoming a living, breathing haze of virus particles.

Within a few more days, macrophages sweep the infection into the capillaries of her skin, starting with a few *herald spots* on her face and scalp, before spreading in turn to her back, arms, chest, hands, legs and finally her feet. The rash is denser at points where her clothing is tightest, where bra or belt or knicker-elastic presses against her skin. At first, the spots are red and flat *macules*, but then cell death and swelling create raised *vesicles*, filled with clear fluid. She starts to experience a prickling sensation in her skin, like bad sunburn, but involving every part of her body's surface.

By the time Parker enters hospital, her spots are stuffed with enough pus and cellular debris to produce *pustules*. She now harbours huge quantities of the virus in her spleen, lymph nodes, liver, bone marrow and kidneys. Variola virus is spilling out into her tears and her urine. The viral offensive is in full swing and the viral army has seized the heartland of the country that is Janet Parker.

33

A UNICORN ON THE LAWN

DEBORAH SYMMONS WAS BORN IN 1954. Her mother was a teacher and her father a company director.[1] She grew up in Buckinghamshire and was taught by nuns at St Bernard's Convent School in Slough in nearby Berkshire. She was the first medic in the family and, for her undergraduate medical training, she chose Birmingham, because it was just the right distance from home and offered continuous assessment—and the young Deborah did not like the pressure of final exams.

After five years as a medical student, the newly qualified Dr Symmons started her medical career on a memorable date, 7-7-77, when she took up a surgical house job at the Birmingham General Hospital with Mike Baddeley (a pioneer of bariatric surgery). Six months later, she started a medical house job in the professorial unit at the Queen Elizabeth Hospital, working for Professor Raymond 'Bill' Hoffenberg, a charismatic, tall and athletic South African endocrinologist, who had worked with Albert Schweitzer and had had to flee his homeland on account of the Apartheid regime. Birmingham had taken the bold step of appointing Hoffenberg to the William Withering chair of medicine in 1972. Now, five years on, Bill had proven his worth locally and nationally as a clinical-academic mover and shaker and made a strong impression on the 23-year-old Deborah.

Without much forethought, the young Dr Symmons stumbled into her fateful role as Senior House Officer in Infectious Diseases job after an impromptu discussion with Alasdair Geddes, in which she asked whether she could have a job in Infectious Diseases and he simply replied 'Yes'. The plainspoken Hoffenberg expressed his disapproval, making it clear that he thought she should instead have gone straight on to a general medical rotation.

AND SO, ON Tuesday 1 August, 1978, after a fortnight's unpaid holiday, Dr Deborah Symmons started work as SHO in Infectious Diseases at East Birmingham Hospital. That month she experienced a minor car crash and other car trouble, but it was what happened at work that made it the most eventful month of her life.

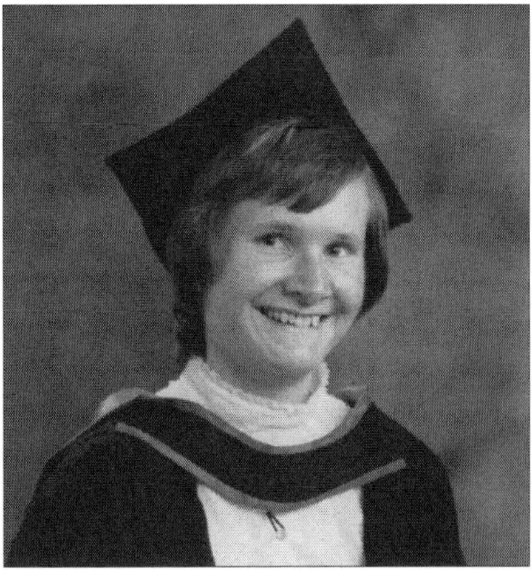

DEBORAH SYMMONS
At her graduation a year before she started work as an infectious disease doctor at the East Birmingham Hospital.
{Source: D. Symmons}

The excitement started with an unusual bout of food poisoning.[2] On Sunday 30 July, an elderly married couple from Yardley in Birmingham, Leonard and Clara Farmer, prepared a meal for Leonard's brother and sister-in-law, Jesse and Betty. Between them, they ate seven and a half ounces of canned red salmon from Britain's best-known brand, John West, garnished with some salad. They noticed that the salmon tasted slightly odd.

A few hours later, first Leonard and Clara and then Jesse and Betty fell ill with a dry mouth, blurred vision and vomiting. An astute junior doctor, Adrian Hastings, recognised the symptoms as botulism: a rare form of paralysis caused by a toxin from the bacterium *Clostridium botulinum* ('Botox' is now better known for its use in the cosmetic industry).

The botulism patients were admitted to East Birmingham Hospital early on Monday 31 July. By the next day, they had been treated with antitoxin and hooked up to ventilators in the intensive care unit. Although the four patients fell under the care of the infectious diseases team run by consultants John Innes and Martin Wood, Dr Symmons put a lot of effort into looking after them while on call. In coming face to face with botulism, Dr Symmons experienced her first baptism by fire as an SHO in infectious diseases—she was not expecting a second.

OUT IN KINGS HEATH, seven miles southwest of the East Birmingham Hospital, Janet's parents had grown tired of watching over their ailing daughter, as her condition went from bad to worse. They called their own GP, Dr Annis Price, to Myrtle Avenue to see Janet. Dr Price called by early on the morning of Thursday 24 August. She soon decided things were serious enough for a hospital opinion. She asked to speak to the admitting doctor at the local infectious disease unit at East Birmingham Hospital—and was put through to Dr Deborah Symmons.

Dr Symmons was partway through a ward round that morning when the phone call came through. Dr Price explained that she had just seen a woman with a strange rash. She apologised for the fact that she did not know as much about the patient's background as she would have liked, but explained that the patient actually belonged to another local GP, Dr Arundel, and that she had seen Janet Parker as a temporary resident at the home of the patient's parents.

Dr Price explained that Mrs Parker had already been seen by Dr Arundel, who had suggested chickenpox, and by another GP, who had suggested a drug reaction. But Dr Price did not think the rash was quite right for chickenpox. She described it over the phone: a vesicular rash all over the body, almost confluent on the face, where the blistered spots were starting to look umbilicated (i.e. dimpled in the middle, so that they resemble the umbilicus).

Dr Price said she would appreciate a second opinion and asked whether someone from the hospital could pop round to see Mrs Parker on a domiciliary visit. In response, Dr Symmons explained that this was normally done only for suspected cases of smallpox or Lassa fever (a deadly viral haemorrhagic fever first described nine years earlier in Nigeria).

'Oh,' replied Dr Price 'it's nothing like that—she's British and hasn't been out of the country for five years!' With smallpox apparently out of the running, the SHO agreed that Janet Parker should be admitted to hospital and arranged for an ambulance to bring her to the East Birmingham Hospital.

IN THE 1890s, BIRMINGHAM Corporation paid just under £5000 for a 23-acre site in Little Bromwich, then a rural location to the east of the city.[3] Here, they built a new isolation hospital, used initially just for smallpox patients, later extended to cater for patients with measles, scarlet fever, whooping cough, diphtheria and tuberculosis. With the decline of infection and rise of the National Health Service, by the 1960s, Little Bromwich Hospital was turned into a general hospital, although it maintained an infectious disease unit. In 1963, Little Bromwich Hospital merged with the nearby Yardley Green Hospital to become the East Birmingham Hospital.

Over the next two decades, the hospital mushroomed in size, with demolition of old blocks and extensive new construction. On 24 August 1978, more than eight decades after its launch as a smallpox hospital, East Birmingham Hospital played host to an unexpected new case of this old disease.

Janet made the nine-mile journey to East Birmingham Hospital in an ordinary ambulance. At three o'clock that afternoon, during visiting time at the hospital, she was wheeled into Ward 32 in the infectious disease unit.

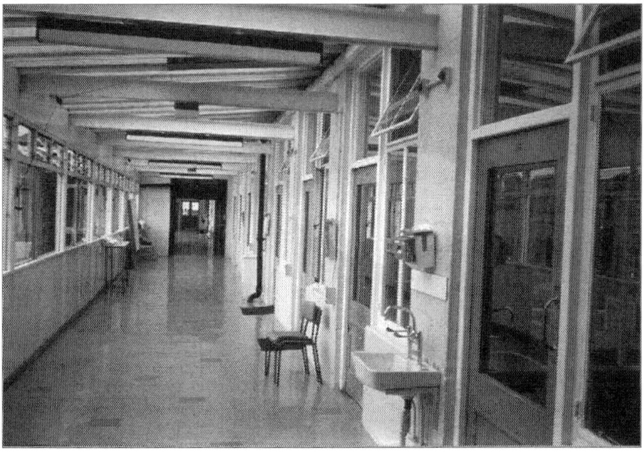

WARD 32 AT EAST BIRMINGHAM HOSPITAL.
{Source: Dr Graham Beards CC BY-SA 3.0}.

The unit provided no-frills accommodation for patients in need of isolation. Janet entered via a two-metre-wide corridor lit on one side by sunlight that streamed through a row of austere metal-framed windows set above some insubstantial panelling. The ceiling sported a series of low-hanging metal joists and a flimsy roof. Along the dark side of the corridor sat a suite of single rooms, built from brickwork, painted yellow, but free of any plaster. Each room had a red door and a set of multiple metal-framed windows facing the passageway, with a window on the opposite side of the room providing daylight. The ambulance drivers wheeled Janet Parker into a single room. As they left, the ambulance drivers asked Dr Symmons whether they should regard the case as infectious and decontaminate their ambulance. She said 'yes'.

Dr Symmons had to finish off seeing another patient before she could see Janet Parker, but by 3.30pm she was ready to see her latest admission. The young doctor's first impression was that Janet did not seem too unwell in herself, but the rash looked horrific. She took a careful history and, with a degree of foresight, donned latex gloves before performing a detailed clinical examination and taking some blood for testing.

Dr Symmons started a set of medical notes for the patient, broadly adopting a format known as the Problem-Oriented Medical Record or the SOAP note (the acronym stands for *subjective, objective, assessment, plan*).[4] In neat handwriting, Dr Symmons documented the presenting complaint: *Widespread umbilicated vesicular rash*. She then summarised the HPC—*the history of the present condition*—noting, alongside the history of the flu-like illness and rash, that Janet now felt so weak she could no longer stand up on her own and her limbs felt stiff. Janet also reported that she had had a slight cough for the last couple of days and was experiencing a vague itch, but was not in pain. Janet was confident that no new spots had appeared in the last two days. She let Dr Symmons know that she worked at the Medical School and reported that she had been vaccinated against smallpox in the 1960s. However, there was no mention of the fact that anyone was working on smallpox at the University.

In writing up her physical examination, Dr Symmons recorded: *Covered in a vesicular rash—most pronounced on the face. Lesions ½ cm containing a white fluid with an erythematous margin. More advanced lesions umbilicated with darkened centres. No crusts. Lesions present on genitalia and in the hair. No lesions in the mouth. Febrile.*

The rest of the physical examination was normal. Under the heading *Assessment* two options were listed:

? Erythema multiforme 2° to drug reaction

????? Variola

Blood test results[5] were entered into the notes, showing that Janet Parker had anaemia and a raised white cell count, with an unusual profile suggesting her bone marrow was struggling to cope. The level of protein in her blood was lower than usual and she had cold agglutinins (a kind of antibody active only at low temperatures). The results also suggested a mild degree of renal failure. All this was consistent with a severe infection.

About an hour later, Dr Symmons was joined for a ward round reviewing recent emergency admissions by three colleagues: the other SHO in Infectious Diseases, Dr Judith Fothergill[6], a research registrar Dr Peter Davey, who was doing an MD on how antibiotics damage the ear, and the Professor of Tropical Medicine, Hugh Morgan. They were all puzzled by Janet Parker.

HUGH MORGAN WAS A SHORT, quietly spoken Welshman[7], with deep Christian convictions, who had been Professor of Medicine at the University of Khartoum in the Sudan from 1952 to 1968. In this role, he had criss-crossed the country in a truck-cum-trailer that acted as a mobile clinic and laboratory, ministering to the medical needs of the local population. His services to medicine and medical education in Africa culminated in the award of a CBE in 1966.

By 1978, Morgan had been in Birmingham for over ten years, where his clinical experience overseas and his good grasp of Arabic proved valuable in dealing with immigrants from the Tropics and Middle East. Now sixty-two years old, bald on top, with a wide-domed forehead, a warm friendly smile and an unthreatening avuncular demeanour, Morgan was close to the end of a long and distinguished career. His juniors saw him as a bit eccentric, particularly as he accosted them with phrases like 'you don't work *for* me: you work *with* me!' His memory was starting to falter—the nurses had already nicknamed him 'the absent-minded professor'. Sadly, a few years later, in retirement, his forgetfulness was to be transformed into full-blown Alzheimer's disease. But that day in August 1978, the decision over what to do with Janet Parker fell to him.

There is a saying among medics that 'when you hear hoof beats, think horses, not zebras'.[8] This is applied as a corrective to those who have spent more time with textbooks than with patients, to prevent doctors jumping straight to the rare small print stuff when making a diagnosis. The three GPs who had seen Janet Parker had obviously been working to this rule. And not unreasonably: the newspapers had announced the last known case of smallpox the year before, and, although the WHO smallpox eradication team were still cautiously on the lookout for new cases in faraway tropical climes, in suburban Birmingham in the summer of 1978 smallpox was not even a zebra; it was the equivalent of a unicorn on the lawn in front of them!

Hugh Morgan did not make a decision right away. While Dr Symmons went off to admit another patient, Morgan and his colleagues continued on the ward round, reviewing new admissions on the children's ward. Half an hour later, once the ward round was over, Morgan, Symmons and other doctors again met up and turned again to the problem of Janet Parker. With the possibility of smallpox still in the air, Professor Morgan declared to his colleagues 'I don't suppose for a minute that it is, but we had better set the wheels in motion'. They called in the local community physician, Dr Mukund Jamnadas Khetani, who agreed that this could *not* be smallpox. Nonetheless, Khetani suggested that they should seek an opinion from Birmingham's designated smallpox consultant, Alasdair Geddes.

Geddes had held this position since he had returned from Bangladesh in 1973. In his role as smallpox consultant, Alasdair had been called out around half a dozen times over the past five years to examine suspected cases of smallpox. All had turned out to be false alarms: either bad cases of chickenpox or non-infectious conditions like erythema multiforme and Stevens-Johnson syndrome. Yet each time, he had been paid the princely sum of twenty pounds.

At 7.30pm, the Welshman Hugh Morgan phoned the Scotsman Alasdair Geddes and asked him to come in and see what he called 'a lady with an unusual rash who worked in the east wing of the Medical School'. Morgan might have fleetingly raised the possibility of smallpox, but for him it still did not make any sense—after all, you don't get unicorns on the lawn in England!

34

THE DIAGNOSIS

ALASDAIR GEDDES IS JUST opening a bottle of wine when the phone rings.[1] A few moments later, he jumps into the car. During the six-mile journey from his home in sedate suburban Solihull to the East Birmingham Hospital, his mind is racing over the facts. He knows the new patient works in the East Wing of the Medical School. Unlike Hugh Morgan, Alasdair also knows that Henry Bedson is working on smallpox in the very same wing—one of only thirteen laboratories in the world still holding stocks of smallpox.

On arrival at the hospital, Geddes takes care to don gloves, a gown and a mask, before he enters Janet Parker's room. As soon as he enters the cubicle, his suspicions are confirmed. A less experienced infectious disease physician would have consciously and doggedly worked through a checklist that differentiated smallpox from the far more common chickenpox:

- Has the patient being suffering from a high fever for one to four days before the onset of the rash and is she suffering from prostration, headache, backache, chills, vomiting, and/or severe abdominal pain—which would all fit with smallpox?
- Are the spots deep-seated, well-circumscribed, firm and hard (*shotty*)? Are they *pearly*, round and filled with clear fluid (*vesicles*) or pus (*pustules*)? A yes to all these questions indicates smallpox. Or, instead, are the spots superficial, soft and oval in shape, like dewdrops—indicating chickenpox?
- On any one part of the body, such as the face, or arm, are all the spots slowly maturing and all at the same stage of development (all vesicles, or all pustules), indicating smallpox? Or are they appearing in fast-developing crops at different stages of maturation within the same region—as seen in chickenpox?
- As the spots evolve, have they become umbilicated or started to merge into one another to become confluent? Both features favour a diagnosis of smallpox.
- Is the rash *centripetal*, concentrated on the torso,

suggesting chickenpox? Or *centrifugal*, worse on the extremities, particularly on the palms and soles, suggesting smallpox? Has the rash spared the armpits compared to nearby skin? Another hallmark of smallpox.

But, from the end of the bed, even before examining her, Geddes *knows* that this is smallpox, with the lightning bolt of recognition that psychologists call Gestalt—an expert seeing the diagnosis as a whole rather than as the sum of its parts. Geddes also has a unique insight into the context, which shifts the balance of probabilities—a diagnosis of smallpox made perfect sense, given that the photographer works in the very same building that houses the poxvirus laboratory. No longer a unicorn on the lawn, in this context, the smallpox virus is simply a horse that has bolted from its stable.

ALASDAIR'S SUSPICIONS are confirmed as he interviews and examines the patient. He diligently documents the details of Janet's movements within the two-three weeks leading up to the onset of symptoms and confirms that she has not been out of the country or in contact with any obvious cases of any relevant infectious disease. Since she has been ill, she has been into work for just one day and has been in contact with just friends and family since then. She has not been into the animal house for over a month. She was vaccinated against smallpox in 1966, when variola minor hit Birmingham that year.

As the daylight fades on that fateful August evening, Geddes examines the entire surface of Janet Parker's skin, documenting the distribution of the rash. Running his fingers over her rash, he feels the hard shotty pearls, which, despite their savage appearance, are neither hot to the touch nor tender.

Alasdair Geddes makes his own careful notes on the patient's condition:

On examination the patient was febrile and complaining of aching in her limbs but fully conscious and lucid. Her temperature was 101°F. There was a generalised vesicular/pustular eruption on all areas of skin including palms of hands and soles of feet. Lesions were principally round with surrounding erythema. The rash was semi-confluent on the face.

On such visits, Geddes always brings along a little box containing needles, a syringe, scalpels, a little tube and a slide, so that he can take samples whenever needed. Geddes uses the contents of his box to take specimens of fluid from three of Janet's vesicles. Now all he needs to do is get the specimens into the hands of the duty virologist.

The smallpox research lab at the Medical School also serves as the Regional Diagnostic Smallpox Laboratory. There are four virologists on the duty rota: Professor Henry Bedson (who got back just two days ago from his holiday cottage in Llangynog in mid-Wales), Dr Alexander 'Sandy' Buchan, Dr Gordon Skinner and Dr Rob George. Geddes consults the rota: Bedson is on call tonight.

Geddes rings Bedson at home and, after an opening greeting, exclaims: 'I have a suspected smallpox here, Henry, and it's a lady who works as a photographer at the Medical School'. For a long moment, the line goes quiet, as Bedson absorbs the full ramifications of what has been said to him. If his colleague's suspicions are true, this smallpox can have come only from Bedson's very own laboratory.

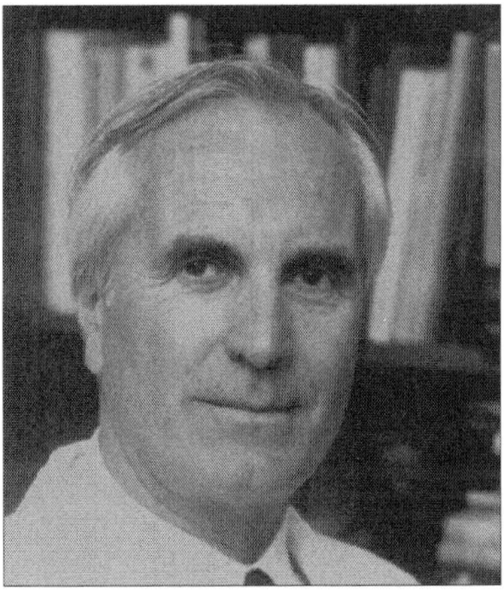

ALASDAIR GEDDES
The Birmingham infectious disease consultant who diagnosed Janet Parker's smallpox
{Source: A. Geddes}

AROUND 9.00PM, GEDDES SETS OFF for the Medical School, accompanied by Deborah Symmons, who, although now off-duty as a doctor, remains intensely curious as to what is wrong with Mrs Parker. Less than half an hour later, they meet Henry Bedson outside the Medical School, which looms dark and daunting. Bedson unlocks the imposing outer door. The two middle-aged men enter the building with their eager young accomplice. Geddes hands over the samples, which Bedson prepares for examination under the electron microscope.

Bedson goes on alone to feed the preparations into the electron microscope. There is tension in the air, when, a few minutes later, Symmons and Geddes join Bedson in the microscope room. They find Bedson silent, deathly white, hunched up, peering at the microscope screen.

Geddes asks Bedson what he has found. Bedson doesn't answer—instead, he sits mute and motionless, transfixed, unable to draw his gaze away from the horror in front of him. Geddes gently pushes the virologist to one side and looks for himself. There on the screen are the brick-shaped particles, which Geddes knows are characteristic of poxviruses. And not just one or two—with bricks strewn across the field of view, the image that springs to Alasdair's mind is that of a building site.

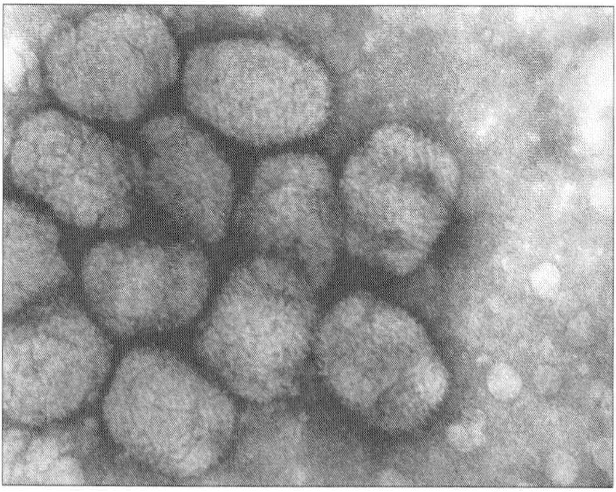

ELECTRON MICROGRAPH OF VARIOLA VIRUS

Something very similar greeted Henry Bedson when he examined material from Janet Parker.

{Source: CDC Public Health Image Library #2292}.

So, the diagnosis is no longer in doubt. This *is* smallpox and, to Bedson's horror, the source is almost certainly his own research lab. The distraught virology professor inoculates some chick chorioallantoic membranes in the hope that he can isolate and characterise the virus that is running amok through Janet Parker's tissues. In the meantime, Geddes rushes to the phone to pass on the news to Dr William 'Willie' Nicol, Medical Officer for the Birmingham Area Health Authority, and arranges to meet him at East Birmingham Hospital. Geddes also phones Hugh Morgan, who has already set in motion plans to re-open the smallpox hospital in the Warwickshire village of Catherine-de-Barnes. In a moment of brave naiveté, Dr Symmons—just over three weeks into the job and knowing next to nothing about smallpox—volunteers to go with Janet Parker to the smallpox hospital at Catherine-de-Barnes. She is told that won't be necessary—at least for now. However, as we shall see, the destinies of the doctor and her patient were to remain entwined.

35

MEETINGS AND CONTACTS

PATIENTS GO TO HOSPITAL to get well, not get sick. From the infection control viewpoint, regular normal hospitals are the worst place on Earth to house smallpox patients. As 'temples of illness', they are home to hundreds or thousands of patients, often highly vulnerable, crowded together, providing tons and tons of fresh flesh for the variola virus to colonise. Janet Parker's admission to East Birmingham Hospital creates a public health emergency that needed urgent action. Those caring for the hospital's patients strive to obey the first tenant of the Hippocratic Oath—*primum non nocere* or *first do no harm*—by protecting them against smallpox.

As we have seen in Brighton and Bradford, Wales and London, after importation into Western countries, transmission of smallpox within hospitals has been an all-too-common problem, accounting for over half of the cases in post-war Europe.[1] As a result, Janet Parker is no longer seen as just a patient; she is now viewed as a dangerous bioreactor, sixty kilograms of human flesh and blood brewing up billions of copies of the world's most fearsome virus. She sat at the centre of a cloud of airborne virus particles, capable of infecting vulnerable face-to-face contacts within a two-metre-radius, with the risk of subsequent onward transmission wreaking devastation on a much wider scale. Janet Parker should be got out of the East Birmingham Hospital as soon as possible and everyone and everything that has been in contact with her there needs to be followed up immediately.

So, at around 10.00pm on the day of her admission, Janet Parker leaves the East Birmingham Hospital in a special smallpox ambulance. With her, goes all the bedding from her cubicle in Ward 32. Less than half an hour later, she arrives at Catherine-de-Barnes Hospital.

It must have been gone eleven o'clock when Alasdair Geddes and his SHO, Deborah Symmons, arrives back at the East Birmingham Hospital after their visit to the Medical School. As the midnight hour strikes, Geddes and Symmons are thrust into the midst of an *ad hoc* emergency meeting dealing with the crisis. Among those present are Hugh Morgan, Judith Fothergill, Willie Nicol and his close associate, Dr. Surinder Bakhshi (Birmingham's Medical Officer of Environmental Health), plus Dr. Jim Hutchison, Director of the hospital's Public Health Laboratory, some nursing officers and a hospital administrator.

Willie Nicol takes charge of the meeting: a big bear of man with a large frame and solid round head, bald on top and fringed with tufts of grey hair. Nicol's mellow well-to-do Glaswegian accent[2] and baritone voice project an air of quiet authority and placid imperturbability that commands the attention of the room. That day he is probably impeccably dressed as usual, in his best Saville Row suit,[3] with a tight collar and tie holding back an emerging double chin.

Nicol is Glasgow-trained and has served in the Royal Naval Volunteer Reserve before settling into Public Health, first in Edinburgh and then, from 1949 onwards, in Birmingham.[4] He became the city's Deputy Medical Officer of Health in 1960 and Area Medical Officer of Health in 1974. He is a veteran of Birmingham's 1966 smallpox outbreak. By 1978, he had become a much-respected member of the Birmingham medical scene, inspiring loyalty and respect from his colleagues, while also leading a lively social life, often out drinking with members of the city's police force. To add to his distinguished image, he sometimes sports a monocle.

Earlier that evening, Nicol has already made the decision to close the East Birmingham Hospital to new admissions and minimise any movements in and out of Wards 32 and 31. He has also phoned Janet Parker's husband Joseph and arranged for him to stay right where he was, with his in-laws in Myrtle Avenue. Within the hour, the Community Medical Officer, Dr. Mukund Khetani, arrives at the house, vaccinates Joseph and the Witcombs, quizzes them on movements between their two houses and places them in quarantine.

That night, Nicol designates Bakhshi as Outbreaks Liaison Officer and sets up an Emergency Committee, which includes Geddes, Bakhshi, Mr Payne, the hospital administrator, Dr John Innes (a Consultant in Communicable Diseases) and a Senior Nursing Officer. Deborah Symmons is impressed at how well people from different backgrounds and professions are working together with such efficiency. Questions fly around the room. What should the press be told? Who were the contacts? Who was responsible for each group of contacts?

The meeting is adjourned at 1.00am and all the doctors present then line up with arms bare to be vaccinated. Around the same time, Ian Farrell, a microbiologist from the hospital's Public Health

Laboratory, has Janet's room and the ward lift fumigated with formaldehyde to kill any remaining smallpox virus particles. Those who have been in contact with Janet while she was in the hospital have to bag up all their clothing so it can be sent for incineration—this includes their stethoscopes, name badges and Judith Fothergill's favourite pair of shoes! At 2.00am, Drs Symmons and Fothergill both take baths and wash their hair in the doctors' mess, much to their sleeping colleagues' annoyance. They then grab some well-deserved sleep.

WORRY. ANXIETY. FEAR. Millions of susceptible people within a two-hour drive. For those at the epicentre of the outbreak, this was their JFK assassination moment: the largest public health emergency since the 1974 Birmingham pub bombings. All those involved in managing the outbreak would remember those few days in the late summer of 1978 for the rest of their lives. This time the enemy was not the provisional IRA, but a virus resurrected from the dead.

Deborah Symmons is up and out of bed by 6.30am. She quickly sets about gathering a list of all the patients and visitors who had been on Wards 31 and 32 during Janet Parker's short, seven-hour stay. This proves tricky, as at least a quarter of the patients were immigrants from South Asia who spoke little or no English.

At 9.00am, the Emergency Committee reassemble at East Birmingham Hospital. Nicol makes it clear that all the medical and nursing staff involved in Janet's admission to the hospital should be interviewed with immediate effect. He gives the order to re-open the hospital to new admissions, but makes sure that wards 31 and 32 are kept closed to admissions and there are to be no discharges.

Again the questions fly back and forth. Luckily the answer to one question—is there enough vaccine—is clear: Jim Hutchison's laboratory alone has 60,000 vials of smallpox vaccine, enough to immunise 180,000 people. But how are contacts to be notified? Who should vaccinate them and where? And what about people working in the hospital. How many of them should be considered contacts?

Dr Symmons wracks her brains to come up with fresh candidates for direct contacts of Janet Parker: a man who came to fix the bedpan washer, the ambulance men who delivered patients, the physiotherapists, the hospital chaplain, the GPs who had seen Janet Parker out in the community. She spends most of that hour ducking in and out of the meeting, making and taking phone calls.

At the end of the meeting, Nicol jumps into his car and makes the 15-minute drive back to his office in central Birmingham. Nicol's work at the hospital is over for now, but Dr Symmons spends the rest of the day vaccinating patients, nurses and other hospital patients. After another long day, she makes it home at 8pm, with some vaccine in hand for her flatmate Mary, who has just suffered the hassle of having her car stolen.

36

SAVING A CITY FROM SMALLPOX

TALL BUILDINGS MAKE a statement about the aspirations of the cities that host them: New York's early-twentieth-century skyscrapers; Dubai's twenty-first-century towers in the desert; the verticality of Hong Kong and Shanghai; the Shard piercing the London skyline. Birmingham proclaimed itself a modern metropolis in the 1960s, with a phase of high-rise development that threw up numerous concrete box-shaped towers, providing office accommodation or social housing. The tallest of these, right in the heart of the city's business district, was the Alpha Tower, a hundred-metre-tall office block designed in a modernist style by George Marsh of Richard Seifert & Partners.[1]

Alpha Tower was built between 1969 and 1973 to house the headquarters of the television company ATV and remained the city's tallest tower block for more than three decades. An iconic symbol of the new Birmingham, it featured heavily in the 1973 Cliff Richard film *Take Me High*.

That Friday in late August 1978, the thirteenth floor of Alpha Tower was home to the headquarters of the Department of Health and Social Security (DHSS) and the Birmingham Area Health Authority (AHA), so it was from here that Surinder Bakhshi was faced with the task of saving Britain's second city from smallpox.

SURINDER SINGH BAKHSHI ('Surinderjit' to his friends) came from a Sikh family that originated in the Ras Koh Hills in what is now Pakistan's Baluchistan province.[2] When the British took control of German East Africa after the First World War, they took over the railway line that connected Lake Tanganyika to the coast. Expansion of the railway drew in new labour from elsewhere in the British Empire—and so Surinder Bakhshi's parents left their ancestral home to become inhabitants of East Africa.

Bakhshi was born in 1937 and grew up in Dar es Salaam, a bustling port on the eastern coast of Africa. He and his family were part of a substantial Indian community that ran much of the region's economy. In 1960, Bakhshi travelled a thousand miles inland to enrol as a medical student at Makerere University in

Kampala, Uganda. Here, he imbibed the heady cultural and political excitement driven by the University's fellow students, who included eminent writers such as Paul Theroux and V. S. Naipaul and future presidents of Tanzania, Uganda and Congo.

After graduating in 1965, Bakhshi married his childhood sweetheart and, on completing house officer jobs on the coast, moved nearly two thousand miles south and west to become medical officer in the Zambian town of Mongu, at the eastern edge of the Zambezi flood plain. He found it dull. The only excitement came from a local ceremony known as the Kuomboka[3], in which heavy drumming marked the river journey from the king's dry-season palace on the flood plain to his flood-season palace up on higher ground. In Mongu, Bakhshi never encountered a case of smallpox or any major outbreaks of disease—instead the main medical problem was snakebites. The *British Medical Journal* came three months late.

Bakhshi spent three years in Mongu, but always felt he was destined for better things. By the light of an oil lamp, he wrote letters to all and sundry—including the Ford Foundation and the Rockefeller Foundation—looking for an opening. After badgering his bosses in Lusaka, he was given responsibility for immunisation programmes in the Zambia, so he got to travel more widely. His lucky break came when the Population Council, a Rockefeller project in New York, agreed to sponsor him for a Masters in Public Health in Michigan. As part of the package, he took the chance to travel around the world with his wife and young child, visiting Ethiopia, Pakistan, Thailand, Malaysia and Hawaii, before arriving in Michigan.

The MSc complete, the return journey took the Bakhshis to the UK, France, Turkey and Egypt. Back in Zambia, Surinder became a regional medical officer and came face to face with cholera among refugees from Mozambique. Still keen to broaden his horizons, his attention turned to the UK, where his parents had now settled. He took up a registrar job in Kingston-upon-Thames, which started with a two-month orientation period in Exmoor. A short while later, he obtained a senior registrar job in Gloucestershire, living in a nurse's cottage in Slimbridge, close to Jenner's home in Berkeley.

Young and ambitious, Bakhshi soon felt ready to try for his first consultant position. Colleagues advised him to apply for a position as Medical Officer for Environmental Health in Birmingham and he did so for interview practice, never expecting to get the job.

When he arrived at Alpha Tower for his interview, Bakhshi came face to face with the gratuitous racism of the time. After asking at reception for directions to the AHA offices, he was told that 'people like him' could not use the lift and he was forced to walk up thirteen flights of stairs. The subsequent two-hour interview was intimidating, with over twenty stakeholders in attendance. Luckily, the interviewers spent more time talking to each other than to Bakhshi. After the interview, Bakhshi was sent out for a walk and then sent home, while the panel deliberated. Only the next day, did they finally offer him the job.

In his new role, Bakhshi soon won the respect and affection of his colleagues in Birmingham, even the prejudiced Alpha Tower receptionist. During his first year in post, Bakhshi grappled with an outbreak of hepatitis B associated with an acupuncturist. He spent his weekdays in Birmingham, but returned to the family home in Gloucestershire at weekends. He was given an office in the Medical School just down the corridor from Bedson's, but the two men never met.

IN THE EARLY HOURS of Friday 25 August 1978, in post for little over a year, Dr Bakhshi receives a phone call, informing him that smallpox has arrived in his city. At 10am, with spectacular views across Britain's second city, Willie Nicol's Alpha Tower office plays host to a meeting of the Control of Smallpox Outbreak Advisory Committee, which includes Bakhshi, Geddes and Bedson.[4]

They spend most of the morning reviewing their options, interrupted by a brief visit to the nearby conference room, where Nicol makes statements to the press: 'There is a strong presumption that the disease has been picked up from the laboratories.' *The Daily Express* goes on to describe the Medical School as a 'Doomwatch medical unit'.[5]

The outbreak committee starts with two main tasks ahead of them: detecting and preventing any additional cases of smallpox among contacts and investigating how Janet Parker has acquired the infection in the first place. Their efforts focus on three settings: the city's community, the East Birmingham Hospital and Birmingham's Medical School. Bakhshi takes over operational management of the community and public health efforts, while Nicol works with the authorities at the hospital and Medical School.

They have three kinds of weapon in their battle to contain smallpox. First, individuals can be quarantined and put under surveillance—and because smallpox has a predictable incubation period, this does not need to start until eight days after exposure. Second, they can offer immunological protection—anyone who has not been recently vaccinated is going to need a shot in the arm of vaccinia virus, while the least protected will also benefit from anti-vaccinial gamma-globulin, an injectable antibody preparation that provides short-term but immediate protection. Third, thee final weapon in the anti-smallpox arsenal is an antiviral drug, *methisazone*. This shows activity against poxviruses, but it remains uncertain whether it brings benefit to those exposed to smallpox.

According to the recently published *Memorandum on the Control of Outbreaks of Smallpox*,[6] primary contacts are defined as people in contact with Janet Parker during the infectious period (which is supposed to have started 24 hours before her first symptoms) or with contaminated objects. *Category A contacts* have had face-to-face contact with Janet Parker (within two metres), while *Category B contacts* are people who have been in the same room or other enclosed space with Janet during her period of infectivity, but have not come close enough to warrant Category A status.

However, with a tally that eventually reaches over four hundred Category A contacts, Nicol, Bakhshi and their colleagues make the pragmatic decision to adopt a more fine-grained classification, which split Category A cases into *close contacts* and *remote contacts*.[7] The seventy-five *Category A close contacts* include household contacts, which are the easiest to identify and the easiest to deal with. There are the four relatives (Joseph, Fred, Hilda and Hilda's sister), the three GPs (Dr Arundel, Dr Horry and Dr Annis Price) and the two neighbours (Mr and Mrs Rowley). All are placed under quarantine at home and visited that day by Bakhshi, who gives them human anti-vaccinial immunoglobulin and methisazone. The following day, health officials fumigate the Parker house and cars.

Category A close contacts also include colleagues at work, staff from the poxvirus laboratory at the Medical School and all those who have come into contact with Janet in the course of her admission to East Birmingham Hospital (including medical and nursing staff, ambulance men, Environmental Health Inspectors and several dozen laboratory and public health staff). Any that have not been vaccinated in the last five years are vaccinated immediately, then given the immunoglobulin and methisazone.

Those classified by Nicol as *Category A remote contacts* include the rest of the Medical School's Microbiology Department staff, patients, and visitors to the East Birmingham Hospital Infectious Diseases Ward on 24 August, refuse collectors, newspaper and milk delivery boys and some television and newspaper reporters that have visited potentially infected premises.

Category B contacts include—amongst others—staff and recent visitors to the East Wing of the Medical School housing the Microbiology and Photographic Departments. *Category C contacts* include anyone who works in the Medical School or in East Birmingham Hospital and others who may have had similar peripheral exposure.

IN ENGLAND, WHEN the banks close, the country closes. The 1871 Bank Holidays Act established four bank holidays, including a bank holiday Monday in August.[8] For the English, the August Bank Holiday represents the last gasp of summer, before school holidays end, autumn leaves start to fall and the nights draw in. During such holidays, the human resources of the NHS and local authorities are depleted. The August Bank Holiday weekend also marks the start of Europe's largest street festival, the Notting Hill Carnival. That weekend in 1978, the weather is sunny but cool, struggling to top 20°C.

Despite the handicap of a bank holiday weekend, over the coming days, the full force of Britain's National Health Service is deployed to prevent or contain an outbreak. The Outbreak Committee meets every day from 26 August to 16 September 1978, bringing together decision-makers and smallpox experts to formulate policy and review progress.

Bakhshi takes a number of bold steps to ease the lives of his workers.[9] He contacts his superiors in the local authority and establishes that his budget is effectively unlimited for the duration of the outbreak. He requisitions three floors of the Intercontinental Hotel, which sits next to Alpha Tower. He contacts the city's black cab taxi service and says that they are now contracted to the local authority, so that those managing the outbreak (particularly young women) can get around and get home safe and unhindered. He arranges for food to be supplied to the outbreak team, together with liberal supplies of wine and beer for those working late into the night.

A Central Control Operational Centre is set up in Congreve Passage in Birmingham city centre and is linked to operational centres at the Birmingham Medical School and East Birmingham Hospital. Twenty-five telephone lines are made available within the Operational Centre. Bakhshi and other senior officers are supplied with electronic pagers, so that they are contactable at all times. Staff from CDCC, the Communicable Disease Control Centre in Colindale in north London, provide advice and take away some of the heat in communicating with the outside world. Doctors from outside the city volunteer their services. In total, an estimated sixty doctors, forty nurses (including twenty health visitors), eighty-five environmental health inspectors and staff, six disinfection officers and ninety administrative, clerical and support staff take part in the citywide effort. Those caught up in the effort take up their new jobs and responsibilities with enthusiasm, working hard long hours.

A frantic search begins, using GP's records, the radio and newspapers. Britain's second city is combed for contacts, who are then isolated from the rest of the population. Within twenty-four hours most of the principal contacts across the region, the country and even those who had travelled overseas have been accounted for. Two contacts from the Medical School are located in the USA and West Germany.

Reg Wickett, a 53-year-old hospital engineer, who has been working in a ward close to Parker, is tracked down to Poole in Dorset, while Nursery nurse Angela Tudor is forced to terminate her holiday in Cornwall.[10] A 22-year-old physiotherapist contact of Parker, Cathy Hyde, is forced to cancel her 100-guest wedding to 25-year-old Alan Plant and instead goes into quarantine in Harborne.[11]

BY BANK HOLIDAY MONDAY, over five hundred people have been vaccinated. However, the week that follows brings confusion, with muddled advice about the need for smallpox vaccination for British holidaymakers travelling overseas and a rush for jabs. By 1 September, ten countries start demanding vaccination before Brits can enter.[12]

Surveillance is enforced for sixteen complete days from the date of last exposure to Janet Parker. Medical staff take responsibility for the surveillance of Category A contacts, while Category B contacts are looked after by health visitors. Close contacts are subjected to immediate quarantine and daily surveillance, while more remote contacts are placed under surveillance, but quarantined only from the eighth day after the date of first exposure to the eighth day after the last exposure.

In total, 328 contacts are placed under quarantine at home or in hospital. A handful of contacts, including Janet's husband Joseph Parker, are released from quarantine on 6 September. However, for most contacts, quarantine begins on 1 September and ends at midnight on 9 September. Forty-five close contacts remain under surveillance for four additional days.

The East Birmingham Hospital's Ward 31 is used for the quarantine of some of the hospital staff. Those put into quarantine include ten doctors and thirty-five nurses, plus hospital porters, engineers, a clergyman and a paperboy—although for reasons that are unclear, eleven refuse collectors, although classified as Category A, are excluded from quarantine.[13]

For the duration of the quarantine, the hospital runs on a skeleton staff. By the end of the outbreak, 1,820 contacts at the East Birmingham Hospital have been vaccinated, including over a thousand of the hospital's staff. An additional 1,602 are vaccinated at a central vaccination clinic in Congreve Passage (just across from Birmingham Museum and Art Gallery), co-ordinated by South African doctor, John Mokuena, together with Dr Mukund Khetani and a nurse administrator Doris Hinsley. On top of that, 481 contacts from the Medical School receive vaccinations.

An extra 12,079 vaccine doses are issued for use by General Practitioners, Industry and Hospitals during the outbreak. Mass vaccination of the public is actively discouraged but vaccination is made available to travellers to countries that insist, against WHO advice, on international certificates of vaccination.

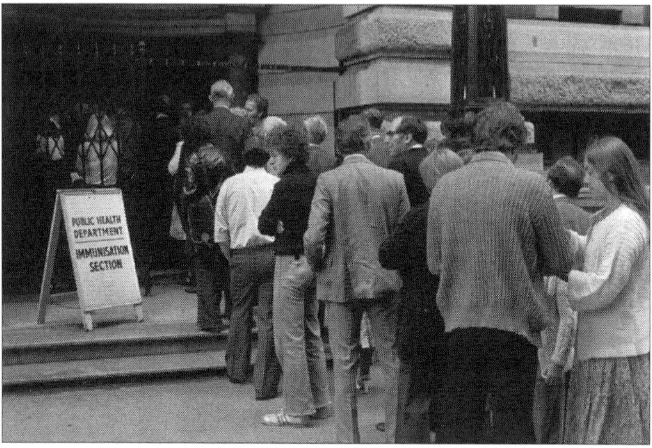

QUEUING TO BE VACCINATED

Outside the vaccination clinic in Congreve Passage, Birmingham

{Source: Birmingham Mail}

Across the city, Category A Contacts isolated at home are kept under surveillance by four teams of doctors and nurses organised geographically, while outside Birmingham, surveillance is organised by the local medical officers of environmental health. Seventy-five of those treated as Category A close contacts are, in fact, merely contacts of suspected cases, rather than direct contacts of Janet Parker; these indirect contacts are released from surveillance as soon as the relevant direct contact is cleared of the disease. Examples include sixteen people who came into contact with the GP Dr Annis Price.

Surveillance includes oral measurement of body temperature with a single-use, disposable thermometer, which together with any relevant symptoms is reported daily to a designated Smallpox Contacts Telephone Number. The Public Health authorities chase up anyone who fails to return a daily health report. All General Practitioners, Casualty Departments and Emergency services in Birmingham are reminded to bear in mind the possibility of mild or atypical smallpox in the city. Patients with a rash are told to avoid GPs and hospitals, but instead receive home visits from a dedicated team. Alongside Janet Parker and her parents, eight additional contacts are admitted to Catherine-de-Barnes Hospital during the outbreak and all staff at the isolation hospital are put into quarantine.

A massive effort is mobilised to offer social support to those under quarantine. They are given access to a 24-hour telephone help line, while the authorities arrange to supply food, remove waste and even deliver newspapers. Some take the imprisonment stoically. For example, Janet's husband Joseph declares: 'Being confined to the house will not unduly worry me. The worst thing is the waiting and not being able to visit Janet. I'm confident I can cope. Luckily the freezer is well stocked and any other food I need is being left by a friend on the doorstep.'[14]

Bakhshi receives occasional reports from the police and nosey neighbours about people skipping quarantine, but takes a relaxed approach. Sometimes things do go wrong— after a boy, Romi Jacobs, is treated for gastroenteritis at East Birmingham Hospital, he, his mother Susan and their friends Rachel and Nigel Andre are placed in quarantine.[15] However, within days, both families are forced to break their quarantine when officials failed to bring them food.

FROM A DISTANCE OF over three decades, it is hard to gauge the public mood in Birmingham and in Britain during those fateful days in late August and early September 1978. According to Bakhshi, throughout the smallpox incident, public confidence in the medical authorities remains high and interruptions to life and leisure in the city are kept to the minimum. For him, Birmingham seems more like a friendly village than a city. Individuals may be in quarantine, but the city is not. Life goes on. The shops are open. The outbreak team are happy to stamp paperwork with 'safe to travel'. Bakhshi refuses help from the military in enforcing quarantine and gives the go-ahead for the opening of the British International Motor Show at the National Exhibition Centre in October 1978. The local authority bill comes to more than £200,000, but they are happy to pay it, as the price for avoiding the catastrophe of a protracted and uncontrolled outbreak.

The Labour government is preoccupied at the time with plans, never realised, for an autumn election. In a cartoon in the Daily Express from 1 September, Prime Minister James Callaghan proclaims 'I am not worried about smallpox. I'M worried about an outbreak of Socialism in the Labour Party between now and Election Day...'[16]

On 26 August 1978—the same day that the smallpox story first hits the headlines—a new pope is elected. By 28 September, he is dead.[17] On 16 October, Birmingham is declared free of smallpox[18]—but with three dead. To tell their tragic story, we must turn our attention first to the Medical School and then to the smallpox hospital.

37

THE MEDICAL SCHOOL

THE PRACTICE AND TEACHING of medicine in Birmingham date back to the eighteenth century.[1] In the 1760s, John Tomlinson, first surgeon to the Birmingham Workhouse Infirmary, gave seminars in medical education. In the 1770s and 1780s, William Withering, founding father of pharmacology and a member of the Lunar Society of Birmingham, served as physician to Birmingham General Hospital and settled in Edgbaston. Local surgeon, William Sands Cox, established the first medical school in the city in 1825, which later in that century received patronage from Queen Victoria.

The current Medical School building at the University of Birmingham has a certain presence, but it is hard to call it attractive. William Doe, Dean of the Medical School around the turn of the millennium, unsympathetically described it as 'having just missed Art Deco'. The building sits next to the remains of a Roman fort, on a site donated by the chocolate-making Cadbury family in 1930. Building work on the Medical School and adjacent Queen Elizabeth Hospital began in 1933 to a design by the Scottish architect Thomas Arthur Lodge and was completed by 1938.[2]

Both the Medical School and hospital are fashioned from a dirty light-brown brick that contrasts badly with the much warmer red brick of the main university buildings. There is a pretence at grandeur in the imposing masonry of the Medical School's front entrance, where a rectangular extension—capped with a sculpture by the local artist William Bloye depicting Asclepius, the god of healing, and the University coat of arms[3]—frames a massive off-white porch, which in turn surrounds three tall metal-framed windows that sit above a gigantic doorway. Above the doorway, large metal letters proclaim MEDICAL SCHOOL, while, on either side, sit solid metal torches that would not look out of place in Hitler's Olympic stadium, which was built around the same time.[4]

The school's two four-storey East and West Wings sprawl with gawky angularity either side of the entrance, their frontages punctuated by a dozen rectilinear metal-framed windows. In 1978, the ground floor and lower ground floor of the East Wing are home to the Department of Medical Microbiology, with its smallpox laboratory. Above on the first floor, sits the Department of Anatomy in which Mrs. Parker works.

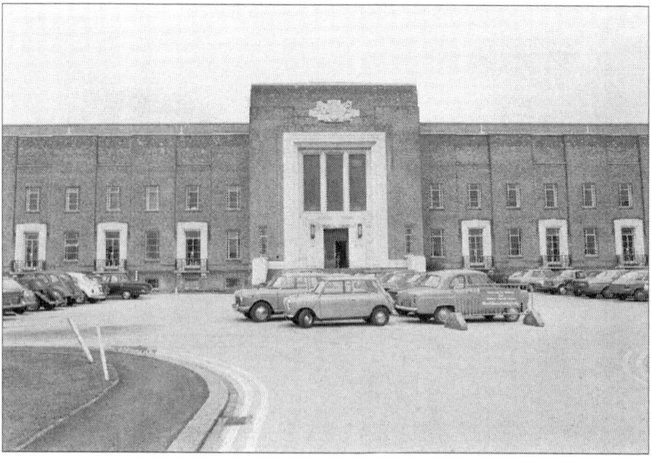

ENTRANCE TO BIRMINGHAM MEDICAL SCHOOL
As it looked in 1978.
{Source: *Birmingham Mail*}

Let us do an imaginary fly-through into the Medical School as it was in August 1978. We proceed through the front entrance to reach the main lobby. We turn right into a poorly lit corridor that takes us into the East Wing. On the right, along that corridor, sits a suite of high-ceilinged offices and meeting rooms, clad in impressive oak, with leafy views that look out across the lawn to University station. In one of these offices hangs an imposing portrait of William Withering. Under that portrait sits Professor Brodie Hughes, sixty-five-years old and Dean of Medicine. Thin-faced and large-eared, with a sagging chin and craggy, lined complexion, he carries an air of quiet authority.[5]

A surgeon and son of a surgeon, Brodie Hughes has been in Birmingham since 1945, when he took control of the neurosurgery unit at the Queen Elizabeth Hospital. He has been a Professor of Neurosurgery for thirty years and is well known for his pioneering work on Parkinson's disease and for servicing all his own highly complex stereotactic equipment. In his leisure time, he puts his manual dexterity to good use in cabinet making, gardening, fly-fishing, sketches and watercolours, fiddling with electronics and playing the oboe.

An adept committeeman, Hughes has been at the helm of the Medical School for the past four years. He is respected for his objectivity, lucidity and sense of proportion. Although patient with junior staff, he sets high standards for himself and for his colleagues and can sometimes come across as sharp-tongued. His bookshelves carry the library of a well-read civilised gentleman.

Hughes is master of the tactically inappropriate remark, delivered to create controversy or merely to cater to his quirky dry sense of humour. Children like his unconventional manner, even though Hughes himself is childless. He has married late in life—just seven years earlier—but it is a happy marriage.

As the smallpox storm is about to break, Hughes has less than a week left in post, preparing for a comfortable retirement in the sleepy Suffolk market town of Saxmundham, close to his beloved Aldeburgh classical music festival.

AT 8 O'CLOCK ON the morning of Friday 25 August, Brodie Hughes receives a message from his Professor of Virology, Henry Bedson, that they need to discuss a matter of the utmost urgency.[6] Twenty minutes later, Hughes is at his desk in the Medical School and shortly afterwards, Bedson lets the Dean know that one of the Medical School's employees, Janet Parker, has been admitted to Catherine-de-Barnes Hospital with suspected smallpox. Hughes decides that all work in the Medical School's smallpox reference laboratory should cease immediately and that the door to the lab should be locked. Hughes insists that notices be displayed at either end of the Medical Microbiology corridor, explaining the risks and restricting access to members of the department. He gives the job of compiling a list of all Medical Microbiology staff to Mr. Hill, a senior administrator from the neighbouring Department of Anatomy. Hill is asked to document the whereabouts and state of health of all concerned and to determine who was in close contact with Janet Parker between 8 and 11 August.

At 9.45am Hughes briefs Professor Owen Wade, soon to be his successor as Dean, and they agree to work together on the problem. At 12.30pm, Wade speaks on behalf of the Medical School to two reporters from the *Birmingham Mail*, but takes care to stick to generalities.

At two o'clock that Friday afternoon, Hughes meets Willie Nicol and Alasdair Geddes at the Medical School. They fill him in on the details of what has happened to Janet Parker and on the morning's discussions. The three men confirm that all work should cease in the smallpox laboratory. However, Nicol and Geddes reassure the Dean that, in their opinion, it was not necessary to arrange for all staff in the Medical School to be vaccinated. Nicol shares plans for setting up a Committee of Inquiry into the origin of Parker's infection.

Henry Bedson joins them and the four men—Hughes, Bedson, Geddes and Nicol—accompanied by the Anatomy administrator Mr Hill, visit the Department of Anatomy looking for the photography room where Janet Parker works. They find the room at the end of a second floor corridor, facing a courtyard. Leading off this room, they discover a windowless dark room, equipped with an Xpelair fan and what looks like an air-conditioning unit. They step outside and take a look at the exterior of the building, formulating ideas about possible routes of infection. Their gaze settles on an extract duct coming out of the first floor smallpox lab—a blue section of metal tubing about eighteen inches long, located a third of the way up the wall of the building about forty feet from the room where Parker works. Next to it sits a large ventilation duct, pumping air into the quadrangle.

Hughes ensures that the two rooms in which Parker works are locked and fumigated later that afternoon. After discussion with Henry Bedson, they all agree that any additional specimens for smallpox diagnosis should no longer be processed locally, but instead sent to the Central Public Health Laboratory in Colindale, London. Mr Hill reports that all available members of the staff of the Department of Anatomy are to be vaccinated later that afternoon and confirms that he has made arrangements to trace several people not on duty, including a close contact of Mrs. Parker's said to be on holiday with his parents in Ilkeston, Derbyshire.

At 3.30pm, Hughes and Bedson provide university officials, including Owen Wade, with an update. Hughes and Wade divide up the rest of the afternoon's work between them. Hughes briefs two representatives of the ASTMS union, while Wade meets two visitors from the Health and Safety Executive.

That evening, Wade is sufficiently worried to phone Bedson at home at 10pm to ask when they would know for certain that they really were dealing with smallpox. He is not happy when Bedson says laboratory confirmation will not come for another 48 hours.

EARLY ON THE MORNING of Saturday 26 August, Brodie Hughes visits the Medical School to check that precautions are in place to close the ground floor corridor outside the pox lab.

At one end of the corridor, Hughes is pleased to find the double doors leading to the corridor have been locked and the swing barriers within the corridor padlocked. He is also pleased to see a notice forbidding anyone other than departmental staff from entering. At the other end of the corridor, Hughes finds a line of metal lockers blocking entry, together with a similar notice.

During the course of that Saturday, Hughes speaks to Geddes and Nicol and satisfies himself that all is going well with their investigations and that staff in the Medical School have been helping with their enquiries.. Although all work in the pox lab has ceased, they agree that Bedson will be allowed to enter the lab the following day to open the eggs he has inoculated with material from Janet Parker.

At 10.30am the next day, Hughes meets Geddes and Nicol at Alpha Tower, who stress that it is not necessary to close the Medical School, but that the corridors in the east wing of the Medical School should be fumigated.

That day, Bedson's observations of the eggs confirm the diagnosis of variola major, the most severe form of smallpox. Bedson usually chairs the University Pathogenic Organisms Group, but it is felt that he should not do so while investigations on his own laboratory were under way. Instead, that evening, a pathologist, Professor Robert Curran, is asked to chair an ad hoc meeting of the Group without Bedson.

The Group agrees it is okay for the Department of Medical Microbiology to open for work as usual on the Tuesday after the bank holiday weekend. They point out that a number of contractors have worked in the Medical School during the period when Parker acquired her infection and agree to let the Health Authority know.

ON THE MORNING of the Bank Holiday Monday, Hughes visits the Medical School and is pleased to see that notices have been placed in the front hall, letting people know that a member of staff has contracted smallpox and when and where vaccination is available. Some of the staff are already there, waiting to be vaccinated.

That morning, a young technician in the Medical School's Educational Services Unit, Patricia Muddyman, contacts her employers with vague and implausible claims that Janet Parker had visited the Medical School after 11 August and that she and Janet had been in close contact. Later in the day, Muddyman resurfaces at the Medical School, now complaining of a headache and fever. She is sent home and told to avoid contact with others. A few hours later she is admitted to Catherine-de-Barnes Hospital, even though a diagnosis of smallpox is thought unlikely.

At 2.00pm, a member of the University's senior management team, Professor North, chairs a meeting of academic and technical staff in the Dean's room. They are told that the diagnosis of smallpox has been confirmed, that several areas have been fumigated and that an inquiry team has been set up under the chairmanship of Liverpool infection expert Barnett Christie. They make preparations for a return to work, agreeing to ask heads of departments the following morning to fill in a questionnaire on Parker's potential contacts, focusing on staff on annual or sick leave. The Dean's office prepares a pamphlet to give to all Medical School staff, informing them of the precautions taken and assuring them that it would be business as usual everywhere, apart from the Department of Medical Microbiology itself. Copies are run off on the Medical School's Roneograph—a kind of printer used to duplicate type-written sheets before photocopiers became common.

38

PERSONAL INTERLUDE

THE GHOSTS OF BIRMINGHAM PAST

Alongside DA Henderson, I had another hero early in my career as a microbiologist: a remarkable bacteriologist from Stanford, Stanley Falkow, who is revered as a pioneer in the use of molecular approaches to study how microbes cause disease. By the 1990s, Falkow had started an apostolic tradition, tutoring a series of younger scientists, who went on to tutor the next generation of scientists. As a result, everyone in the field is just a few handshakes away from Falkow—in my case, I did a PhD with Gordon Dougan, who did a postdoc with Stan.

Another of Falkow's acolytes, David Relman, first came to my attention in 1992, when he and Falkow published a ground-breaking paper using DNA sequencing to identify the unculturable bacterium that causes a devastating intestinal infection called Whipple's disease.[1]

In the early 2000s, I was lucky enough to collaborate with Relman on sequencing the genome of the Whipple's bacterium[2] *and I met him several times at microbial genomics meetings over the next few years. By late 2013, I had become the Director of a new Institute of Microbiology and Infection at the University of Birmingham and was looking for a keynote speaker for our inaugural symposium. Around that time, I had also started dipping into the recent biomedical literature on smallpox and was amazed to discover that Relman had been involved in a study published in 2004 in which live smallpox virus had been administered to monkeys.*[3] *Bearing all that in mind, I invited David Relman to speak at the symposium.*

By the time the symposium arrived, I had already accepted a new job at the University of Warwick. Nonetheless, I seized the opportunity to play host to David and arranged a pre-conference smallpox tour for him. David and I met up with Alasdair Geddes at the entrance to the Medical School and then proceeded along the eastern corridor to meet the Head of College, Lawrence Young, who sat reading the journal Nature under a portrait of William Withering in the imposing wood-clad office previously occupied by Brodie Hughes. Lawrence, like me, was working out his notice period before a move to Warwick, so he was at a loose end and joined us as we ventured further into the East Wing.

Alasdair took us to the East Wing's ground floor corridor that used to house the pox lab and we soon arrived at a door that bore an old Bakelite label 'EG34', looking as if it dated back to Bedson's day. As we peered in, the room looked much as it did in 1978. From the nearby stairwell, we looked out of the window and into the courtyard, and a glance at the Shooter Report confirmed that it also looked more or less the same as it did in 1978. As we peered up to the windows on the floor above—where Janet Parker used to work—it seemed as if time had stood still for four decades. And it felt odd discussing science and history in such august company in such a nondescript but eventful place.

Alasdair took for us lunch at the Edgbaston Golf Club, which occupies the former home of William Withering. There we stumbled across another member of the Birmingham medical establishment Sandy McNeish and we all started talking about the 1978 incident.

During those few hours, that morning in the winter of 2013, the ghosts of Birmingham's past—whether from the Lunar Society in the eighteenth Century or from smallpox in the twentieth Century—all seemed very close to us. Then the symposium began and we returned to the twenty-first Century.

39

THE CHRISTIE COMMITTEE

ANDREW BARNETT CHRISTIE was born in 1909, educated in Aberdeen and worked from 1949 till his retirement in 1974 as an infectious disease physician in Liverpool.[1] A whole generation of microbiologists and infectious disease physicians learnt their trade from his elegantly written textbook *Infectious Diseases: Epidemiology and Clinical Practice*. He was a keen sportsman, a lifelong swimmer and an enthusiastic traveller, having written a memoir of his journey around Greece.[2]

During the August bank holiday weekend in 1978, Geddes invited Christie to stay at his home in Solihull and to set up a committee of inquiry into the source of Janet Parker's smallpox.[3]

At 10.30 that Monday morning, Barnett Christie chaired the first meeting of the Birmingham Source of Infection Committee, which included Alasdair Geddes, Professor Mike Brown, a pharmaceutical microbiologist from nearby Aston University; and Dr Edward Lowbury, a bacteriologist-cum-poet from the Hospital Infection Research Laboratory at Birmingham's Dudley Road Hospital. In attendance as observers were local virologists Henry Bedson and his deputy Gordon Skinner.

The committee ascertained that Parker had not been abroad recently, nor come in contact with anyone who had been abroad recently. That meant that they could dismiss importation of infection from abroad and instead focus on a local source. Within that context, they felt that there were three main possibilities: that Parker caught the infection from the smallpox lab itself, or from a missed case (someone ill in early July) or from slides or other material from the Medical Microbiology department that she had handled in the course of her photographic duties.

They started off with the pox lab, quizzing Bedson over the kind of work done there. He confirmed that work on smallpox virus had been underway for most of July, including work involving variola major virus towards the end of the month. He stressed that it was all business as usual, with no change in the kind of work or in the staff doing it for several months. When Bedson described the procedures for disrupting virus particles to yield radioactively labelled proteins, Mike Brown raised a concern that, if not all virus particles were disrupted, an infectious aerosol might be produced. Bedson and the rest of the committee agreed, but stressed that a similar hazard must occur in all pox labs.

The committee established that Bedson's pox lab consisted of two rooms: an outer room, where various poxviruses other than variola were handled and where smallpox virus was stored or incubated; and an inner room where smallpox virus was handled and processed. Bedson made clear that when any variola virus was taken from the inner to the outer room, the door of the outer room was locked. The smallpox lab was ventilated through vents in the door between the inner and outer room. Work was carried out in a safety cabinet from which air was expelled through a filter. Bedson's staff had checked the airflow and the work surfaces from time to time and had never found any problems. Glassware and plasticware were chemically treated and contaminated material was autoclaved within the inner room.

Bedson was asked whether he thought the safety procedures in the pox lab were adequate. He said that a week earlier, before Parker's illness, he would have said 'yes'. After all, the WHO Inspectorate had visited the lab in May 1978 and they had raised only minor concerns, such as the lack of showers, or absence of containment in the outer room. A new purpose-built pox lab would have been ideal, but everyone had agreed that work on smallpox was going to cease by the end of the year.

The committee members turned their attention to Option 2: a hidden case. They established that a register of illness was maintained for all staff within the department and that five people had been off ill towards the end of July, three with colds, one with menopausal symptoms and one with severe morning sickness. They felt that all five should be interviewed and examined as soon as possible. In addition to the scientific and technical staff, there were two cleaners who had access to the outer but not the inner room.

As for Option 3, Bedson made clear that was a non-starter as Parker did no photographic work for the Department of Medical Microbiology and any slides containing smallpox would never have left the department.

The committee returned to the possibility of airborne spread of the smallpox virus and whether the virus might have escaped from the inner room through the vent of the safety cabinet and then entered the photography room upstairs where Janet Parker worked. They knew that a previous smallpox victim Tony McLennan had worked in the very same room as Parker back in 1966 and wondered whether the virus could have survived in the room for the past twelve years. Gordon Skinner pointed out that there had been some recent spring-cleaning in the Department of Anatomy, which might have disturbed pox-laden dust. However, the idea was dismissed when the committee realised that McLennan's outbreak was *variola minor*, but Bedson had just shown that Parker was suffering from the far more serious *variola major*.

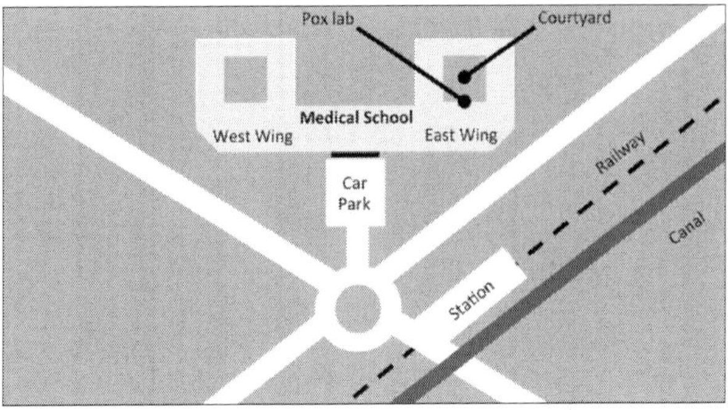

LOCATION OF THE EAST WING IN 1978

The pox lab and photography studio overlooked the courtyard

CHRISTIE'S TEAM TOOK a lunch break, before reconvening at 2.30pm in the Medical School, where they were joined by Christie's colleague from Liverpool, Kevin McCarthy, a smallpox expert and veteran of the investigation into the 1973 outbreak in London. They started the afternoon's proceedings with a tour of the internal courtyard associated with the East Wing of the Medical School.

As with the previous inquisitorial tour of the courtyard three days before, attention soon settled on the blue metal extract duct on the external wall of the pox lab on the first floor. They estimated that the pox lab and the window of Parker's photography room were around 15 yards apart. They confirmed that the inner room of the pox lab had no opening windows, but found that outer room had windows that could open.

The photography rooms had windows that opened wide and they could see that air was sucked in to ventilate the dark room. Ventilators within the windows served the rest of the Anatomy Department, forcefully driving air out into the courtyard. With only a narrow side opening, the courtyard appeared to be shielded from the wind, but they speculated that cross winds could suck air out of the courtyard from above. They noticed pieces of airborne fluff drifting across the courtyard away from the Anatomy and Microbiology side of the building and spied a small green plant fluttering in a different breeze. They concluded that there was obviously air turbulence within the courtyard, but it remained unclear whether it was capable of pushing air—and smallpox virus—into the photography department.

They went back inside, first visiting the photography section of the anatomy department. They confirmed that various fans were sucking into and out of the rooms and used a piece of fluff to show that air was flowing into and around the inner dark room. Next, they visited the pox lab and agreed that the viral strain isolated from Janet Parker should be frozen and, if possible, typed. They contacted Jim Hutchison who agreed to test the air filter from the safety cabinet in a couple of day's time. To cap off their afternoon's work, the committee interviewed Sandy Buchan, the virologist and collaborator of Bedson's, who admitted that he often visited the Anatomy Department and also had access to the outer but not inner room in the pox lab. A long and detailed discussion focused on the potential transfer of variola virus on equipment shuffled between the Anatomy and Microbiology departments, which in the end they concluded was a highly unlikely source of infection.

At 4pm the team of inquiry briefly met Professors Hughes and Wade, before concluding what was to prove their first and only visit to the Medical School. They aimed to meet again later that week.

But the powers-that-be had other plans.

40

BACK TO WORK

THE COUNTRY, THE CITY and the Medical School returned to work the Tuesday morning after the bank holiday weekend. At 10.00am, Professor North chaired a second meeting of his university smallpox committee in the Medical School.[1] Those present included Brodie Hughes, Owen Wade, the University's pathology professor Robert Curran and the Medical School's assistant registrar Alun Roberts.

Owen Wade opened the meeting by noting that officers of the two local unions, ASTMS and NALGO (the National and Local Government Officers' Association), had expressed satisfaction with the University's actions up to that point.

The committee heard that all smallpox virus was now locked away in the deep freeze. They also learned that Pat Muddyman had been admitted to the smallpox isolation hospital for observation. Rumours were circulating that Muddyman had been diagnosed with smallpox and the committee heard that Alun Roberts, as a contact of Muddyman, had been advised to cancel his holiday in France. Wade suggested that a statement be made to staff to clarify that Muddyman was very unlikely to have smallpox. Concerns were also raised about who was in a position to issue orders. Was it the Area Health Authority? Or was it the Health and Safety Executive (HSE): the new-kid-on-the-block quango created by the *Health and Safety at Work Act* of 1974 and eager to flex its muscles.

Hughes discussed the status of Henry Bedson with Professor North and they agreed that Bedson should transfer the bulk of his administrative and other duties to his junior, Dr Gordon Skinner, so that he could contribute to the investigation into the source of the infection. Although Bedson and Skinner agreed to this move, Hughes felt the need to stress that the University was in no way removing Bedson from his position as Head of Department. The Dean was now worried about Bedson's state of mind: in his notes on the incident, Hughes wrote that Bedson was 'clearly deeply concerned about the situation and was very depressed.'

At midday, Wade met with a member of the Medical School maintenance staff and reassured him that vaccinated people could not carry smallpox home with them. Later that afternoon, Wade spoke to Willie Nicol, who asked him to stop people using the Medical School as a thoroughfare between the Queen Elizabeth Hospital and the railway station. Wade arranged for notices to be put up and for a library side door to be locked to prevent commuters passing through.

A little while later, Wade was contacted by the University's Registrar who passed on a rumour from a reporter at *The Times of London* that Janet Parker had visited the London School of Hygiene and Tropical Medicine within the last three weeks. Wade was sceptical but suggested that the information be passed on to Geddes or the Health Authority.

ON THE AFTERNOON of the following day—the Wednesday of that week—Brodie Hughes met with Willie Nicol and two associates from the DHSS, a Dr John Evans and a Mr Jones. Nicol handed over six copies of a report from Christie's committee of investigation, stating that Christie and Lowbury would be happy to discuss the contents with the University's own committees. Nicol reassured the Dean that, in his view, the smallpox stocks held in the laboratory presented no further risk and that no additional steps need be taken for now.

Then Dr Evans dropped a bombshell, making it clear that the Christie committee would be going no further. Instead, the DHSS was going to advise the Secretary of State for Health and Social Services, David Ennals, to run a small informal inquiry through the Dangerous Pathogens Advisory Group (DPAG), chaired by Professor Reginald Shooter, a microbiologist at St Bartholomew's Hospital. Shooter had already agreed to lead the inquiry, which could start in as little as a week's time. But, ever the diplomat, Evans stressed that Ennals might disagree and go for a full and formal public inquiry into the affair.

Evans sought and received an assurance that the pox laboratory would stay closed and nothing in it would be interfered with, nor any work done, such as servicing of ducts, that might destroy evidence. Hughes raised concerns with Evans as to potential conflicts of jurisdiction between an inquiry ordered by the DHSS and investigations carried out by the HSE. Evans reassured him that both had overriding positive powers, i.e. if one said a room must be closed while the other was happy for it to remain open, the room should be closed.

That evening, Owen Wade popped in for a couple of hours to see Bedson at his home. Wade wanted to learn all he could about smallpox, the variola virus and the work that Bedson doing. They went to Bedson's study. Bedson looked exhausted and seemed miserable, certain that he would be 'crucified' because of what had happened to Janet Parker. However, Wade was pleased to find that Bedson—ever the boffin—became much more cheerful once he started to talk about the details of his research.

THE FOLLOWING DAY, Thursday 31 August, there was another 10am meeting chaired by Professor North in the Medical School. Brodie Hughes gave out copies of the report from the Christie committee and let them know about the soon-to-be-set-up Shooter Committee. The pox lab was to remain closed and in its present state until the Shooter team had visited.

There was discussion of the emerging turf war between the AHA, DHSS and HSE. Positions seemed to be hardening across the board, with the HSE stoking union fears by raising a prohibition notice forbidding the University from doing any more work on smallpox and the AHA's Willie Nicol now demanding that anyone who had been working in the pox lab be quarantined. The committee heard that Dr John Evans at the DHSS was keen to settle what he called the 'rank' issue between the various organisations. It was agreed that copies of the HSE's prohibition notice would be given to the union reps.

Concern was raised about the difficulties of restricting access to the Medical School, with fourteen doors into the building, many of them fire escapes that could not be sealed. It was agreed that arrangements should be made for staff who fell ill to be seen immediately and all those who wanted the vaccine to receive it.

Straight after the meeting, Owen Wade rang Willie Nicol to get the go-ahead on setting up vaccination clinics, only to discover that the person he had in the frame for doing all this, Gordon Skinner, was about to go into quarantine. Instead, the job fell to the University Health Service. A few minutes later, he spoke to a couple of microbiologists at the HSE and at his behest they agreed to co-operate with the AHA on control measures in the Medical School.

After lunch, Wade spoke to the medical students, who were due to resume their studies after the holiday break. He told them about the smallpox incident and the measures underway to mitigate harm, but was greeted by healthy mock-indignant boos when he said that lectures would go on as normal.

At 4.30pm Wade spoke to John Evans at the DHSS, who informed him that the turf war had been resolved: orders in future would come from the health authorities rather than the HSE. Evans also gently floated a list of candidates for the Shooter Committee, which included Robert Williams, Director of the UK's Public Health Laboratory Service, Oxford microbiologist Sir David Evans, former director of the National Institute for Biological Standards and Control, an MRC scientist Dr Robinson and former president of the Royal Society of Medicine, Sir Gordon Wolstenholme.

41

THE LAST SUPPER

AS AUGUST DREW to a close, William Nicol concluded that all staff in the Department of Medical Microbiology might have been exposed to smallpox through Janet Parker or through whatever route she had caught the disease.[1] He therefore decided that all the staff should be quarantined at home for sixteen days from 30 August. Among those put under quarantine was the one local virologist who knew most about smallpox: Professor Henry Bedson. Effectively under house arrest, Bedson might have concluded that he was being blamed for Janet Parker's infection.

Around the same time, the HSE decided to close Bedson's pox lab. They issued an order banning smallpox work in Birmingham, at least until the recommendations of a 1975 working party had been enforced. The local branch of the ASTMS had been considering a walkout, but with the lab closed they called off industrial action, while still complaining about lack of consultation.

Bedson saw the writing on the wall and made a statement to the press that day that work on infectious strains of smallpox was unlikely to restart in Birmingham. The University of Liverpool also announced that it would destroy all its stock of the smallpox virus. The HSE fumigated, then sealed Bedson's pox laboratory. They weren't really thinking about what they were doing—in the process, they destroyed the viral cultures established from Janet Parker's samples, hindering any attempts to establish precisely what kind of virus had infected Parker!

With Birmingham's own Smallpox Reference Laboratory out of action, the Government had to turn to virology services outside the city. The DHSS in London quickly called Kevin McCarthy back from Liverpool, asking him to take skin scrapings from Janet Parker, in the hope of re-isolating the virus and determining what kind of poxvirus it was.

What followed on the afternoon of Thursday 31 August can only be described as a farce. The DHSS insisted that McCarthy and the specimens he was to collect should travel under police escort, fearful that the smallpox samples might present a risk to the public. McCarthy made an uneventful outward journey by road from

Liverpool on the M6 motorway. As he left the motorway, he was met by a police officer on a motorbike, who travelled with McCarthy to Catherine-de-Barnes Hospital. As soon as they arrived, the policeman attempted to say 'goodbye' to McCarthy. He changed his mind only after McCarthy had pointed out that a police escort was really only relevant *after* the samples had been collected.

McCarthy entered the hospital and took skin scrapings from Janet Parker, who had now been in hospital for more than five days. McCarthy expected the police officer to escort him all the way back to his virus lab in Liverpool, only for the policeman to say that was not what he had been told to do. Initially, he offered to show McCarthy the way back on to the M6, only to discover that there had been an accident on the motorway, causing a long tail back. He therefore suggested that the virologist should leave Birmingham to the west of the city via the M5 motorway. He escorted McCarthy part of the way to the M5, only to abandon him at five o'clock at the heart of the rush hour in Digbeth in the middle of the city.

McCarthy was not keen to fight his way through the rush hour, so he decided to call in and see his old friend and fellow virologist Henry Bedson at home in Harborne, just a few miles south of the city centre. Henry had been confined to his house, starting quarantine the evening before. As McCarthy dined with Henry and his family, there was a delicious irony in the *supposedly potentially infectious* (but, after repeated vaccinations, actually highly immune) Bedson being confined to his home, while the *actually infectious* samples of smallpox sat outside in McCarthy's car unguarded on a drive in suburban Birmingham.

One thing is certain: as he left the hospitality of the Bedson home, McCarthy had no idea that he just participated in Bedson's last supper. Farce was about to give way to tragedy.

42

THE NEW DEAN

I became Dean of the Medical School at one minute past midnight on 1 September 1978. By midday Professor Bedson, the Professor of Medical Microbiology, had cut his throat and I had shut half the Medical School.
Owen Wade (1996) *When I Dropped the Knife.*

THE NEW MONTH BRINGS regime change at the Medical School in Birmingham.[1] At one minute past midnight on 1 September, Brodie Hughes steps down as Dean. The man who takes over, Owen Wade, was—as his obituary was later to report—'no ordinary man': a hard-working, straight-talking, cheerful, extrovert Welshman, capable of keeping many balls in the air at the same time.

Born in Penarth, a seaside resort near Cardiff, fifty-seven years previously, Wade has already confronted many challenges that would have floored the 'ordinary man'. As a teenager, he assisted his father in surgical operations. As a medical student, he delivered a baby on the platform of Warren Street tube station in London. He gained a first at Cambridge and in war-torn London completed his obstetrics exam hiding under the table with an examiner, fearful of an approaching V-bomb.

A few years later, as a Lecturer in Birmingham, Wade showed steely resolve as the first medical researcher to perform the risky procedure of cardiac catheterisation on a normal subject, deftly threading a plastic tube into a living, beating heart. In his late thirties, he moved to Belfast, where he revived an ailing pharmacology department.

Within a few years, driven on by the thalidomide tragedy, he has become a world authority on the safe prescribing of drugs and their adverse effects. In 1971, Professor Owen Wade moves back to Birmingham to set up the Department of Clinical Pharmacology and Therapeutics.

Now, on 1 September 1978, Wade enters the Dean's oak-clad office and assumes responsibility for the Medical School—a post that is to test his leadership and communication skills to the limit.

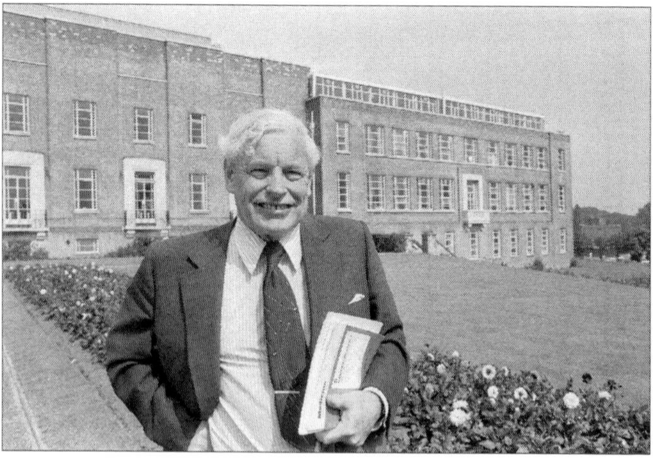

PROFESSOR OWEN WADE
Dean of Medicine, outside the
East Wing of Birmingham Medical School
{Source: Birmingham Mail}

43

THE MOST UNKINDEST CUT OF ALL

SEPTEMBER BEGINS IN BIRMINGHAM with clouds in the sky and an autumnal chill in the air. On Friday 1 September, the sun rises a little after 6.00am.[1] As Henry Bedson and his wife Pat stir from their slumber at their home in Cockthorpe Close—a quiet cul-de-sac in the well-to-do south Birmingham suburb of Harborne—they find themselves at the eye of the storm. Henry has been stuck at home since the night-before-last under quarantine and no longer able to play a hands-on role in managing the smallpox incident. In the meantime, the news media have been badgering the Bedsons with numerous phone calls

Considering the strain they are under, the Bedsons have slept well—Henry got up just once in the night to fill a hot water bottle.[2] Now that Henry no longer has to go into work, they grant themselves a treat and have breakfast in bed.

A little later that morning, Henry and Pat Bedson decide that they have had enough of being stuck in the house and need to get some fresh air. Like most suburban house-owners in Britain, they have a garden, with a lawn and a garden shed. They go outside to work in the garden. Around ten o'clock that morning, the phone rings and Pat goes indoors to take the call, which turns out to be from one of her friends. Henry somehow gets hold of a kitchen knife.

NO ONE CAN KNOW precisely what thoughts were going through Henry Bedson's mind that morning. Pat can see that her husband is weary and concerned, but she doesn't think he is depressed. He has never been one to wear his emotions on his sleeve—if someone says something that upsets him, he goes quiet, but only those who know him well can work out why.[3] Although he has no history of mental illness, over the previous week, plenty has happened to disturb the balance of Henry Bedson's mind.

The fact that Janet Parker has caught smallpox from his lab is bad enough. However, on top of that, at the meetings about the smallpox incident, there has been some blokey banter about them 'having to clear up the mess that you have created for us, Henry'.[4]

This might have seemed light-hearted to the speaker, but must have hit home with Henry. And now Willie Nicol's insistence on mass quarantine of all staff in the Department of Medical Microbiology has added to the weight of responsibility on Bedson's shoulders.

When Owen Wade tells his wife Margaret that Bedson has been confined to his home, she responds angrily: 'Why don't they take him and stick a knife in his back. That man needs to be in action and working with his colleagues in such a crisis. He is the last man on this earth to get smallpox!' Nicol himself later claims that he had 'warned people in high places' that Bedson was at risk of self-harm.

Effectively under house arrest, Bedson is frustrated that he cannot make a greater contribution to sorting things out. But worse than the sense of isolation and inability to sort things out are the intrusive phone calls. From eight in the morning till late at night, Henry and Pat have been harassed by the press, with as many as forty phone calls in the run-up to that fateful morning.

Although the Regional Health Authority has offered to take calls for him, Bedson insists on answering them himself, so that no one has any grounds for believing in a cover-up. The callers insinuate that if Bedson doesn't answer their questions, they will have to conclude the worst. The continual intrusions grind him down, as he has to repeat the same information over and over again to one caller after another.

A LITTLE AFTER TEN that morning, Henry Bedson is found in the locked garden shed with his throat cut. Pat is confronted with the aftermath of an act of gut-wrenching violence—Bedson has used considerable force to create an 8-inch wound in his neck, cutting into his windpipe, his jugular veins and even into his carotid arteries. Henry is unconscious, but still alive.

Pat rushes back into the house to phone for help. First, she calls her family doctor. Then, the phone starts ringing. She answers it to find a Birmingham radio journalist making an inquiry. She asks him to get off the line. She slams the phone handset down, then picks it up again, praying for a dialling tone. Instead, she hears a voice saying, 'She wants us to get off the line as she has an urgent call to make'. Three times she thrusts the phone down and snatches it to her ear again, before she has a clear line and can call an ambulance. Fortunately, they confirm that her GP has already called one.

Pat calls the Medical School and a neighbour to take care of her 10-year-old daughter Sarah. At the Medical School, Owen Wade hears the news at 10.40am from Mr Roberts, the Assistant Registrar of the Medical School, who calls him out of a meeting.

An ambulance arrives for Henry, with police escort, and takes him to Birmingham Accident Hospital. The police attempt to visit the house, but decide they cannot enter a household under quarantine. Only after Henry has been taken off to hospital, does Pat find a bloodied kitchen knife in the shed. She then sets off for the hospital herself.

As the ambulance makes the three-mile dash along the Hagley Road, the ambulance men rush to replace the fluid that Bedson has lost. As Bedson is rushed through Casualty, staff recoil in fear, scared he might infect them with smallpox. As a sign of the panic, the unit is later fumigated.

Bedson receives a transfusion of several units of blood. The eminent vascular surgeon Professor Geoff Slaney (later to be Sir Geoff and President of the Royal College of Surgeons) makes a heroic effort to save Bedson's life by suturing the main arteries of his neck, even though the blood loss has starved Bedson's brain and other organs of oxygen for a prolonged period. After the operation, Bedson is put on life support.

At the hospital, a reporter confronts Pat, trying to get her into an interview room. Meanwhile, Owen Wade and his wife are also inundated with calls, many of them inappropriate or even childish. Was Wade at Henry's bedside? Was Mrs Bedson there? Was it true that Bedson had cut his throat because he knew he had smallpox?

Pat returns home to find the house besieged by reporters and photographers. Kevin McCarthy and his wife come down from Liverpool to provide moral and practical support.

THE NEXT DAY, PAT finds a suicide note from her husband in the garden shed: 'I am sorry to have misplaced the trust which so many of my friends and colleagues have placed in me and my work and above all to have dragged into disrepute my wife and beloved children. I realise this act is the least sensible thing I have done, but it may allow them to get some peace.'

Henry Bedson survives the weekend on life support. During the Sunday lunchtime, Pat Bedson pops round to visit Margaret and Owen Wade. Margaret lends a sympathetic ear as Pat expresses concern that they might have to stop the life support for Henry, but stresses she was determined to see things clearly and objectively for the sake of their children. Pat makes it clear that the 'very ignorant man' who has put Henry into quarantine has quite literally killed him.

At 11.00 on the morning of Tuesday 5 September, Pat makes a visit to Henry's bedside in the Accident Hospital's Intensive care unit. Shortly after noon, the TV channel ATV approaches Owen Wade at the Medical School to claim, erroneously, that Henry Bedson has died. Wade, stuck down by grief, dons a black tie.

Later that afternoon, Pat Bedson, accompanied by Kevin McCarthy, visits Wade at his home and informs him that Bedson is still alive, albeit critically ill and unconscious on a ventilator. In typical English fashion, Wade makes a pot of tea, which all three of them share—numbed by the horror of what has happened, but also faintly amused at the absurdity of the situation. A little later, Wade meets some ATV reporters at the Medical School and asks them to make a public announcement, apologising for the error, but nothing like that happens.

The next day, tests show that Henry Bedson is brain-dead and at 10.20am his life support is turned off. He has become the first casualty of Birmingham's 1978 smallpox incident. Owen Wade immediately pays tribute to Bedson's work in television interviews, stating that 'His death adds one more medical man to the many who have died to make life better and safer for us all. We must all be unutterably sad at this tragic death.' He also writes to the surgeon at the Accident Hospital who has been caring for Henry, thanking him and his colleagues for all their efforts, while also pointing out that he is unutterably sad about Henry, but that his admiration for Pat is unbounded.

An inquest is held into Bedson's death two day's later. A verdict of suicide is recorded. However, the Birmingham coroner Dr Richard Whittington pulls no punches in blaming the press, stating 'I do feel that the inquiries repeatedly being made to his household must have been an important factor in producing Professor Bedson's mental state of exhaustion. I only hope that some people, or perhaps some press organisation or association, can develop some mechanism whereby families in this sort of situation, when they reach a time of great personal distress, can be protected from these inquiries and given some help to deal with them.'

The coroner adds: 'If anybody feels that a complaint should be made to the Press Council, I am quite prepared to provide the notes of evidence of this court to support any complaint by any person to the Press Council'. In response, journalists covering the case deny any wrongdoing and a later Press Council inquiry finds no evidence of improper press behaviour.[5]

Owen Wade later writes: 'Henry should have cut the telephone wires not his neck.' Unfortunately, despite Bedson's death, Birmingham's smallpox tragedy is far from over.

44

AT THE HELM

OWEN WADE HAD HIS hands full for the month that followed, working twelve to fourteen hours a day, juggling media enquiries, union anxiety and anger, orders from Willie Nicol and investigations by the Shooter committee. He took care to document the myriad concerns that crossed his desk—plus the countless meetings and phone calls—in a 55-page diary[1], which was subsequently typed up neatly for posterity. The problems were generally political, rather than medical.

Shortly after Bedson's incident in the shed, Wade returned to his office to find a telephone message that Nicol had issued an order, telling him to close the East Wing of the Medical School and seal all the doors apart from the front entrance. Wade was not at all happy with this, as just a few hours earlier Nicol had stated that the restrictions already in place were 'Draconian' and to do more would be obsessive. Particularly galling was the fact that a representative of the ASTMS had announced the order over the radio at 11.00 that morning, before Wade was even aware of it.

One hard man confronted another, as Wade raised multiple concerns with Nicol over the coming days: policy by diktat was unreasonable; who would look after the animals; what about fire escapes? Wade was concerned that changes in policy from Nicol's AHA, together with the HSE's prohibition notice, were giving the unions a rod to beat the Medical School with.

Although Nicol would not yield on closing the East Wing—only later would he admit privately that he did it to placate the unions and against his better judgement—Wade's daily phone calls wrung concessions from his Glaswegian antagonist: yes, Nicol would agree to provide a statement that the circumstances had not changed; yes, Wade could visit some of those in quarantine, so long as he kept quiet about it; yes, Wade could open the doors in the West Wing of the Medical School. One key concession was a statement that Bedson had been released from quarantine the day after he had been admitted to hospital and, contrary to rumour, Bedson did not have smallpox.

After an inspection by DHSS man Dr Desmond Robinson on

Saturday 9 September, concerns were raised as to whether smallpox virus could have escaped from the pox lab through cracks in shafts into an adjacent seminar room and into the rabbit facility on the floor below. An effort was made to get Hugh Morgan to ask Janet Parker whether she had ever been in the seminar room, but she was too ill to answer.

Robinson insisted that the Medical School's laboratory rabbits be killed, which greatly upset the local virologist Gordon Skinner. The rabbit room was then fumigated, the rabbit carcasses removed in plastic bags and Skinner and his colleagues were forced to incinerate the dead animals.

An audit was performed of the 200-animal-strong monkey colony, showing that forty-seven Rhesus macaques and six baboons had been purchased and appropriately quarantined over the last eighteen months.[2] All the animals were bled, and, in antibody tests, all but one showed no evidence of pox infection—and the one animal with a slightly raised antibody level had been fit and well for three years. It was established that Janet Parker had not visited the monkey colony during July.

Over the coming weeks, the ever-more-stressed-out Des Robinson became ever more assertive in his dealings with the Medical School, while taking care to brief the unions. A lot of fuss was made as to whether the Christie and Shooter inquiries were confidential. The ASTMS objected to Shooter as head of his inquiry, because he was a 'university man'. Wade began to wonder whether Robinson's willingness to disclose information to the unions might be prejudicial to the Medical School, but then scribbled in his diary: 'perhaps "we have nothing to hide" stance is good'. However, he was clear that Robinson had a conflict of interest in serving as secretary to the Shooter Inquiry, helping the DHSS advise Willie Nicol and the AHA, while also allowing the union's views to inform decision-making.

Wade was also forced by the media to confront the possibility that the 1966 Birmingham outbreak might also have originated from the Medical School's pox lab, even though Tony McLennan stated quite definitely that he had not caught his infection this way. Wade soon convinced himself that there was no evidence for this.

IT IS WORTH PAUSING for a moment to imagine what it must have been like for those working in the Medical School and their representatives in the union. The very worst-case scenario had come to pass: one of their members had acquired a terrifying life-threatening illness at work and no one knew how this had happened. And if no one knew how the virus had escaped, how could anyone assure them that they were safe?

But, sadly, encouraged by ATSMS leader Clive Jenkins, the union went well beyond the facts to stir things up. Things became so polarised that the union even complained when Bedson was described in *The Times* as 'an eminent doctor'.

All this came to a head in a meeting at the Medical School in mid-September between 30-year-old Scottish trade unionist Sheila McKechnie[3]—who was Health and Safety Officer of ASTMS—and Owen Wade, Willie Nicol and Desmond Robinson, along with four local ASTMS reps. After Nicol and Robinson said that they were satisfied that the Medical School could be re-opened, McKechnie castigated Wade for not keeping Medical School staff informed—an accusation he countered by saying he had had two meetings with staff that very morning.

A short while later, McKechnie laid into Nicol, asking why the union was not honoured with a copy of the Christie report until ten days after the University had received it. Never one to suffer fools gladly, Nicol was adamant in his response to his fellow Scot that it was a private report and he was entitled to show it to anyone who might be able to help him get to the bottom of the epidemic. He stressed that it was a doctor-to-doctor report and he never had the slightest intention of showing it to the unions. McKechnie then attacked Robinson, saying that the union should have all and any reports as soon as they are available.

The next day, two of the local union reps (who happened to be from the Department of Microbiology) conveyed apologies to Wade for McKechnie's behaviour the previous day. However, then McKechnie stirred things up by phoning to ask whether it was true that a notice had been placed in the Medical School saying that Parker had died from monkeypox. It was not true at all, but in response, Wade spent half the night putting together a statement suggesting that animal pox viruses presented no significant risk to humans.

That was not the end of it: over the next couple of months, McKechnie and her boss Clive Jenkins revealed 'a fine mastery of the art of smear by hypothesis', claiming in interviews that Bedson had been carrying out unauthorised and illegal genetic manipulation experiments to create a vaccine-resistant version of smallpox.[4] Although most of the press ignored their 'alternative facts' and unwarranted scare mongering, fear-provoking headlines proliferated and Owen Wade's wife experienced guilt-by-association when she was 'uninvited' from an exhibition of paintings overs fears of carrying smallpox.

On 28 September, Owen was given the go-ahead by Nicol and Robinson to reopen the East Wing of the Medical School. However, that evening he was forced out of the bath to take an urgent phone call from the University's Vice-Chancellor, Bob Hunter, informing him that they had both been summoned to London the next morning to meet David Ennals, the Secretary of State.

The next day they duly met Ennals, his leg suspended on a stool as he convalesced from an attack of phlebitis. Initially hostile and towing the union line, Ennals soon came around to the University's side when presented with a letter from Desmond Robinson, carrying the DHSS letterhead, stating that he was satisfied that the Medical School need no longer remain closed. However, Ennals insisted that the University meet the ASTMS to explain that there was no remaining danger in re-opening the East Wing.

It took nearly two weeks to arrange such a meeting. But at the meeting, the ASTMS was dismissive of the University's reassurances, with a union man saying they were not prepared to listen to 'experts', as 'experts' might be wrong. The union then staged a walkout.

Eventually, life at the Medical School returned to a kind of normality, despite the continual criticisms from Clive Jenkins. To signal the return of the routine of academic life, Owen Wade gave the president of the medical students' union, Miss Brockensha, the go-ahead for a Freshers' Party in the Medical School's Arthur Thomson Hall to mark the start of the new academic year.

45

CATHERINE-DE-BARNES

CATHERINE-DE-BARNES IS A VILLAGE that sits at the edge of the borough of Solihull, within England's West Midlands.[1] Curiously, there was no eponymous 'Catherine of Barnes'—instead this is a corruption of 'Ketelberne', the name of a local twelfth-century Lord of the Manor. Today, locals have corrupted things further and often call their village 'Catney'. The village expanded in the eighteenth and nineteenth centuries, thanks to the building of the Grand Union Canal, which connects Birmingham and London and provides an attractive backdrop for Catney's only pub, The Boat Inn.

Henwood Lane is a straight narrow road that connects the village centre to Henwood Hall Farm, about a mile to the south. Initially it runs parallel to the canal, before crossing the waterway, as the canal swings westward. Even today, the lane is flanked on either side by open fields. It was here, in this secluded rural setting, that the Solihull and Meriden Councils built a fever hospital in 1907 for isolating patients with infectious diseases such as diphtheria, typhoid fever and smallpox.[2]

The hospital was situated to the west of the road, about five hundred yards south of the village centre. Its twenty-acre grounds included a gatehouse, a central quadrangle and two large two-storey blocks, surrounded by one-storey buildings, suitable for housing patients in isolation. In total, it could house ten staff and sixteen patients.

In the 1950s, as the prevalence of infectious diseases waned, the site was redeployed as a convalescent home for ailing mothers, who had given birth at Netherwood Maternity Hospital in Solihull, and even occasionally served as a maternity hospital. In the late sixties, two developments led to the re-designation of Catherine-de-Barnes Hospital as an isolation hospital: a new maternity block was built at Solihull Hospital and Birmingham's Witton Hospital was decommissioned as a smallpox hospital and, as we have seen, was burnt down in May 1967.

By 1978, even though there was growing confidence that smallpox had been eradicated, Catherine-de-Barnes Hospital was still being maintained exclusively for patients suffering from proven or suspected smallpox. Between cases, the hospital was left empty but maintained in good working order by resident caretakers, ready to take patients at an hour's notice.

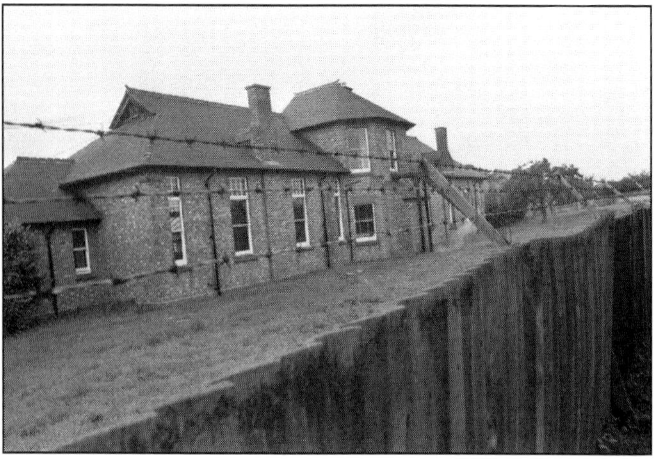

CATHERINE-DE-BARNES HOSPITAL
Seen across the barbed-wire perimeter fence
{Source: Birmingham Mail}

Leslie and Dorothy Harris took over the care of Catherine-de-Barnes Hospital in 1967. They spent the next eleven years of their working lives cleaning, maintaining, waiting for a calamity that nobody wanted to happen. On Thursday 24 August, 1978, a little before midnight, their worst nightmare comes true: Janet Parker arrives, stricken with smallpox. Over the days that follow, Janet is looked after by two live-in nurses, fully vaccinated and wearing protective clothing, who work lonely and stressful alternating shifts, largely devoid of the companionship of colleagues. A hospital porter comes across with Janet to support the hospital during her stay. The consultant Hugh Morgan visits each day, but sleeps at his own home. Janet is the sole occupant of a ward capable of taking many more patients. The severity of her illness means that she remains largely restricted to her bed for the duration of her stay.[3]

Morgan takes two photographs of Janet Parker during her stay in the hospital. One shows the rash on her legs, with the pustules on the feet no longer islands, but instead coalescing to form peninsulas of pus within the skin.[4]

The other photograph, too distressing to reproduce here, shows a full-frontal view of Janet Parker's face, covered by a grisly, friable, pearly 'mud-pack' of coalesced spots, flanked here and there by small patches of unaffected skin. The reddish hue of her diseased face is mirrored by the pink of the NHS blanket that covers her body and is thrown into stark contrast by the fresh white pillow, which supports her weary head. Through sore eyelids, she gazes out of half-open eyes, oblivious to the photographer, staring listlessly at some distant point, to one side of and behind the viewer. Her expression reveals a sorry, sad, exhausted resignation. Her long grey hair, roughly swept back from her face on three sides, suggests a languid abandonment of any need to keep up appearances. She looks much older than forty.

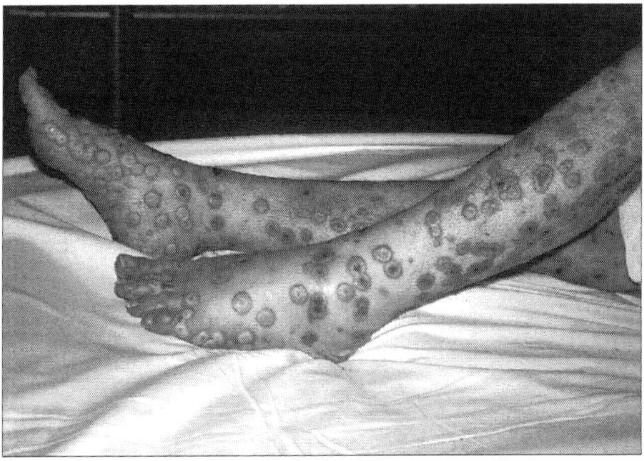

SMALLPOX RASH ON JANET PARKER'S LEGS
Note umbilicated spots, with coalescence of spots on the feet
{Source: A. Geddes/H. Morgan}

JANET PARKER'S FIRST NIGHT in hospital is described as 'fair' in her hospital notes. Hugh Morgan records that she seems slightly confused in the morning, but has no complaints apart from the itching. Janet's rash is maturing, with some new small red spots, but many of the older spots are developing centrally placed dots (becoming *umbilicated* in the medical jargon). One of the spots on Janet's right upper eyelid has ruptured overnight, provoking a nasty red eye. That first Friday, she is given a radio, some chloramphenicol eye drops and some antihistamine tablets to help with the itching.

Janet's second night in hospital is more disturbed. She claims that she fell out of bed in the night, but the ward sister says that she was watching Janet all night and this simply did not happen. However, come the Saturday morning, despite sporting a fever, Janet appears to be rational, comfortable, even cheerful. There are no new red spots and all the spots have at least reached the stage of forming blisters (become *vesicular* in the jargon), with some forming dark scabs. None have burst and started weeping fluid, although some of them, particularly on the hands, are very tense. Hugh Morgan notices a couple of spots in her mouth. There is a mild heart murmur and her heart seems to be enlarged. When Henry Morgan examines her chest, he detects a hint of pneumonia on the right side, but with the basic facilities available in the isolation hospital, he cannot confirm his suspicions with a chest X-ray.

Luckily, by the Saturday afternoon, the congestion in that right lung seems to have cleared and Janet is clear-headed enough to complain about hospital food, as she takes some soup, some cold drinks, a cup or two of tea and a little soft food.

By the time she starts her first Sunday in hospital, Janet is generally feeling a lot better, with her fever down and the spots on her face feeling less tense and becoming crusty. The spot on her right eyelid has dried up, but the red eye is still a problem, making it hard for her to read. She is also still having trouble getting air right down to the bases of her lungs, particularly on the right. She feels giddy when she sits up for any length of time and slips back down in the bed. By the afternoon, she is complaining of a slight cough. That evening there is virological confirmation that Janet has variola major. She is given an oral antiseptic gel, Bonjela, for the sores in her mouth. She sleeps well that night on a sheepskin blanket.

Monday 28 August brings continued improvement: the sore eye is more comfortable and the spots are drying out; the heart murmur and lung congestion less marked; she is drinking well and seems a lot more with it, as she discusses recent events.

Over the next couple of days Janet still seems to be doing OK. On Tuesday 29 August, *The Guardian* describes her condition as 'showing signs of improvement'. The right eye is still playing up: she can see through it well enough to count fingers but not read. Hugh Morgan seeks advice from the eye hospital, who suggest that Janet starts on steroid eye drops, in addition to the antibiotic drops. The rash on Janet's back is now developing into a mass of yellow crusts that start weeping, particularly over the shoulder blades and other pressure points. They also stick to her hair.

On Tuesday 29 August, Janet's neighbour Millicent Rowley is admitted to Catherine-de-Barnes hospital, feeling a little unwell, but she is soon given the all clear and discharged the next day. Janet's colleague from work, Patricia Muddyman, is admitted with a rash, although no one really thinks she might have smallpox. She stays for a week before being sent home.

On the Wednesday and Thursday nights, Janet doesn't sleep well and starts to feel uncomfortable, although she says she is not in pain. She is switched to a strong sedative, chloral hydrate, to help her sleep. She still has a cough. Her ankles start to swell and become a little tender. On the right-hand side, the swelling persists even when the skin is depressed with a finger (*pitting oedema* in the jargon), suggesting that she is accumulating fluid.

ON FRIDAY 1 SEPTEMBER, Dr Deborah Symmons starts her time in quarantine by joining Hugh Morgan in looking after Janet at the isolation hospital. Unlike Dr Morgan, Dr Symmons lives in at the hospital. As a side issue, she has to help caretaker Leslie Harris cope with his poorly controlled diabetes.

The hospital is run according to strict protocols, with a 'clean side' where drugs and provisions are delivered without exposing delivery men to risk, before the goods are transferred through a kind of air lock to the 'dirty side'. Dr Symmons has to grapple with the lab equipment sent from East Birmingham Hospital to perform blood tests on her patients. In the meantime, Leslie and Dorothy do all the cooking, cleaning and portering for the patients and staff held captive in Catney.

Leslie soon fires up the hospital's incinerator to cope with soiled bed linen and other potentially infectious material. His work is doubled when a paramedic, Malcolm Tomlinson, brings Leslie the blankets that covered Parker in the ambulance. Getting them there has been no simple process: Tomlinson has been vaccinated and has had to wear some old clothes, a surgical cap, mask and gloves to drive to the isolation hospital—and on arrival, he is forced to abandon his vehicle, which is fumigated.[5]

NOW OVER A WEEK into her hospital stay, on Saturday 2 September, Janet is still very weak, even though she is sleeping better. There are now raw areas on her back, which are being treated with flannels soaked in an antiseptic, potassium permanganate. That day, they install a special air mattress for her, which helps prevents bedsores.

The spots below Janet's lip have now cracked open and are

bleeding. The swelling and tenderness that started at the ankles has moved up to encompass her calves. The vision in her right eye seems slightly worse. She is asking for the bedpan every hour, but passing just small amounts of urine. She receives a pep talk, telling her how well she is doing and encouraging her to keep her limbs moving and her lungs inflated.

On Sunday 3 September, Janet's father, Fred Witcomb, is admitted to the hospital, into the male ward across the corridor from Janet's female ward. Fred and his wife Hilda were put into quarantine a few days earlier and he is now complaining of slight nausea. As there is no phone at the Witcomb's house, if Fred deteriorated the only way his wife could tell anyone would be by breaking her quarantine, so he is brought in as a precaution. Also admitted that day is Reg Wickett, an engineer who had been working at the East Birmingham Hospital when Janet was admitted. He has had to cut short his holiday after a police call-out and is now suffering from flu-like symptoms, which are thought to be vaccine-related.

That weekend Janet Parker continues to deteriorate. She has a cough and is short of breath when she exerts herself. She feels very weak and has completely lost her appetite. She appears to be depressed and seems to be giving up on life. The rash on her face is still cracked and bleeding and has started to affect her nose, so she has to breathe through her mouth. She feels like her back is on fire. Her buttocks have also become sore. They look clean but are starting to smell of ammonia, probably because of a bacterial infection. She is still anaemic and the high urea level in her blood suggests her kidneys are not working properly. Janet is told that the swollen ankles are probably a sign that she needs to eat more to keep protein levels up in her blood.

Despite these setbacks, on 4 September Janet's condition is described as 'satisfactory' by *The Guardian* and 'comfortable' by the *Daily Express*. On 5 September, *The Guardian* repeats the term 'satisfactory'.

At just after 7 o'clock on the morning of Monday 5 September, Dr Symmons is called to see Janet Parker, who is having difficulty breathing. Janet has had a bad night, feeling frightened all the time, and has been struggling for breath for the last half an hour. Dr Symmons listens to Janet's chest and makes a diagnosis of left lower lobe pneumonia. She starts an intravenous drip and gives Janet a combination of injectable antibiotics, together with an oxygen mask.

Later that morning, Deborah Symmons and Hugh Morgan

respond to an emergency call to attend to Janet's 71-year-old father, Fred, who has collapsed pulseless in his room. Their attempts at resuscitation are hampered by Morgan's lack of familiarity with the resuscitation procedures and general clumsiness. Fred Witcomb is declared dead. A provisional diagnosis is made of a heart attack, perhaps brought on by the stress of the situation.[6] However, the diagnosis has to remain provisional, because no one wants to have a post-mortem performed when he may have been incubating smallpox.

That afternoon, Janet is given six units of *purified protein fraction*, a sterile solution of proteins prepared from pooled human plasma, interspersed with a diuretic to make sure she doesn't become overloaded with fluids. She perks up a bit. Her husband Joseph is offered the opportunity to visit her, but turns down the offer, saying it would only alarm her. He makes it clear that he doesn't want Janet to know what has happened to her father.

The next day, Wednesday 6 September, Janet's breathing is easier, but she now has diarrhoea. The vision in her right eye is still bad, but her ankle swelling has improved somewhat. Her bladder is full and has to be relieved by passing a catheter. Later in the day, she falls out of bed while trying to disconnect her drip. The anaemia is getting worse and Dr Symmons considers the possibility of a blood transfusion.

On Thursday 7 September, Janet has perked up again after a good night's sleep. Her lungs are working well. She has a urinary catheter in place and is passing large amounts of urine. She is having a new antiseptic, silver sulfadiazine, applied to the rash on her back, which she finds very soothing. Unfortunately, she is now completely blind in her right eye and the left eye is gunked up with secretions from her sores. She is given a transfusion of two units of blood, carefully warmed to avoid the cold agglutinin antibodies clumping in her bloodstream.

The next three days see new arrivals at the Catherine-de-Barnes Hospital, each of whom goes into a separate bungalow.[7] Cheryl Hall is a 23-year-old virology technician at East Birmingham Hospital, who handled samples from Janet Parker and has developed a rash; she is discharged five days later. Next comes Janet's 70-year-old mother, Hilda Witcomb, who is admitted with a rash that is thought, at first, to be vaccine-related. Ann Whale is a 30-year-old ambulance driver, who took Janet Parker from East Birmingham to the hospital and now has a rash. She is discharged three days later.

46

NINE ELEVEN

JANET PARKER BEGINS her third week in hospital on Friday 8 September, having been unwell for four weeks. She starts the day confused and paradoxically seems weaker following the blood transfusion. Her face is painful and sticky, oozing pus. Her limbs are stiffening up and painful. Her hands are now starting to swell up like her feet.

She gets worse as the day progresses, appearing to give up the struggle to stay alive. That evening, she is seen by Dr John Innes, a consultant physician at the East Birmingham Hospital, who suspects that Janet's copious urine production is evidence that she is suffering from acute renal failure.

Janet's condition worsens over the weekend. She appears depressed and keeps repeating the phrase 'shame, shame'. Her face looks terrible—a caked mass of congealed scabs. She is now completely blind. Her pulse is fast and weak. She has developed another bout of pneumonia and the pattern of her breathing becomes shallower with disconcerting pauses between breaths. She stops responding to questions.

Dr Symmons has a word with Joseph Parker, pointing out that they are running out of treatment options. At Sunday lunchtime, a nasogastric tube is passed into Janet's stomach in the hope that it can be used to administer nourishing fluids. She is now delirious, making involuntary picking or grasping movements with both arms. That evening, there is some improvement in air entry into her lungs, but she is making only poor respiratory movements. She has passed three litres of urine that day.

At 3.50am on 11 September 1978, Dr Symmons is called to see Janet Parker for the last time. She finds her patient pulseless and not breathing. Janet has fixed and dilated pupils. Dr Symmons declares her dead. A vicious virus has killed for the last time. The ward sister informs Joseph Parker as well as Janet's brother by phone.

The next day, the West Midlands Coroner Dr John Brown holds a brief inquest into Janet's death behind closed doors at the Catherine-de-Barnes Hospital.[1] Dr Brown and Professor Morgan inspect Janet's body in the hospital mortuary. Morgan confirms her identity. They shower before and after the viewing. The Coroner rules out a post-mortem on grounds of safety and signs a cremation certificate.

Fred Witcomb is cremated on 14 September and Janet Parker's funeral is set to take place the following day four miles away from the hospital at the Robin Hood Crematorium in Solihull.[2] Undertaker Ron Fleet is shocked when he arrives at the Catherine-de-Barnes Hospital to find Janet Parker's pox-ridden body on the floor of a garage, away from the main hospital building, packed in disinfectant-soaked sawdust and wrapped in a transparent body bag.[3] Working on his own, with no one at the hospital keen to help, he is forced to manhandle the body into his van, terrified that the bag might split. En route to the funeral, the undertaker's cars are given an escort by unmarked police vehicles in case there is an accident. All other funerals were cancelled that day, as smallpox's last victim is cremated. Afterwards the crematorium is thoroughly cleaned.

Back at the hospital, Deborah Symmons is given the task of disposing of all of the hospital's unused morphine by smashing vials on the 'dirty side', while a local policeman watches from the safety of the 'clean side'. With Janet Parker dead, Deborah Symmons assumes she will now be given the all clear to go home.

However, plans change, when Deborah admits to having a single troublesome spot on her shoulder. She is fairly sure it is just acne, but she thinks she had better mention it anyway. Hugh Morgan diligently aspirates material from the spot, which is sent off for testing at the Central Public Health Laboratory in London. Only after a vexatious forty-eight hour wait—still holed up in Catherine-de-Barnes—is Symmons finally declared free of infection.

As she walks out of the hospital, a friend and fellow medic picks her up and drives her back to her flat in Birmingham. Dr Symmons arrives home to a pleasant surprise—her bosses have arranged for someone to cover her work in her absence, so she is granted ten days off work before returning to her usual job.

For the remaining four months of Deborah's infectious diseases house job, nobody mentions smallpox or makes the slightest fuss about the extraordinary experience that she and her colleagues have just lived through.

JANET PARKER WAS NOT the last case of smallpox. That unfortunate honour goes instead to her mother, who acquired the infection from Janet Parker sometime in mid-late August. Hilda is vaccinated and given anti-vaccinial antibodies on 24 August and is given the anti-viral drug methisazone a day later.[4] Fluid from one of Hilda's blisters is examined by Dr M. Pereira, at the Public Health Laboratory in London, who confirms the diagnosis by isolating smallpox virus.[5] Hilda Witcomb's illness runs a mild course and she is discharged free from infection on 22 September, having missed the funerals of her husband and daughter.[6]

Smallpox has made its last stand in Birmingham and, unlike the last time it visited the city in 1966, it has been snuffed out after infecting just two individuals (maybe three if Fred Witcomb was also infected). But, as life returns to normal in Birmingham in the autumn of 1978, two persistent questions still hang in the balance: how has Janet Parker caught smallpox and who was to blame for this unhappy incident?

Part Five

The Investigation

47

A POX IN THE DUCTS

Vituperation: the act of vituperating; severely blaming or censuring; criticism or invective which is sustained and considered to be overly harsh; abuse, severe blame or censure.

THE UNITED KINGDOM is an unbalanced sort of place, with most of the wealth and influence concentrated in the southeast of England and particularly in London. This lack of balance is reinforced by the use of the language: the counties surrounding London are termed the Home Counties, while the rest of the country can be dismissed as merely 'provincial'.

It is thus no surprise that, when smallpox presented a problem in Birmingham, the UK's London-centred political establishment was not going to trust a bunch of 'provincial' medical academics, such as Christie and McCarthy from Liverpool or Geddes and Lowbury from Birmingham, even if some of them had direct experience of smallpox or of variola virus. No—instead the establishment's answer was to send up a crack team of investigators from London, drawn from the great and the good of the medical establishment.

David Ennals, Secretary of State for Social Services, had no appetite for an expensive QC-led formal Public Inquiry so soon after the Cox Report on the 1973 smallpox outbreak. So, he settled for a compromise, setting up an informal inquiry, held without input from a lawyer and behind closed doors, away from public or professional scrutiny.

The man that Ennals chose for the job was an establishment figure: 62-year-old Professor Reginald 'Reggie' Shooter.[1] He was the son of a Methodist preacher, educated at a private boarding school, at Gonville and Caius College, Cambridge and at St Bartholomew's Hospital ('Barts') Medical School, London. Shooter was a bacteriologist, with an interest in hospital infection and, since 1972, he had been Dean at Barts—a prestigious hospital dating back to 1123. As further evidence of his apparently impeccable credentials, he had given advice, albeit fleetingly, to the London School of Hygiene in 1973 on how to deal with their smallpox incident.[2] Plus, he was chair of the Dangerous Pathogens Advisory Group (DPAG), which had been formed in the wake of the Cox report.

On 30 August 1978, while Henry Bedson and Janet Parker were still alive, David Ennals asked Reggie Shooter to lead an investigation into the 'occurrence' of smallpox in Birmingham. Reggie faced a few days of turf warfare, with twenty-five different bodies clamouring for representation on the investigation.[3] He soon saw off these distractions and settled on a team of five mostly establishment figures, all of them men, to serve as members of his investigation team.[4]

Probably the loudest of the bunch was left-leaning 54-year-old Yorkshireman and gastroenterologist, Chris Booth.[5] With an Iraqi wife ten years his junior[6], a reputation of being both charming and outspoken, he fancied himself as an anti-establishment figure. Booth had risen up the ranks to become director of the Clinical Research Centre at Northwick Park Hospital in north London and was, for that year, president of the British Society of Gastroenterology. Along with Chris, came his deputy at Northwick Park, the 53-year-old virologist David Tyrrell, who had worked at the UK's Common Cold Unit from 1957-1967.

The third man on the team, 69-year-old retired bacteriologist Sir David Evans, was another establishment figure: he had become a Fellow of the Royal Society in 1960 and had been knighted the year before. Although Evans was now based at the Dunn School of Pathology in Oxford, he had until recently served as Director of the UK's National Institute for Biological Standards and Control.

The fourth member was another knight of the realm: 62-year-old bacteriologist Sir Robert Williams, who was director of the Public Health Laboratory Service and President of the Royal College of Pathologists. Perhaps to add a common touch to such a distinguished crew, the fifth of Shooter's companions was Mr J. R. McDonald, a senior technical officer from the Central Public Health Laboratory in Colindale, London.

Two secretaries served the team: the DHSS man Dr Desmond Robinson (who, as we have seen, was also busy issuing instructions to Owen Wade), along with a Mr Owen Thorpe. The World Health Organization sent Joel Breman, a veteran of the eradication campaign, to act as an observer, but he was able to attend only the first three meetings. The HSE was represented by Mr E. J. Morris, while the Trades Union Congress was represented by a specialist in occupational medicine, Dr E. Owen.

Remarkably, there was no representative from the British Medical Association, the Association of University Teachers or the

University of Birmingham, and none of the UK's smallpox experts were invited on to the team. Also, unlike the 1973 inquiry led by the barrister Philip Cox, Shooter's witnesses were not interviewed under oath, nor represented by their own lawyers.

The Shooter committee held eight formal meetings between 30 August and 21 December 1978 and between these meetings, Shooter and his colleagues made multiple visits to the Medical School in Birmingham.

SHOOTER'S TEAM, FEELING the full force of union anger and public anxiety, clearly saw it as their job not just to fix the *problem* of how Janet Parker acquired her infection, but also to fix the *blame*, at every level, for what had happened. The narrative description of their self-styled 'Scientific Investigation' occupies a mere 38 pages of their report: the rest of the report's 215 pages are taken up with 'Lessons to be Learned', followed by numerous appendices. Shooter and his men engaged in a furious bout of vituperation, variously pointing the finger at DPAG, the WHO and the University of Birmingham.

Let's start by considering the so-called 'scientific investigation'. Shooter and his fellow investigators did not start their work in a vacuum. They commandeered the report from Christie's committee, while also reproducing verbatim an account of Janet Parker's illness drafted by Alasdair Geddes (without, he tells me, ever seeking his permission). They had a copy of the Cox report to hand and faithfully reproduced its look-and-feel by laboriously describing the built environment of the pox lab and its environs, documenting their findings through copious figures and photographs.

Given that there had been no smallpox anywhere in the world for nearly a year and none in the UK for over five years, they felt safe in concluding that Parker's infection had somehow originated in the pox lab in Birmingham. However, quite how it had reached Janet Parker remained uncertain.

Going over ground already covered by Christie, they considered five potential sources of Parker's infection:

- Option 1: from the pox lab, through the air or from inanimate objects or by direct human contact.
- Option 2: from someone else infected with smallpox.
- Option 3: from the Medical School's primate colony.
- Option 4: from smallpox virus surviving since 1966.
- Option 5: from variola virus deliberately or accidentally removed from the lab.

Option 4 was dismissed early on, when they re-established that Parker was infected with a strain of the *variola major* virus, whereas the 1966 outbreak was caused by a strain of *variola minor*. Scrutiny of laboratory records and a comparison of viral strains isolated from Janet Parker and her mother with other strains of variola virus established that Parker was almost certainly infected by a strain isolated in 1970 from two Pakistani patients—a 3-year-old boy called Abid and an 18-year-old man called Taj—and handled in the Birmingham pox lab in the July of that year, i.e. just at the time when Janet Parker becomes infected.

Option 2—a missed human case—was dismissed after questioning twenty-eight members of the microbiology staff and ascertaining that none had experienced a flu-like illness during July. Blood tests for antibodies indicative of a recent smallpox infection were performed on ninety members of staff from the Departments of Anatomy and Medical Microbiology and all but four were considered to be normal. On interview, it was established that all of the four that tested positive had been vaccinated recently, which accounted for the raised antibody level, and none of the four had had any contact with the pox lab.

Option 3—an infected monkey—could be dismissed as Parker had had nothing to do with the primate colony for the two-to-three months before her illness. In addition, as we have seen, blood tests for antibodies to smallpox were negative on all but one of the two hundred animals, while the one positive animal had been at the Medical School for three years and had remained healthy throughout that time.

Option 5—deliberate or accidental removal of virus from the lab—presented more of a problem. Through investigation of custom and practice in the pox lab, Shooter's team established that smallpox virus stocks were handled exclusively in a small, inner 'smallpox room' EG34a, but stored in a freezer in a larger, outer 'animal pox room' EG34. As the containers were not disinfected on leaving the smallpox room, any smallpox virus left on the outside might be inadvertently transferred to containers housing other viruses, which could then be taken out of the pox lab entirely. Perhaps more worrying was the risk that someone might take the wrong container out of the freezer and so unwittingly remove variola virus from the pox lab and work on it in another part of the Medical School. However, in the absence of any evidence that a gross breach of biosecurity had actually taken place, the committee seemed happy to dismiss this option.[7]

THE POX LAB AND OTHER ROOMS

Air ducts A, B, C and D are shown in grey

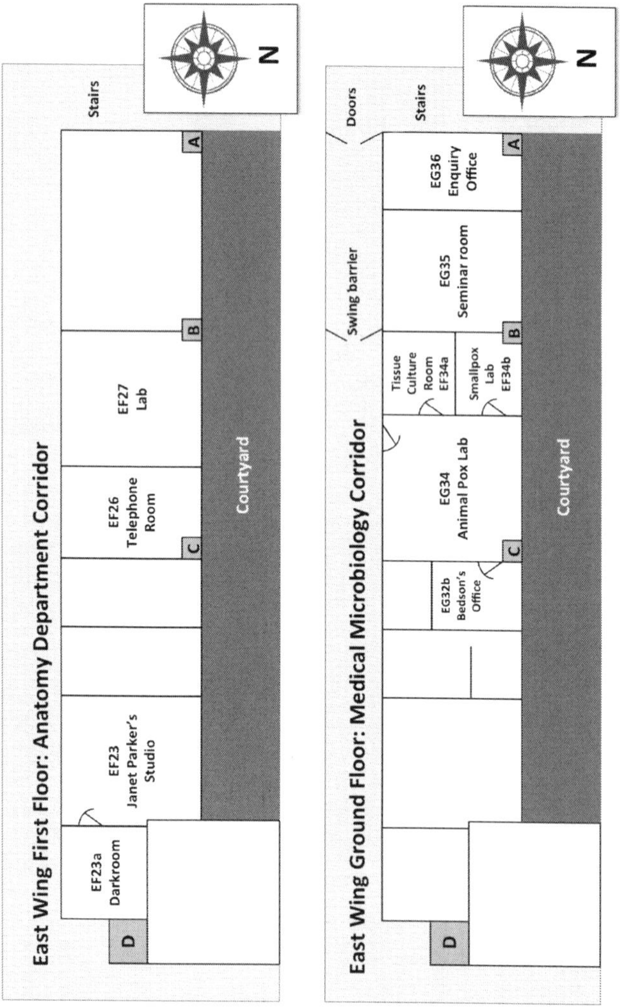

AND SO, HAVING apparently dismissed all the other options, Shooter and his associates focused on how variola virus escaped from the smallpox room, EG34b, the only place where live variola virus had been handled. At 8-feet-square, the room was scarcely big enough to swing the proverbial cat. Nonetheless, EG34b was large enough to house a bench bearing a biological safety cabinet and a foot-operated sink, plus a floor-mounted centrifuge and a portable autoclave. Under the bench there was a loosely sealed plywood-covered inspection panel leading to a service duct (termed 'Duct B' in the report), which ran vertically through the building. The inquisitors commissioned tests on the safety cabinet and its air filter—and found no faults. Similarly, the autoclave passed muster when tested and the centrifuge proved incapable of creating an aerosol.

However, they soon identified lapses in what they considered to be acceptable practice. It appeared that discarded pipettes were not always fully immersed in disinfectant after use. Culture supernatant potentially laden with smallpox virus was stored in a refrigerator in the animal pox room. Containers of smallpox virus were transferred between the smallpox room and the animal pox room without being placed in sealed containers. Staff moved between the two rooms without washing their hands or removing or disinfecting the gloves or special rear-fastening gowns that they wore.

Bearing all this in mind, Shooter's team concluded that smallpox virus might have contaminated the air or work surfaces within the animal pox room. They ram the point home in value-laden language at the end of Chapter 4 in their report: 'The intention of the laboratory's safety measures was the containment of smallpox virus within the smallpox room itself. The result of the *unsatisfactory* procedures taking place was that the animal pox room could become *heavily contaminated*. This represented a *major breach* in containment policy' (my italics).

There was one practice in the smallpox room that upset them more than anything else. Most work on the smallpox virus was carried out in the biological safety cabinet, which sucked air in and away from the handler and ensured that exhaust air was filtered as it left the cabinet. But, when virus particles were harvested from tissue cultures, infected culture medium was sucked out of open Petri dishes on the bench outside of the cabinet using a rubber tube connected to a water pump. The aspirated fluid was sucked into two flasks containing a strong disinfectant, formalin, which would have killed any virus.

However, the committee was concerned that this practice meant that fluid containing the virus could be spilt on the bench or could generate an infectious aerosol during the process of aspiration. Curiously, given the significance they later attached to this process, in paragraph 62 of their report, they qualify their accusation by stating that it is only an opinion: '*In our opinion*, the use of the aspirator outside the safety hood to remove culture fluid from Petri dishes was a dangerous practice.'

Next, the committee homed in on how the virus could have got from the pox lab to Janet Parker, focusing on three potential routes: through the air, by personal contact or by contact with equipment. The movement of air in and around the building was something that they could investigate through hands-on experimentation.

The DHSS man Des Robinson carried out some fairly basic smoke tests in the smallpox room, establishing that, when the adjoining door was open, air could move from the smaller smallpox room EG34b to the larger animal pox room EG34. However, the committee chiefly relied on a report from Dr Owen Lidwell, a former associate of David Tyrell and an expert on aerobiology and infection at the Medical Research Council's Air Hygiene Unit.

Lidwell started off by surveying the pox lab and its environs. He noted that there were four vertical service ducts that ran through the lower ground, ground and first floors of the East Wing before venting out to the courtyard through grilles. It was clear that access panels to the ducts, which were found in adjoining rooms, made no pretence at being airtight. His attention focused on three of the ducts: Ducts B, C and D.

Duct B ran on the ground floor through the smallpox room EG34b, but also opened through an access panel into an adjacent seminar room EG35. Duct C ran on the ground floor through the animal pox room EG34 and then, one floor up, through EF26, used largely as a junk room, but equipped with a telephone that could be used to make external calls (hence the nickname 'the telephone room'). Duct D ran alongside the dark room where Janet Parker worked on the first floor.

Lidwell considered four potential airborne routes of dispersal of smallpox virus particles from the pox lab to parts of the building frequented by Janet Parker.

First, infected air could leak out of the lab, into the corridor and then via stairwells be dispersed throughout the building.

Second, it could leak out into the courtyard through the windows in the animal pox room, EG34, or via the safety cabinet in that room, which had been found to be defective. Drawing on the precedent from Meschede, he reasoned that air from the courtyard could enter open windows on the floor above, into the rooms where Janet had worked

Third, air could pass through Duct B and/or Duct C down into a subway at bottom of the building and then into Duct D, to escape into the dark room where Janet Parker worked. However, this seemed highly unlikely given the very high dilution factor and need for particles to travel against the usual upward flow of warm air.

Fourth, air might be sucked into Duct B and/or Duct C through cracks or openings in the access panels and then travel sideways into the adjacent seminar room, EG35, or upwards into the telephone room.

Lidwell and his two assistants decided to concentrate their efforts on investigation routes 3 and 4. On three separate occasions (21 September, 3 October, 4 October), they performed smoke tests with titanium chloride, each time showing that air was drawn into Ducts B and C from both rooms in the pox lab. They also consistently saw smoke travelling from Duct C into the telephone room EF26. They found airflow from Duct B into the seminar room EG35 and occasionally into a lab, EF27, on the floor above.

On their final visit on 4 October, Lidwell and his assistants performed three particle dispersal tests, which allowed them to quantify the extent of transfer via various routes. A spinning disc was used to generate minute particles of potassium iodide (just 7-microns wide), which were collected on filter papers and detected by placing the filters in a 0.1% acid solution of palladium chloride.

Through this approach they established that particles dispersed in the smallpox room EG34b could leak out through an open door into the larger animal pox room EG34, even if the safety cabinet was operational in EG34b. They also found that particles were transferred from EG34b in appreciable numbers into the seminar room EG35 and into the telephone room EF26. A substantial number of particles also leaked from EG34 into the corridor. They found little or no evidence for transfers from Ducts B and C via the subway or from Duct D into the dark room EF23a.

Lidwell attempted to contextualise his findings by calculating the potential dose breathed in at a site after dispersal of a starting population of a billion particles. Within EG34, the dose was as high as 170,000 particles, but fell in the corridor or seminar room to figures in the hundreds or, in one case, just over a thousand. The potential dose received in the telephone room ranged from just one to eighty-two particles, i.e. a dilution factor of 10-million to a billion to one.

ARMED WITH LIDWELL'S REPORT, the committee focused on Janet Parker's movements. The found no evidence that she had ever visited the pox lab. However, they discovered that Parker had, during the relevant time frame, visited a darkroom and an enquiry office, both situated about fifteen feet away along the corridor from the pox lab. However, lots of other people from other parts of the Medical School must have passed through that corridor too, so they wanted to understand why Janet was the only one to get infected.

They put two and two together when they discovered that Janet Parker was the only person to have made frequent use of the 'telephone room', which shared Duct C with the animal pox room. In the run-up to the end of the departmental accounting year on 31 July, she had used the phone several times a day, day in day out, to order photographic materials. And crucially, Janet Parker had placed a remarkably large number of orders on 25 July, just as the Abid strain of smallpox virus was being handled in the smallpox room on the floor below. As Lidwell had shown leakage of particles in his tests from the pox lab into the telephone room, it now all made sense!

In his report, Shooter does at this point make a cryptic reference to 'some experts who have worked with smallpox virus who would doubt whether airborne dissemination of the virus during laboratory work is a credible route for the transfer of infection'. These unnamed experts in fact included Keith Dumbell and Kevin McCarthy, who were given the chance to elaborate on these options in a subsequent court case. Shooter also accepts that there were no proven cases of airborne spread of smallpox from lab cultures. However, like Lidwell, he is impressed by the supposed precedent of airborne spread from one floor to the next in the hospital in Meschede.

Although the 'pox-in-the-ducts' hypothesis became the headline explanation for Janet Parker's illness, Shooter and his team did also consider the possibility that the smallpox virus had been transferred by direct contact between Parker and someone who worked in the pox lab. They discovered that Parker occasionally did private work, chiefly passport photographs, for staff in the Medical School—but not for anyone working in the pox lab.

However, from staff interviews, Shooter's team identified a potential go-between, who was left unnamed in their report, but identified in the subsequent court case as the young virologist Sandy Buchan. Shooter discovered that Buchan often popped into the animal pox lab without wearing a lab coat or washing his hands. In addition, Buchan had at least once, and maybe twice, consulted

Parker in July in her studio and darkroom. Buchan had been regularly vaccinated, so was presumably immune to infection, but might have provided a route for the transfer of virus on his hands or clothes from the lab to the photographer.

It also turned out that two of Parker's coffee mates occasionally visited the pox lab corridor. However, if that meant they were exposed to smallpox virus, how come they as unvaccinated individuals did not also succumb to infection?

The pox-in-the-ducts explanation also made sense in the light of another disturbing incident—the 1966 smallpox outbreak. Shooter and his team dedicate a whole chapter in their report, plus a lengthy appendix, to investigation of the origins of the outbreak that started with Tony McLennan, who had worked, like Janet Parker, as a photographer in the East Wing of Birmingham Medical School. They established that, although McLennan had no recollection of ever visiting EF26 (the telephone room), he had popped into the adjacent room EF27, which in his day was used as a histology lab. In addition, they established that variola minor virus was handled on the open bench in the pox lab eleven days before McLennan fell ill. Thus, it seemed highly tempting to conclude that a similar pox-in-the-ducts mechanism of dispersal accounted for the escape of smallpox in 1966 and 1978.

IN THE SECOND HALF of their report, Shooter and his team attempt to fix the blame, which, in their words, meant examining 'the circumstances in which the bodies most directly concerned, DPAG, WHO and Birmingham University, had failed to ensure that work with the smallpox virus in the Birmingham University was carried out in conditions of complete safety'.

In the wake of the 1973 London outbreak of smallpox, Philip Cox's team published an Interim Code of Practice in June 1974. The following year, Sir George Godber, a former Chief Medical Officer instrumental in the establishment of the National Health Service, set up a working party on dangerous pathogens, which formulated a comprehensive Code of Practice for labs working with the most dangerous pathogens. Godber's team also recommended the establishment of DPAG to advise those responsible for such labs, which held its first meeting in November 1975.

A few months later, in February 1976, a team from the newly formed DPAG inspected Bedson's smallpox lab. In their judgement, the laboratory and its safety practices complied with the Cox's Interim Code of Practice (apart from not offering vaccination to the whole building), but fell short of proposals of the Godber Working

Party in lacking an air-lock, a shower, changing facilities and a double-ended autoclave. Nonetheless, DPAG was happy to exercise its discretionary powers to relax requirements and allow work on smallpox to continue, citing the reasons for its judgement:

'First, Professor Bedson was a very reputable, experienced and safety-conscious virologist. Second, all smallpox work was restricted to a few named members of staff working under Professor Bedson's personal supervision. Third, a highly efficient vaccination programme was in force in the Department. Fourth, the safety procedures in use were very thorough. Finally, the laboratory served in its diagnostic capacity a large and important area in the Midlands.'

With the benefit of hindsight and full of righteous anger, Shooter and his team begged to differ in the strongest possible terms, railing against the 'mistaken use of the Group's discretionary powers' and dedicating an entire appendix to their own point-by-point assessment of the Birmingham pox lab's lack of compliance with DPAG recommendations.

This was backed up by a series of proposals all prefaced in capital letters with 'WE RECOMMEND', ending with the firm opinion that the country's last surviving smallpox lab, at St Mary's Medical School in Paddington, should certainly be moved out of the metropolis and probably closed down entirely—because 'it seems to us that no matter how good the measures of containment may be in laboratories, it is impossible by these means alone to guarantee safety'.

One has to recognise that Shooter was in a very difficult position here, as he was head of DPAG and this had happened on his watch, so he clearly suffered a conflict of interest in passing judgement. One suspects that a desire not to appear to go easy on the advisory group that he led motivated his highly vituperative approach.

Not content with castigating DPAG, Shooter's team also devoted four paragraphs to the DHSS—berating the lack of regular and frequent inspections of labs handling dangerous pathogens—before turning their fury on the WHO, who had funded Bedson's work and had sent inspectors to his lab in May 1978.

The WHO inspection team had expressed reservations about the physical facilities in Bedson's lab, even though they thought immunisation practices seemed very good. The issues they focused on included mouth pipetting, use of gloves and gowns, lack of bleach as a barrier in sinks and use of table-top hot water sterilisers.

Bedson defended himself in a letter dated 2 June, pointing out that mouth pipetting had not been used with smallpox for ten years and that back-fastening gowns were worn in the smallpox room. He confirmed he was happy to comply with suggestions on the use of bleach and of gloves, 'even though one could argue about the extent to which they affect the safety of the work'.

The WHO response was sent out on 1 August, but Bedson received it only after returning from his holiday in Wales in late August. In the letter, Dr Richardson at the WHO expressed continuing concern over the lack of a shower, the lack of secondary containment in the outer lab where smallpox virus stocks were stored and the uncertain maintenance of the biological safety cabinet. He concluded his letter: 'The laboratory falls short of the WHO Standard and should be upgraded to meet the Standard or should discontinue work with variola at the earliest possible date.'

Professor Bedson replied on 24 August—the very day that Janet Parker was admitted to hospital. He said he was not going to be able to upgrade his lab to meet WHO standards and so he was aiming to complete his studies with variola and whitepox viruses by the end of the year.

Shooter's team found fault not just with the WHO's missed opportunity to close Bedson's lab, but with their failure to express their concerns to the DHSS. They also quibbled with a statement in one of Bedson's letters that he was scaling down work in his pox lab.

The final target for Shooter's fury was the University of Birmingham and in particular, Henry Bedson. Here, Shooter and his men homed in on a number of what-they-saw-as shortcomings.

First was the fact that Bedson had a conflict of duties, in being responsible for safety in the whole Department of Medical Microbiology as well for his own lab. Although there were supposedly two Departmental Safety officers, they were often kept out of the loop as Bedson dealt with issues directly. A key example was an incident the year before in which a tray of vaccinia virus samples was dropped in the lab—Bedson knew about this, but nobody bothered to tell the Safety Officers. Shooter's team felt that it was inappropriate for a Head of Department to be a member of a team performing a safety inspection of his own department. They also did not like the fact that Bedson had been dealing with the WHO's concerns about safety without involving anyone higher up in the University hierarchy or communicating details to relevant meetings.

They also grumbled that, as Head of Department, Bedson had been preoccupied with administration and teaching, rather than overseeing work in his own laboratory. They complained that his staff and students had not received adequate training, because they had not been directly trained and supervised by Bedson.

Finally, they attacked the University's vaccination policy, complaining that vaccination against smallpox was offered only to those in the Department of Medical Microbiology rather than all those working in the Medical School.

Shooter and his team concluded their report with a series of general observations. They made it clear that Janet Parker had been infected by a virus from the lab in Birmingham. They claimed that the smallpox virus escaped 'because measures designed to contain it while it was handled were not fully carried out', even though they had established no lapse in good practice that could be blamed for this. Next, they admitted that they did not *know* how, but they *believed* one of two routes to have been most probable: first, airborne spread through the service duct to the telephone room frequented by Janet Parker, or, second, via direct or indirect transfer from someone who had been in or near the pox lab. In their summing up they claimed that 'the facts speak for themselves' but felt the need to express 'deep concern for the failure to follow the agreed safety rules'. They expressed sympathy for the families of Henry Bedson and Janet Parker.

ON 21 DECEMBER 1978, Professor R. A. Shooter sent a cover letter to the Rt Hon. David Ennals MP, accompanied by a copy of his report. With their elegant and persuasive pox-in-the-ducts hypothesis, Shooter and his colleagues had found a way to allay fears and help bring speculation to an end. However, with their damning allocation of blame, which seeped out into the press and into the court of public opinion, they had ensured that the fears expressed to Owen Wade had come true: poor Henry Bedson had been crucified in time for Christmas.

Fortunately, the facts got another chance 'to speak for themselves'—this time in a court of law—but not before some underhand politics.

48

POXY POLITICS

CLIVE JENKINS WAS BORN in 1926 in Port Talbot, a steel-making town in South Wales.[1] Educated at Port Talbot County School, he started work in a local metallurgy lab at the age of 14. As a young man, he joined the Communist Party and threw his energy into union work, leaving Wales in 1946 to move to the Birmingham office of the Association of Supervisory Staff, Executives and Technicians. By 1961, he had become general secretary of the union, which later became ASTMS. Jenkins saw it as his mission 'to organise the middle classes', promoting trade unionism among white-collar workers. He was good at it—by the seventies, when trade unions were at their most powerful in the UK, ASTMS was the fastest-growing union in the country, counting Janet Parker among its members.

During those heady years of union power, Clive 'the mouth' Jenkins cultivated a flamboyant sense of humour, ensuring he stayed in the public eye, with numerous TV appearances and opinionated newspaper columns to his name. A brash and arrogant millionaire, he was the archetype of the champagne socialist, winning a fortune from property deals and from suing his critics for libel.

Relations between ASTMS and the University of Birmingham were never great, but they took a nose-dive a month after Janet Parker's death, when Jenkins had issued a press statement suggesting that Parker had died not from smallpox, but from some illegally produced genetically modified virus, created in Bedson's lab.[2]

In early December 1978, the HSE informed Owen Wade and his colleagues at the University of Birmingham that they were going to take the University to court under the *Health and Safety at Work Act* of 1974 for not providing safe working conditions for its employees.[3] The first hearing was due to take place early the following year. As a result, the University asked David Ennals to treat the matter as *sub judice* and to withhold publication of the Shooter Report until after the court case. Ennals agreed not to publish, but nonetheless sent copies of the report to the University and to Clive Jenkins. Alongside the copy sent to Jenkins was a letter from Ennals' private secretary saying that it was a 'pre-publication' copy and explaining that the report could not be published before the court case against the University, for fear that it might prejudice the case.

On 4 January 1979, Jenkins handed out photocopies of the report at a press conference, proclaiming 'Publish and be blessed. It must not be hushed up'. He claimed that his copy was not marked as 'confidential' and that Ennals must have known he was going to leak it. Jenkins backed up his decision with the outlandish claim that smallpox had been smouldering in Birmingham for 12 years and that 'lots of people had had it without their doctors realising'.[4] Behind the scenes, Jenkins had been colluding with the Anglia Television Company to produce an exposé on the report until the company's chief executive, Lord Lew Grade, vetoed the plan.

CONFRONTED WITH THE REPORT, Wade and others at the University reacted with horror at what they saw as factual errors and the elevation of hearsay to factual evidence. They were dismayed to see the document co-signed by Dr Owen from the TUC and Mr Morris from the HSE, when these individuals had started out as mere observers. If they had been allowed into the inquiry, why not also representatives of the University or of the doctor's union, the British Medical Association?

Over the next few days, the general news media—and even some scientific journals—fed furiously off the Shooter Report, shredding the reputation of the Henry Bedson and the University of Birmingham. *The Daily Express* carried the headline 'UNSAFE! But the work still went on—until infection killed a woman'.[5] In *New Scientist*, Lawrence McGinty claimed that 'Bedson misled the University, WHO and the DHSS', 'lied about the scale of his work' and 'clearly breached the trust placed in him'.[6]

Such coverage was in no way conducive to a fair trial. As a result, the University asked for the court case to be delayed. On 22 January, the University's barrister, Brian Escott-Cox QC, made a successful application to the Queen's Bench Divisional Court in London for permission to seek a High Court order preventing Birmingham magistrates from hearing the summons brought against the University by the HSE.[6]

On 24 January, Ennals made a statement in the House of Commons making it clear that official publication of the Shooter Report was going to be held up by the prosecution of the University and that, although copies of the report had been sent to interested parties, no permission to publish was expressed or implied. He confirmed that the Government accepted the substance of Shooter's report and clarified that no further work on smallpox was underway in Birmingham or London.

Ennals' opposite number on the opposition benches, the MP for Wanstead and Woodford, Patrick Jenkin, took the opportunity to challenge the Secretary of State, arguing that the Ennals had been expressly and positively told by Clive Jenkins that if he got the report he would publish it, implying that Ennals was disingenuous in pretending that he was withholding publication. In response, Ennals claimed that he had followed the legal advice he had been given, but that Clive Jenkins had been offered a different opinion by his legal advisors.[7]

Despite the media frenzy, with the court case looming, Owen Wade and Bedson's colleagues felt that they should say nothing in response to the leaked report. The media furore soon died down—and, besides, their day in court would come.

49

PERSONAL INTERLUDE

INFORMATION WANTS TO BE FREE

In my early efforts to find out what really happened in 1978, I tracked down a copy of Owen Wade's autobiography in the Medical School library and was surprised to learn that the Shooter Report was not the last word on the topic and that the University had won the subsequent court case. In his book, Wade states that he had placed a copy of the transcript from the court case within the University archives. By early 2012, I had tracked down the University's Cadbury Research Library Special Collections to a basement in the recently renovated Muirhead Tower.

My pulse raced as I was given a cardboard box containing typewritten and handwritten notes from Owen Wade and his wife dating back to the smallpox incident. Borrowing material was out of the question and they made photocopying difficult, so I hastily took photos on my mobile phone.

On my second or third visit to the library, just before I left my old job in Birmingham for a new job in Warwick, someone offered me a copy of the transcript of the trial. At over five hundred pages, it was clear that I was not going to be able to photograph the entire transcript on my mobile phone.

In May 2013, a few months after starting work in Warwick, I sent the Special Collections staff in Birmingham an email asking how much it would cost for me to obtain a photocopy of the transcript and how I might get permission to release all or some of it into the public domain. The second of my two questions set the issue bouncing up to Sue Worrall, Director of the Special Collections, and across to the University's legal team and the National Archive. A fraught few weeks followed, as I attempted just to get hold of a copy of the transcript and to backpedal on the matter of the public release. Eventually, I managed to meet Sue Worrall face to face, who rather awkwardly claimed that I could no longer have access to the transcript—even to look at, let alone copy—as it was uncertain whether the University had the necessary legal permission to hold a copy. I started to wonder whether the University had decided it did not like me dredging up old news.

Back in Warwick, I had a chat with a new colleague, Roberta Bivins, who headed up the local History of Medicine centre. She too had an interest in the history of smallpox and was keen to help. She pointed out that the most effective way to get hold of a copy of the transcript would be to issue a freedom of information request, which the University of Birmingham would have to respond to within six weeks. So, I sent off a quick email, invoking the Freedom of Information Act. A few weeks later, I was sent a photocopy of the transcript without any charge—the information was now free, in both senses of the word!

PART SIX

THE TRIAL

50

CASE FOR THE PROSECUTION

SIR ASTON WEBB WAS the preeminent English architect of the late nineteenth and early twentieth century.[1] His remarkable portfolio includes many of the landmarks of modern Britain, from the façade of Buckingham Palace to the Victoria and Albert Museum, from Admiralty Arch to the Victoria Memorial. He also undertook a sympathetic modernisation of many older buildings, including the medieval St Bartholomew-the-Great in Smithfield, London (featured in the film *Four Weddings and a Funeral*) and King's College, Cambridge. In partnership with fellow architect Ingress Bell, Aston Webb left his mark in Birmingham on two buildings: the original redbrick building of the University of Birmingham (now called the Aston Webb building) and the Victoria Law Courts[2], in Corporation Street, at the heart of Birmingham's legal quarter.

This imposing court building, built from red brick with a green stone-tiled roof, provides an exceptional setting for an exceptional trial. The outside of the building carries a luxuriant façade of deep red terracotta, fashioned from the clay of Raubon in North Wales, which contrasts rudely with the sandy-yellow terracotta that covers the interior. Everywhere, inside and out, the terracotta is decorated with intricate ornamentation. An imposing statue of Queen Victoria guards the main entrance.

The trial of *Robert Kenyon Cook versus the University of Birmingham* opened here in October 1979—not in one of the grand Victorian courtrooms, but in a more modest room in a section of the building rebuilt after bomb damage from the Second World War.[3] Nonetheless, the courtroom was well set-out and decently-sized, at around 30 metres by 35 metres.

Like all English trials, this was to be an adversarial contest, in contrast to the inquisitorial style of continental Europe. A battle was to take place between two opponents: *the Prosecution*, seeking to prove its case beyond reasonable doubt and obtain a guilty verdict, and *the Defence*, which seeks to contest the Prosecution's case, to create reasonable doubt and obtain a 'Not Guilty' verdict. The burden of proof rests with the Prosecution, with a presumption of the Defendant's innocence until proven guilty. Getting at the truth is a by-product of the zero-sum game between the two parties to the trial—when one side wins, the other loses.

Like the majority of criminal trials in England, the case against the University was heard not by a judge and jury, but by three lay magistrates (also known as *justices of the peace*). Such individuals are unpaid volunteers, typically with no formal legal qualifications but who are required to act fairly and with intelligence, common sense and integrity. Sitting in judgement on the case brought against the University of Birmingham were Justices Mr James Ernest Bailey (sitting as chairman), Mrs Shelagh Allen and Mrs Cynthia Barbara Zissman (wife of local tailor, businessman and aspiring politician Bernard Zissman and sister-in-law of an eminent Birmingham solicitor, Maurice Putsman).

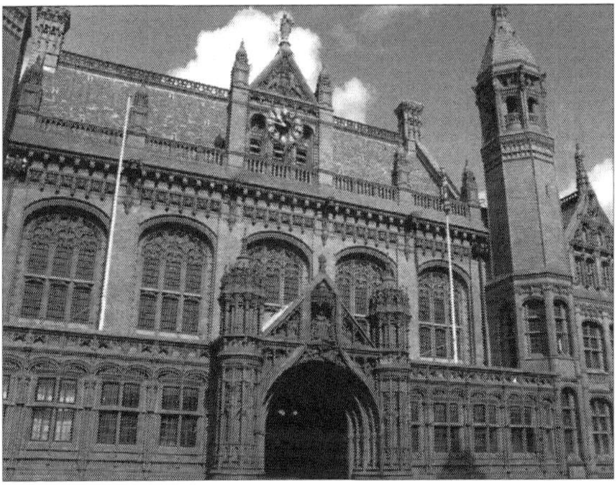

THE VICTORIA LAW COURTS
Site of the 1979 trial
{Source: https://commons.wikimedia.org CC BY 2.0 }

PROCEEDINGS BEGAN AT ten o'clock on Monday 22 October 1979. The magistrates entered at one end of the courtroom to sit high above the rest of the court. Ahead of them and slightly below them, sat the Clerk of the Court, a qualified solicitor there to administer oaths and advise the magistrates on points of law. The barristers sat in a row at ground level facing the magistrates. For this court, they were dressed in lounge suits, rather than wigs and gowns. Behind them sat their instructing solicitors and assistants, accompanied by a mountain of paperwork. From the barristers' perspective, the magistrates were in front and the witness stand was away to the left. However, most of their audience was behind them, in a space for the general public that held thirty or forty people, mostly journalists, taking turns to cover the trial, together with some of the witnesses.

The clerk of the court introduced the Prosecution, the Defendants and their respective teams. The case against the University was brought by Robert Kenyon Cook, one of Her Majesty's Inspectors appointed under the *Health and Safety at Work Act* of 1974.

It was clear at the outset that the legal teams were not evenly matched as the University and their solicitors had elected to pay for a QC (an accomplished senior barrister), while the Health and Safety Executive had taken the cheaper option of instructing a junior barrister. The HSE had initially briefed an outstanding junior barrister, Igor Judge (who went on to become Lord Chief Justice), but Judge—along with his senior colleague Philip Cox QC (of the Cox report)—was tied up in a high-profile trial of four men for the murder of 13-year-old paperboy, Carl Bridgewater. Instead, appearing on behalf of Mr Cook and the HSE was 41-year-old barrister Colin Colston, slightly built, but always well turned out; a quiet, devoted Anglican with an Austrian wife; educated at Rugby, the Gunnery (a private school in Connecticut) and Trinity Hall, Cambridge.[4]

The Birmingham firm of Johnson and Co. acted as the University's solicitors and were represented in this case by their senior partner, Adrian Davis, a diminutive, cultured, astute, hard-working Welshman, who selected two barristers to act for the Defence.

The Defence's main man was 46-year-old Brian Escott-Cox, an eloquent, flamboyant barrister, educated at Rugby and Oriel College Oxford, a QC for four years and a skilful jazz trumpeter with a GSOH.[5] Although he started out with almost no knowledge of smallpox, he had encountered Janet Parker through her appearances in court as a police photographer a few years earlier, which, for him, accentuated the tragedy of her death.

Assisting Escott-Cox was his ambitious junior and former pupil, 29-year-old Colman Maurice Treacy[6], son of an Irish doctor, educated at a Jesuit boarding school and Jesus College, Cambridge and called to the bar in 1971. With his family background, Treacy brought a medical perspective to the Defence team. There was a great rapport between the two Defence barristers, with a shared sense of humour—although how far the younger man minded being called 'Miss Tracey Colman' by his senior remains an open question!

Relations were civil but less cordial between Escott-Cox and Colston. Mindful of the Shakespearean injection that lawyers should 'Strive mightily but eat and drink as friends', Escott-Cox invited Colston home a couple of nights during the trial, but found they had little in common.

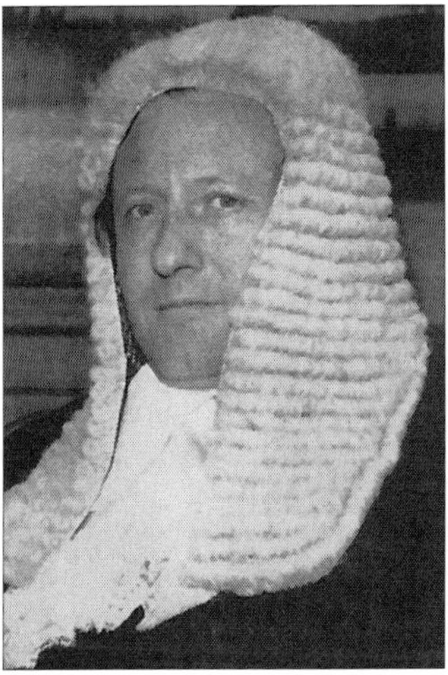

BRIAN ESCOTT-COX QC

Barrister representing the University of Birmingham.
In the trial, he wore a lounge suit rather than a wig and gown
{Source: B. Escott-Cox}

IN THE CHAPTERS THAT follow, the reader is presented with an account of the trial, in which several hundred pages of transcript have been boiled down to just a few dozen. For the first time, what went on in court is being released in full to the public so that posterity can make an informed judgement. However, among all the testimony and arguments presented, the devil is very much in the detail and, inevitably, there are some dead-ends and some repetition. I hope most readers will stay gripped by the narrative, but those less patient can skip forward to the chapter entitled 'Summing up'.

The information against the University—the formal accusation read out in court—was that as an employer, they had contravened the Health and Safety at Work Act, in that they had not 'so far as it is reasonably practicable' ensured the health and safety and welfare at work of their employees in the East Wing of the Birmingham Medical School. In particular, they did not maintain equipment or the working environment or the East Wing as safe and without risk to health and without risk of smallpox infection.

Colston began by asserting that, given the inevitable need for technical discussion about how labs are run, it was preferable for the trial to proceed before the magistrates rather than before a judge and jury. Escott-Cox agreed, citing the 'very great amount of public hostile criticism from different quarters, much of it biased, ill-informed and I am sorry to say politically motivated' and pointing out that derogatory remarks had been made on the radio and in the press in the previous week. It was thus agreed that the trial should be held before magistrates.

Next, Escott-Cox entered a plea of 'Not Guilty' on behalf of the University and the chairman laid out a timetable for the court: a morning session from 10am to 12.45pm and an afternoon session from 2pm to 4pm each day for the length of the case.

COLIN COLSTON PRESENTED HIS opening statement on behalf of the Prosecution, assisted by a bundle of papers presented to the magistrates. After a brief description of smallpox, Colston proceeded to spend most of the day reading out to the court relevant sections of the Cox Report and the associated Interim Code of Practice from 1974, the Godber Report from 1975, the University's own guidance on handling of smallpox viruses, the DPAG inspection report and associated handbook and the WHO inspection report and associated correspondence.

Such documents are dry enough when sped-read silently. To have to listen to them turned into a four-hour-long monologue must have amounted to a slow death by boredom! Colston closed the first day's proceedings with a laborious run-through of the physical environment of the pox lab, requiring no fewer than sixteen photos, together with an enumeration of the personnel attached to the lab and a brief description of Janet Parker's working environment.

New Scientist journalist Lawrence McGinty reported that a barrister he knew was already betting against the HSE by the end of Day One, after Colston had 'bored the pants off the magistrates' with his opening statement.

COLSTON OPENED DAY TWO with a rambling description of laboratory practice in the pox lab. Then, around half an hour into the day's proceedings, the barrister stated that he was going to present in summary form some, but not all, of the criticisms of lab practice relevant to the Prosecution's case. At this point he was challenged by Escott-Cox, who asked that the Prosecution make clear *all* their criticisms before witnesses were called—and cracked the first joke of the case: 'I do not want him to keep something up his sleeve, whether or not he is wearing safety garments'.

Colston made clear that his criticisms of lab technique focused on the movement of staff between the inner smallpox room and the outer animal pox room for various purposes—to use an incubator, a fridge, a freezer and a centrifuge—and the fact that they did this without changing gowns or gloves. He also criticised the movement of live smallpox virus between the two rooms other than in a sealed container and the fact that some work was done on live smallpox virus in the inner room on the open bench rather than in a safety cabinet—in particular, the aspiration of fluid from infected tissue culture dishes using a vacuum pump. The Prosecution also claimed that the positioning of discarded equipment next to the service duct, named Duct B in the Shooter Report, was unsatisfactory.

Colston then tried to change the subject—but in response, Escott-Cox again waded in with the objection that all the criticisms should be outlined at the outset. Colston claimed the purpose of the opening speech was not to rehearse every aspect of the evidence, because if they did that, 'instead of having to listen to the monotony of my voice for a day and a bit, we would be here for a week'! The chairman backed Colston's position.

Colston's outline of the Prosecution's case continued: a strain of the smallpox virus named Abid had somehow escaped from the lab to infect Janet Parker; the windows in the outer lab could not be closed completely; and the safety cabinet in that lab did not work properly.

Colston reported that smoke tests showed that airborne particles could under certain circumstances escape from the labs and enter the corridor outside; enter Duct B and from there escape into the adjacent seminar room; and enter Duct C and travel upwards to telephone room EF26. Now, despite his earlier dull ramblings, Colston at last commanded the court's full attention, as he backed up these claims with vivid photos showing smoke billowing into and out of the ducts. Even the Defence QC could see that the photographic evidence presented was, in his own words, 'hot stuff'.

Colston alleged that the University must have foreseen the danger of airborne spread of smallpox, otherwise why would they have insisted that people working nearby, but not actually in the pox lab, were offered vaccination against smallpox.

Colston made clear that the *Health and Safety at Work Act* set out various duties and that the Prosecution did not have to establish that the University of Birmingham had failed under every possible category: failure under a single heading, say of equipment or working environment, would suffice. He started to explain the meaning of *reasonable practicability*, but Escott-Cox made clear the Defence was not going to reply on that concept.

Attention briefly focused on the first witness, Robert Kenyon Cook, who confirmed that he lived nearby in Dorridge, worked at the HSE headquarters in Birmingham and had served a prohibition notice to the University on 30 August 1978, prohibiting further work on smallpox. He then withdrew from the stand.

51

BEDSON'S STUDENT

MID-MORNING ON DAY TWO, at the Prosecution's request, Dr Linda Harper, Bedson's former PhD student, was sworn in and took the stand. She confirmed that she had started work in the Department of Medical Microbiology at the Medical School in 1974 and had worked under Bedson's supervision for more than two years. Colston questioned Dr Harper on her working habits and those of Professor Bedson. Harper made it clear that the professor visited his lab every day, scrutinising lab notebooks and discussing results of experiments. She explained that although Bedson did not have hands on experience of all the techniques they were using, he provided criticism that she always found helpful. She confirmed that two other women—Mrs Jennifer Durham and a research assistant Mrs Bate—carried out research in the pox lab and that Dr Gordon Skinner came into the lab about once a week to access the stock of vaccine or to perform diagnostic work.

Colston then grilled Dr Harper from mid-morning to mid-afternoon on the details of every experimental procedure she undertook in the pox lab: inoculation and harvesting of virus from eggs and from cell culture; how she worked out how much infectious virus was present in a sample; disposal of infected cell culture medium in formalin; the toing and froing between the two labs; the use of gowns and gloves; the recently adopted technique called *electrophoresis* as an approach to fingerprinting viruses. Linda Harper confirmed that the outer door was always locked when work on smallpox was underway, but that the door between the two rooms in the pox lab was left ajar when material was in transit between the two settings. They established that the process of aspiration of the potentially infected culture medium took place a couple of times a week and was performed on the open bench in the smallpox lab, EG34b.

In the last hour of Day Two, Colston questioned the witness on what instructions she had received with regard to safety. Dr Harper remembered discussing the lab's set of safety rules with Professor Bedson and Mrs Jennifer Durham, but could not quite remember when. She confirmed she had access to the departmental information book, which provided additional safety information. She listed those who had access to the pox lab—aside from those already mentioned, this included Miss Anita Dickerson (now called Mrs Bate), the cleaners who emptied the bins first thing each morning and Dr Sandy Buchan, the virologist who worked in a lab across the corridor and who visited the animal pox lab most days to discuss the progress of the electrophoresis research. However, she made it clear that Buchan never set foot in the smallpox room EG34b. On top of that, there was the occasional visit by maintenance men and some engineers who serviced the centrifuge.

Through his relentless examination of the witness, Colston established that, although there were notices and swing barriers in the corridor outside to discourage unwanted visitors, there would have been nothing to stop him making his way to the pox lab and opening the door to the animal pox room whenever it was unlocked. However, Dr Harper made it clear that anyone that did that would be immediately challenged and vaccinated right away, if not already immune. However, she confirmed that no such event had ever happened.

Colston pointed out that one of the University's own safety documents stated that 'All open work with smallpox virus is restricted to the safety cabinet within 34B' and then asked whether aspiration fell within that restriction. Dr Harper replied, 'Yes. Aspiration is open work.' Colston caught the witness out by saying 'But from what you told us it was done on the bench?' Next, they established that she had never discussed this matter with Bedson, even in the run-up to the WHO inspection.

Colston asked whether the volume of work in the pox lab had increased between the WHO visit in May 1978 and the following August. Dr Harper was adamant: the *volume* of work did not increase; the only *change* was that they worked with some additional strains—twenty-two strains obtained from Professor Keith Dumbell on 26 May. They then worked through Harper's lab notebooks, establishing which strains she had been investigating on which days. Dr Harper confirmed that she had been working with strain Abid on 21, 25, 28 and 31 July and finished up fingerprinting the strain by electrophoresis on 3 August.

Colston declared that he had finished his examination-in-chief and the court adjourned for the night.

AS DAY THREE BEGAN, Colston briefly explored two new matters with the witness. First, he asked Dr Harper when the practice began of autoclaving gowns in room EG34b. She could not remember.

Second, he asked about the windows in EG34 and established that they were sometimes opened when the weather was hot, but not when virus work was underway, because that needed use of a Bunsen burner and the flame would be blown about by the draught from an open window.

Then began the cross-examination of Dr Linda Harper by Mr Brian Escott-Cox. He put her at ease, establishing her credentials as a lab worker, who had started work in a path lab at the age of fifteen.

Then he went straight to the heart of things, with a quick-fire succession of questions about Bedson. Q. Was he very safety conscious? *A. Yes, and a very meticulous worker.* Q. Was he a perfectionist in health and safety procedures? *A. Yes*. Q. Did he have a reputation for this in the Medical School? *A. Yes*. Q. Was his lab, by comparison with other labs, immaculately clean and tidy? *A. Definitely yes*. Q. Did his enthusiasm for work in the lab wane after he got his chair? A. *Definitely not. He was very intimately involved in the research that was going on*. Q. Did the time he spent there fall away? *A. Obviously, he had to spend time on professorial duties, but nonetheless he was in the lab every day*. Q. Working a really important amount of time in the lab? *A. Well, if he had not been there, we could not have done the experiments.*

Next, Escott-Cox batted away some of the aspersions cast by Shooter and his team, establishing through cross-examination that there was no truth whatsoever to the idea that Bedson's interest in the lab or the safety standards therein fell away in the couple of years before the smallpox outbreak. It also became clear that Bedson was a man who made himself available to his staff.

Next, the Defence team determined that all the techniques in use in the pox lab were long established and did not vary from year to year. The only exception was electrophoresis, which represented a significant advance in that it simplified the work of the lab and meant that the scale of the work was reduced in terms of amount of virus needed. Thus, far from the rushed scale-up of work envisaged in the Shooter report, there had actually been a reduction in work on smallpox. There was no increase in hours worked or work documented in the lab notebook. Everyone worked a nine-to-five day. There was no rush and no shortcuts on safety. In fact, safety had tightened up after the WHO visit.

Escott-Cox also deftly demonstrated that the pox lab was in no way cramped, given that it was roughly the same size as the courtroom, but was home for most of the time to only three people, and they all knew and respected each other and the rules to which they were working. A great deal of effort went into making sure doors were locked and safety cabinets left on when work was underway on smallpox.

Next, the barrister asked the witness to deal with what he rather fancifully called an 'October hare' (i.e. the equivalent of a March hare in October): the presence of sticking plaster used to seal up holes in the biological safety cabinet in the smallpox room. Dr Harper explained that this had been put in place after the outbreak to seal the cabinet during fumigation and was nothing whatsoever to do with the normal state of affairs before the outbreak.

Next, Escott-Cox and his witness confirmed that Bedson had implemented the policy of aspirating infected liquid on the open bench, rather than in the safety cabinet. Although Dr Harper did not know precisely why, she was sure it was done that way for a reason.

The senior barrister on the Defence team then seized on an insight from his junior colleague, Colman Treacy: given that the photos submitted by the Prosecution were taken some time after the outbreak, how far did they reflect the usual state of affairs in the lab? In particular, how did a bunch of used pipettes end up so skew-whiff in a half-filled bucket? Dr Harper explained that the pipettes had been disinfected in canisters and had been put in the bucket only later during a post-outbreak clear up. She made it clear that disinfectant supplies were always maintained to an adequate level.

Escott-Cox argued that lab staff were motivated not to contaminate the outsides of containers, not just on grounds of safety, but on grounds of good scientific practice, because cross-contamination between one strain and another would ruin the experiments. He also raised the point that for electrophoresis experiments, the smallpox virus had been labelled with radioactivity. He asked Harper if she had ever witnessed cross-contamination and she responded with 'never'. Escott-Cox closed his cross-examination by getting Dr Harper to confirm that she and Bedson had met on the Monday after Janet Parker's smallpox was recognised and had gone through her lab notebook, scrutinising every procedure in an attempt to identify a source of the infection—and they had drawn a blank.

With Dr Harper still in the witness box, Colin Colston started to re-examine her, clarifying some of the points raised during cross-examination by the Defence team. What kind of criticisms did Bedson make of what she did in the lab? She replied that Bedson would really snap your head off if you sat on the write-up table in the animal pox lab, because you might contaminate it from your white coat. Colston asked her for details of improvements to lab safety after the WHO visit. She could recall use of bleach in sinks, but not much else. Next, they confirmed that she had not been around for the DPAG visit and had no idea what was going on when they visited.

Colston asked for details of what Bedson did in the lab and Linda Harper's response was 'diagnostic work'. When asked about the state of the opening in the safety cabinet before the application of the sticking plaster, her slightly impertinent response was 'the hole was a hole'. Colston revisited the matter of radioactive labelling of virus and got Harper to confirm that aspiration of the infected cultures went on the same way whether radiolabelled or not. She also explained that buckets of disinfectant were set up and removed every 24 hours and the extraction fan in the safety cabinet could be switched on and off only from within the lab.

Linda Harper was dismissed from the court.

52

COMMON SENSE?

THE NEXT WITNESS, George Harper (no relation to Linda), informed the court of his credentials as deputy director of the Microbiological Safety Reference Laboratory at Porton Down and his interest in aerobiology and containment of airborne pathogens. He soon also made it clear that he was deaf in his right ear.

Mr Harper described the tests he had carried out on the safety cabinets in the pox lab in mid-September 1978. He had used spores from a harmless bacterium[1] and had found that the cabinet in the smallpox room, EG34b, passed all the tests applied to it.

However, when George Harper examined the larger animal pox room, he found the windows open and, despite clambering up on to a bench, he could not get them to close completely. On direct questioning, he made his opinion clear: it should not be possible to open the windows and the room should remain sealed. Mr Harper confirmed that the safety cabinet in the outer lab did not function properly, as the volume of air passing into it was only half what it should be and infectious particles were somehow escaping via the exhaust pipe.

Colin Colston led the discussion on to the general issue of airborne infection. He presented Mr Harper with a paper on the Meschede smallpox outbreak and asked if he had read it. George Harper confirmed that he had read the paper and agreed that it showed that smallpox had spread two floors upstairs from a patient with no traceable face-to-face contact between that patient and subsequent cases. Colston noted that the Meschede paper cited a paper of Mr Harper's from 1961: *Airborne micro-organisms: survival tests with four viruses.*

Together they worked through Harper's paper, which established that aerosolised vaccinia virus could remain viable for an hour in the air. Escott-Cox complained that none of the recent topics had been covered in statements previously served to the Defence, so the court agreed to adjourn for an extended lunch break while Escott-Cox prepared for cross-examination. After lunch, Colston briefly asked the witness to clarify that there were two different models of safety cabinet in use in the pox lab.

THE FLOOR NOW OPEN for the Defence to cross-examine George Harper, Escott-Cox fell upon the witness like a lion upon a gazelle. The QC forced Mr Harper to agree that the safety cabinet in the smallpox room was a widely used model, approved by Harper's own employer, and, so, no criticism could be levelled at the University for using it.

Next, the University's barrister focused on the Meschede paper, asking the witness to explain why it was significant. The witness said that he assumed that this was because one was trying to establish how smallpox had occurred in Birmingham. The barrister pointed out that this had not been pertinent in 1970, when the paper was published, and so asked what made it significant enough to be published back then. George Harper responded by saying because it was a well-documented case of something that had long been suspected, namely the airborne spread of smallpox.

The QC circled his prey with repeated interrogation on why this was considered significant, accusing the witness of 'not grasping the nettle' and not answering questions. The barrister pointed out that the need for such a paper presupposed that the matter of airborne spread was *in doubt*. He pressed the witness on whether he knew that long-range airborne infection with smallpox was possible. The witness admitted that he did not. Mindful of the need for guilt to be established 'beyond reasonable doubt' in a criminal court, Escott-Cox finished up this line of enquiry by highlighting uncertainties in the use of language in the Meschede report, with airborne spread described only as 'most probable' or 'very likely' rather than certain.

The barrister asked the witness to confirm he was aware of the recommendations in the Cox Report. Escott-Cox was clearly taken aback when poor George Harper admitted that he had never read the report, responding in disbelief: 'I am sorry, Mr Harper, I either misheard you or misunderstood you?'

Over the next few minutes, the barrister established that neither the Cox Report nor the Godber report required that labs handling dangerous pathogens should be hermetically sealed. The witness responded that he took his advice from the DPAG handbook, needling the barrister with 'if you are familiar with that'. The barrister batted a sure-footed response back: 'We are very familiar with them; they passed this laboratory as safe for work'.

Mr Harper read out the sections of the DPAG recommendations that detailed the need for such labs to be maintained at negative pressure and 'sealed so as to permit fumigation'. Escott-Cox drove a wedge into DPAG's language, claiming that the way it was phrased implied that a lab could be left unsealed when not being fumigated.

George Harper fought back by saying that such labs needed to be sealed to maintain negative pressure. The barrister responded by pointing out that the lab in Birmingham was not built on 'Godber lines' (presumably meaning it had no airlock) and so, given that there was no question of maintaining negative pressure, why should it be sealed? Mr Harper fell back on 'it would seem to me to be a very common sense precaution to take', which evoked the response from the barrister: 'so common sense that it is neither in Cox nor Godber?'

In the final moments of his cross-examination, Escott-Cox turned his attention to George Harper's 1961 paper, highlighting caveats over the effect of light on virus survival and asking point-blank: 'Do you say that this particular paper that you produced assists the Justices in this case in this court in assessing the viability of airborne smallpox viruses in the Birmingham Medical School or not?' The exhausted witness responded with a single word 'no' before withdrawing from the courtroom.

THE NEXT WITNESS CALLED by the Prosecution was a petite blonde woman, Mrs Jennifer Durham, who had worked in the pox lab at Birmingham for eleven years. She confirmed everything that Linda Harper had already said about the state of the lab, the nature of the work and the health and safety precautions. When pressed on how often and for how long Bedson himself worked in the lab, she refused to put a time on it, saying it varied from half an hour one day to half a day the next. Unlike Linda Harper, she could recall an instance—but just once in eleven years—of someone coming into the pox lab unannounced and having to be vaccinated. However, when pressed on her recent work, she made it clear that she had not been handling the Abid strain at the time relevant to Janet Parker's infection.

Late on that first Wednesday afternoon, Mrs Durham was cross-examined by Escott-Cox, confirming earlier testimony that there was no increased pressure to get work done in the run-up to the Parker incident and that Bedson was extremely safety conscious and even a bit of a disciplinarian. She made it clear that she worried about safety herself, but never found cause to raise any concerns with Bedson.

The cross-examination continued into the Thursday morning. Again, Escott-Cox used this witness to confirm that there was no falling away of Bedson's input into his lab or the safety standards therein and that even the most junior member of his research team, the 18-year-old Anita Dickerson, received adequate training and supervision. Escott-Cox brought up an experiment into safety in the lab that had been carried out in November 1974, which involved infecting a large number of tissue cultures with smallpox in the safety cabinet and then swabbing surfaces across the lab. Apparently just two putative poxvirus cultureswere recovered, both from a swab of the floor.

Colston resumed his examination of Mrs Durham, who informed him that aspiration of tissue culture medium was actually quite a rare procedure, perhaps used in only 2% of the sessions dedicated to harvesting virus from tissue culture. Colston questioned her repeatedly on how often the pox lab was left unattended and unlocked during lunchtimes. She offered an estimate of probably once a week.

By mid-morning, Mrs Durham had been dismissed and the third member of Bedson's research team was sworn in: Mrs Anita Susan Bate, *née* Dickerson. Colston established that Bate had initially started work in October 1977 in the Bacteriology Department at the Medical School before moving to the animal pox lab in March 1978. She had received a ten-minute safety talk from Dr Gordon Skinner on starting work with bacteria and later received instruction on safety in the pox lab from Jennifer Durham.

Another session followed, devoted to describing techniques already covered by Linda Harper and Jennifer Durham, plus another technique called *immuno-electrophoresis*. Bate admitted to working on her own in the smallpox lab on one occasion. She also confirmed that Bedson visited the lab most days, but left direct supervision of her work to the other two in his team. She reported that she saw Bedson himself working on the bench on three separate occasions and that the amount of work underway did not change much during her six month stint in the lab.

A short cross-examination of Mrs Bate by Escott-Cox revealed that she had received additional safety training during a half-day induction course and then meticulous training and supervision in the lab from Mrs Durham.

53

COFFEE MATES

NEXT ON THE WITNESS stand in quick succession were two of Janet Parker's coffee mates from the Department of Anatomy. The first of these, Mrs Glenda Millar, confirmed that she knew Janet and often visited Parker's studio EF23, where they stored things for their coffee club. Mrs Millar took the court on a virtual tour of the Anatomy Department, which was on the floor above the pox lab. She explained how the so-called 'telephone room', EF26, had become an unlocked junk room.

Mrs Millar had been vaccinated as a baby, but had not been offered vaccination at the Medical School. She occasionally visited the corridor outside the pox lab to get a key to a cold room in the basement. In the couple of months before the outbreak, she also had to visit Sandy Buchan on that corridor to borrow glass plates and a chemical. When questioned by Colston, she confirmed that she had passed through the corridor's swing gates outside the pox lab and had not been challenged or asked about her vaccination status.

Escott-Cox asked why should she be challenged as she had good reason to be there and together they established that no one in their right mind would go into the pox lab without good reason. She said that she was not aware the union had ever raised the question of vaccination before the smallpox incident.

Next, fellow coffee-club witness and medical artist, Norman Fahy, described the studio and dark room he shared with Janet Parker in EF23 and EF23a. He confirmed that their own phone could not be used to make external calls and so they occasionally used the phone in EF26. He had not been offered vaccination until after Parker's diagnosis of smallpox.

Next came Catherine Jeffries, who had worked in a lab on the same corridor as Parker and Millar. She confirmed that EF26 had become an unlocked storeroom that she used to visit almost every day to get books or equipment or to use the phone. She explained that the phone in EF26 was also used by post-doctoral researcher, Colin Dawson, and 'more than once' by Janet Parker. Like the other two, Mrs Jeffries had not been offered vaccination until after the event. She confirmed that she had visited the ground floor of the

East Wing, but not gone through the barriers in the pox lab corridor.

Aggressive cross-examination by Escott-Cox questioned whether Mrs Jefferies just 'thought' that she had seen Parker use the phone on more than one occasion or was 'sure' of this. She confirmed that she did not just *think* so: she was *sure*. The Defence barrister raised uncertainty about the timing, but he and the witness reached agreement that this use of the telephone happened some time after mid-June, even if it was unclear precisely when.

54

AN INSPECTOR IS CALLED

DURING THE LATTER HALF of that first Thursday afternoon, for reasons that are unclear, the Prosecution read out a written statement from DHSS medical officer Dr Sheila Waiter, confirming that she had signed off approval of Bedson's lab in 1976.

Next, an inspector was called to the witness box. Michael Griffiths was, like Robert Cook, one of Her Majesty's Inspectors of Factories employed by the HSE in Birmingham. Under examination from the Prosecution, Griffiths stated that he, with his colleague Miss Needham, had first visited the Medical School from 5pm to 7pm on Friday 25 August 1978, the day after Parker's smallpox had been diagnosed. They initially met representatives of the University and there was some discussion as to whether the corridor outside the pox room should be fumigated. Bedson said that logically that meant fumigating the whole Medical School, which he judged unnecessary.

When it became clear that one of the University's men, McCracken, had been into the pox lab corridor, despite not been vaccinated for many years, Bedson insisted on vaccinating him there and then. Griffiths took the opportunity to get himself revaccinated by Bedson. For the last half hour of his visit, Griffiths met two representatives of the union. As that Thursday in court came to a close, Griffiths described how he had returned to the University on the Tuesday after the Bank Holiday Monday and in the afternoon met Bedson and others at a meeting of the Christie committee.

ON THE MORNING OF Friday 26 October, Colston interposed a new witness, Dr Owen Lidwell—even though he had not yet finished with Mr Griffiths—as Lidwell had made a special trip to the court from his home in Dorset. Colston took Lidwell through his CV: BSc and DPhil from Oxford and nearly forty years working on airborne infections for the Medical Research Council.

Colston summarised the evidence that had been presented to the court on movement between the smallpox room and the animal pox room, noting that the adjoining door was left ajar during such movements, but kept shut when work was underway. Lidwell confirmed that he had conducted investigations for the Shooter Inquiry based on very similar assumptions.

There was discussion on how accurately the particles in Lidwell's particle dispersal tests mimicked what happens with biologically active particles. Lidwell admitted that there was a wide range of particle sizes generated in nature, but felt that his approach was, if anything, likely to underestimate dispersal of infectious particles. When pressed on whether smallpox material would have been capable of dispersal along the same routes as his test material, he gave an unambiguous response: 'Certainly'.

Through a series of photos and a question and answer session, the Prosecution and their witness recapitulated the results of Lidwell's smoke tests the year before, showing suction of air into and out of Ducts B and C and explained how the dispersal test was performed across three storeys of the building. This laborious oral run-through of the tests and their results was terminated after the Defence asked to be allowed to view the evidence in printed form.

The first printed table (Table 2 in Lidwell's section of the Shooter Report) showed that, with the safety cabinet in the smallpox room switched off, particles escaped in appreciable amounts into the corridor, the seminar room and the telephone room EF26. However, dispersal into the corridor and telephone room fell dramatically when the safety cabinet was switched on. The conclusions from that table were that the ratio of the particles in the telephone room to the number in the pox lab stayed in the same narrow range of around 100 to 1 across all Lidwell's experiments.

Attention shifted to the next of Lidwell's tables in the Shooter Report, which reported the potential dose of particles inhaled by someone in each location for each billion (i.e. thousand million) particles dispersed in the smallpox room. The figures ran from 20,000 in the animal pox lab to a thousand in the seminar room, a few hundred in the corridor and fourteen in the telephone room.

When asked about what this meant, Lidwell pointed out that this was a physical calculation and only a physiologist could determine what was significant clinically. He claimed that if only a million particles had been released in the smallpox lab, a person in the telephone room would have only a one in a million chance of inhaling any particles at all—it is hard to follow his logic here; perhaps he was confusing a US billion with a UK million? After a few minutes more discussion, they adjourned for lunch.

After lunch, Lidwell was cross-examined by Escott-Cox, who scored his first point by getting the witness to admit that the covers on the ducts had been removed and replaced between the time of the outbreak and the time of his tests and that this could have had a substantial effect on the outcome of his tests, if there had previously been a much better fit. He scored his second point by reminding the court that the door between the smallpox lab and the animal pox lab was kept *closed* while work was underway, but that Lidwell's tests had been undertaken when it was *open*. Lidwell admitted that if the fan in the safety cabinet were running and the door was closed, he would regard the possibility of escape into the pox laboratory or into the ducts 'as being minimal'.

Escott-Cox argued that the large cloud of particles created in Lidwell's experiment bore no relationship to the accidental escape of a minute quantity of liquid in the practical running of the lab. Lidwell pointed out that the number of virus particles in a suspension might be of the order of millions to hundreds of millions per millilitre. The barrister responded that even to put a single millilitre into the air by accident, one would need to start with an enormous quantity of fluid. Lidwell acknowledged that his numbers represented an unlikely extreme and that he could not come up from personal experience with any procedure that would generate anything other than a very limited aerosol.

The Defence then attacked his statements about the ducts acting as flues because they contained warm air, as Lidwell had not measured the temperature in the room or in the ducts. Lidwell had marked a photo of EF26 with a comment that the length of the telephone lead precluded use of the phone anywhere apart from on one side of the room, close to Duct C. Escott-Cox suggested that it was possible to use the phone on the other side of the room, standing with your back to the door. Lidwell asked if anyone had actually tried to do that and was rendered speechless, when the barrister said he had done it himself and therefore Lidwell's inference was just not true.

After a few more questions, Lidwell withdrew and Griffiths returned to give an account of his visits to the University. He described Bedson as both extremely co-operative and so upset that he could scarcely get his words out. On cross-examination he retracted his earlier claim that Bedson told him it was longstanding practice to vaccinate anyone who had gone through the swing barriers into the corridor outside the pox lab. Then, after what must have seemed like a long week, the court adjourned for the weekend.

That Friday the newspapers reported a statement from WHO Director-General Halfdan Mahler that 'smallpox had been crushed—not only in the Horn of Africa and on the African Continent but throughout the world.'

55

WITNESS FOR THE PROSECUTION

IT IS SAID that a soldier's life is long periods of boredom, interspersed with short moments of sheer terror. As we have seen from the first week of the trial, life in a courtroom is also characterised by long stretches of tedium—but, then, come short moments of excitement, which light up the room—as happened when, at last, the true experts on smallpox were called to the stand.

But we are getting ahead of ourselves. The court hearing on the second Monday began with some humdrum testimony from Edgar Morris, a principal scientific officer from the Centre for Applied Microbiological Research at Porton Down. He confirmed that he had accompanied the previous witness, Michael Griffiths, on his trips to the University of Birmingham and that among the first thing he had noticed was the absence of an airlock, shower, changing facilities and of mechanical ventilation of the smallpox room needed to create negative pressure. He claimed that even in a safety cabinet, gowns could become infected by splashes and that infectious particles could thus be dispersed into the air in rooms EG34b and EG34 and thence outside the lab. He made clear that aspiration of liquid from infected Petri dishes on the open bench was 'a bad practice'.

Morris reported that Bedson had told him that nothing out of the ordinary, such as spillages, had happened in his lab in the run up to Parker's illness. He said Bedson made clear that he had not personally supervised the lab workers at that time. Bedson had also confirmed that the filter on the safety cabinet was three years old and had not been tested recently. Morris claimed that Bedson also stated that one of the staff in the lab had discussed work with Janet Parker, but had not identified the individual.

Escott-Cox then spent a few minutes cross-examining Edgar Morris, getting him to confirm that he had not performed any tests himself on aspiration and aerosols and to agree that the less equipment in a lab the better for cleaning and disinfection and that moving infectious material into and out of a safety container during transport might increase the risk of it being dropped.

The witness withdrew and the court adjourned for three hours.

LAWYERS SAY THAT ONE bad witness for the Prosecution is worth two good witnesses for the Defence. One might have thought that the Prosecution would have sat down with their next expert witness ahead of the trial and taken him through the Shooter Report and asked him whether he agreed with its findings. However, that clearly had not happened. Instead, the courtroom was shocked when—mirroring the Agatha Christie play *Witness for the Prosecution*—someone called to assist the Prosecution gave testimony that gravely undermined their case.

At the time he took the witness stand, Professor Keith Dumbell was probably the world's leading expert still actively working on the smallpox virus and it is clear that he commanded the respect of the courtroom. The 57-year-old professor had worked alongside Allan Downie, Barnett Christie, Kevin McCarthy and Henry Bedson in Liverpool, where he and Downie had pioneered growing poxviruses on hens' eggs and he and Bedson had devised a temperature-based test for differentiating between related pox viruses. He now held the Chair in Virology at St Mary's Hospital in London and, like Bedson, Dumbell had served on DPAG from its inception.

Things began quietly and uncontroversially, as Dumbell launched into a description of the viral isolates grown from Janet Parker and her mother, detailing their unusual behaviour when grown on layers of cultured human cells known as HeLa cells. In this setting, most strains of variola virus caused small regions of cell growth and death, which looked down the microscope like crazy paving topped with little knobs of dead cells. By contrast, the viruses from Parker and Witcomb caused the cells around each focus of infection to fuse together into a continuous sheet (a *syncytium* in the jargon). Dumbell explained that he himself had seen this strange behaviour only in one other strain, isolated from Pakistan and termed 'Abid' after the patient it was isolated from. However, he seemed to remember that a Japanese doctor had described the same phenomenon in isolates from India and Bangladesh. Dumbell made clear that this was not enough to say that the Parker and Abid strains were identical, merely that they were indistinguishable using such techniques. He confirmed that strain Abid had been transported from his lab to Bedson's lab in Birmingham in May 1978. The Prosecution concluded their questioning of their own witness and Dumbell was turned over to be questioned by the Defence.

As he cross-examined the witness, Escott-Cox first made clear that, although it was probable that the Parker strain was Abid, this was by no means certain. Next, he elicited a eulogy to Henry Bedson from the witness, confirming how important Bedson's work was, how dedicated he was and how meticulous Bedson had been in dealing with lab work and safety.

Next, Escott-Cox asked Dumbell about the practicability and desirability of vaccinating all those who worked in the same building as a pox lab, as opposed to just those working in it. The professor said that it was usual practice to vaccinate all those who came into regular contact with those working in the smallpox lab, including colleagues and family contacts, but where you went after that was an open question. He said that, although vaccination was offered to members of other departments in London and Liverpool, this was not made a condition of work. He also pointed out that the justification for providing vaccination—a procedure not wholly without risk—for those not closely involved in the work had diminished as the chances of encountering smallpox in the outside world had plummeted thanks to the eradication campaign.

Dumbell confirmed that DPAG had recently inspected his own new purpose-built smallpox lab, just as they had inspected Bedson's, and had passed it as satisfactory, despite Dumbell's lab having no air lock or shower and smallpox samples having to be transported to a room outside the dedicated smallpox room for storage.

Dumbell described his own experiments on viruses and cotton to defend the practice of not changing gowns during transit of samples, drawing on evidence that repeatedly removing the gown was more likely to liberate infectious particles than leaving it on. He reported his own unpublished experiment on a couple of storage boxes from Bedson's lab, in which he washed out the boxes with culture medium and then showed that no smallpox virus could be recovered from the fluid.

Dumbell, like earlier witnesses, made it clear that just because Bedson had expanded his stock of viruses, this did not entail a greater volume of work—on the contrary, the introduction of electrophoresis had meant a reduction in the scale of viral culture. Similarly, he explained that there was no need for Bedson to hurry his work, as space in Dumbell's lab was assured. Dumbell rammed home the importance of Bedson's work for humanity, in providing tools that could distinguish smallpox viruses from related poxvirus isolates from animals.

Escott-Cox asked the professor how smallpox spread from one human to another. Dumbell pointed out the paradoxical behaviour of this infection. On the one hand, even within the intimacy of the household, as few as a third of susceptible contacts of a case acquired infection, suggesting that smallpox was not very infectious.

On the other hand, there were many examples of people acquiring smallpox after only fleeting contact with a case, suggesting it was highly infectious. Dumbell provided two potential explanations: either susceptibility varied greatly between potential victims or infectiousness was discontinuous over time, with only intermittent release from patients of a large infectious dose.

The barrister asked about the potential for long-range airborne transmission. Dumbell said he remembered the case of a seaman bringing infection into the UK, being confined to an isolation hospital and then infection somehow spreading to a seven-year-old boy who lived between half a mile and a mile away from the hospital. Dumbell pointed out that airborne infection seemed implausible, as why would such a route single out just this one boy out of the hundreds of others who lived within the same radius of the hospital. He said that substantial transfer of material, perhaps even carriage by an animal, was a more likely explanation for transmission over a distance than carriage on the air.

When asked if he thought there had been any potential for airborne spread from his own old lab—where smallpox samples were handled on the open bench—Dumbell dismissed the idea, pointing out that he had swabbed his own benches and tried to culture smallpox virus from them, but had been unsuccessful. Plus, there had been very many years of trouble-free work on smallpox without safety cabinets in Liverpool and in the Public Health Labs in Colindale, based on very simple safety rules.

When Escott-Cox asked him how long the smallpox virus remained viable in the environment, Dumbell reported that if left suspended in fluid, you could expect to lose 90% of the virus every day, but that in dry scabs, it might last longer—perhaps as long as three months.

However, what was supposed to a witness for the Prosecution, fatally undermined the Shooter Report and the Prosecution case, with his quiet but firm dismissal of the pox-in-the-ducts hypothesis, which to him seemed 'highly implausible'—given the one-in-a-million dilution of particles and the minute amount of virus that could be aerosolised in a tiny burst droplet, when even concentrated stocks held only ten million viral particles per millilitre and most of the work was done on much more diluted material. The smallpox expert shot down Shooter's just-so story: 'as a practical consideration I cannot accept it'.

After this, Dumbell was re-examined by the dumb-founded Prosecution, with Colston asking his own witness 'if we discount that, with what does it leave us?'

The answer: 'It leaves you with a puzzle.'

'Perhaps as an expert in smallpox, you can help us try to solve it?'

'I think... one would look first of all for more direct personal contact.'

'...what are you envisaging?'

'Theoretical unauthorised entry... to the laboratory'.

After that, Colston pressed his witness for an opinion on whether leaving the pox lab empty and unlocked perhaps for one lunch hour per week was 'good key control', to which the answer was 'no'. He also forced him to agree that by his own arithmetic, only around 2% of the viability of a virus stock would be lost during the half hour taken to perform the particle dispersal experiment. Then, after some further discussion about the potential for airborne spread and variable transmissibility of smallpox, an exasperated Colston exclaimed 'It seems to be the sort of thing, which works in a rather unexpected way, certainly so far as a layperson is concerned?'

The barrister's exasperation must have increased when Professor Dumbell said that he regarded aspiration of tissue culture fluid from Petri dishes on the open bench in a smallpox lab as 'a pretty safe procedure' and saw codification of safety procedures into written sets of rules as something needed only in large institutions, i.e. of little importance in Bedson's three-person research team.

Colston asked why Dumbell had created a policy of offering vaccination to people from other departments, to which the professor responded by saying he had not started the policy, which pre-dated his arrival, and in any case it made no more sense to vaccinate those inside the building, but far removed from the lab, than to vaccinate passers-by on the street outside. The conversation veered grumpily though discussion on use of gowns, during which Dumbell pointed out that the system for working with dangerous pathogens in UK labs was 'nicely called *voluntary*'.

The afternoon's proceedings closed with an unusual intervention from James Bailey, the chairman of the three magistrates, asking whether Dumbell had had to upgrade his lab procedures after censure from the WHO and DPAG; Dumbell made clear the answer was no and day six of the trial came to an end, with the Prosecution's case seriously holed beneath the waterline.

DAY SEVEN OF THE TRIAL began with testimony from Dr Robert Harris, a virologist of nearly thirty years standing, former head of the Microbiological Research Establishment at Porton Down, and now a consultant in microbiology to the HSE. He had served on

Godber's working party and on DPAG.

Colston led Harris into confirming that, after the Cox report, it was clear to the scientific community that work with smallpox should be performed in a safety cabinet but that cost considerations seemed to hinder this. Harris admitted his surprise at this, 'Because I did not think you could measure the cost of a life against the cost of a safety cabinet'. At this point, the barrister for the Defence leaped up, asking the witness to confine his answers to the questions and stating bluntly: 'he is not here to preach.'

Harris made clear that in his opinion a smallpox lab should be sealed and subject to negative pressure. However, he refused to lay down a rule as to how often a lab coat should be changed and, in an about-face, admitted that the counsel of perfection of using a clean gown, autoclaved after use, for every procedure might be not be feasible on cost grounds. However, he made it clear he was 'appalled' by the fact that in Birmingham 'the key policy obviously did not work' and that he disapproved of moving smallpox samples between labs other than in sealed containers.

Having sat through Dumbell's testimony, Harris made clear that he did not agree with the smallpox expert—for him, airborne spread in Meschede and Birmingham was a real possibility: 'It could have been by sitting over an air duct that had opened into a place where she happened to be. It could have been.' However, he accepted that precisely how Janet Parker came into contact with the smallpox virus 'will probably never be known'. He also was at a loss to explain why Bedson chose to carry out aspiration outside a safety cabinet.

By the time Harris was cross-examined for the Defence, it was clear that this particular witness had riled Escott-Cox, who laid into his adversary Colston for once or twice describing himself as working for the Crown—instead of for the HSE—and he pointed out that Harris also worked for the HSE and so was not an independent expert witness.

Escott-Cox attacked Harris's credentials, noting that the witness had no medical qualifications, which evoked the spirited defence: 'Nor, might I add, had Louis Pasteur, the founder of microbiology!' The QC pointed out that the witness had no experience with smallpox patients in the field, which evoked the response: 'No, but I usually employed people who had.' Escott-Cox needled Harris, suggesting that such individuals would be better qualified to talk in the court than he was. His fist slamming into the desk, the obviously livid Harris shouted back: 'how has seeing a case of smallpox got anything to do with this?' When asked if he was going to slam his fist down again, Harris said he would leave such behaviour to the barrister.

There followed an angry exchange in which the QC argued that airborne transmission of smallpox was not taken seriously even after Meschede, as evidenced by a lack of reference to the phenomenon in the Cox report. In response, the witness claimed that the point of containment in the lab was not to prevent long-distance airborne transmission, but to stop any release of the virus.

The Defence barrister forced the witness to agree that DPAG was allowed to exert discretion in whether or not to relax certain precautions in certain situations and that Harris had been a member of DPAG when it had approved Bedson's lab. Harris pointed out that this was a consensus decision, rather than a unanimous one. However, the barrister made it clear that Birmingham was not unusual, as such discretion had been exercised at a number of similar centres.

Escott-Cox made it clear that the precautions in place for lab work on dangerous pathogens at Porton Down were exceptional, largely due to the unusual nature of their work on biological warfare. He pointed out that despite these precautions, there had been at least two episodes of laboratory-acquired infection at Porton: one involving the agent of plague, the other the Ebola virus. The barrister asked the witness to agree that even in the best-run establishments, there was scope for human error, which drew the response 'whether a man pricks his finger or not is beyond the question of discipline'.

Harris was briefly re-examined by the Prosecution and then a little before midday on the seventh day of the hearing, the witness withdrew and a deflated Colin Colston declared 'Sir, that is the case for the Health and Safety Executive'.

56

DOWNIE FOR THE DEFENCE

ALLAN DOWNIE WAS BORN in 1901 into a family of fishermen on the remote coast of Aberdeenshire, but broke with family tradition to embark on a remarkable medical career. As a young doctor, he worked under bacteriologist John Cruickshank in Aberdeen, before a move to Manchester introduced him to poxviruses. In the 1930s, while in New York, he worked alongside Oswald Avery—the Canadian-American physician-scientist, who used bacteria to show that DNA is the 'stuff of life'. However, Downie soon returned to poxviruses, making the surprising discovery that the vaccinia virus used for smallpox vaccination was not actually the cause of cowpox. In 1944, Downie arrived in Liverpool to take up a chair at the University and went on to make a pivotal contribution to research on smallpox that underpinned the WHO eradication campaign.

At the grand old age of 78 and twelve years retired, Allan Downie was called as the first witness for the Defence in the Birmingham smallpox trial. Brian Escott-Cox began by establishing Downie's credentials: a Bachelor of Medicine, a Doctor of Medicine, a Doctor of Science; a founder member and Fellow of the Royal College of Pathologists; a Fellow of the Royal Society; a pioneer in developing diagnostic approaches to smallpox; and someone who had studied the release of smallpox virus from patients at the bedside in Madras.

Next, the barrister asked the elderly professor about working on smallpox on the open bench. Downie confirmed that this had been customary until the Cox Report. Downie was asked for his opinion of the pox-in-the-ducts hypothesis and responded by saying that he judged it unlikely, as there were more plausible routes that had not received due attention. Downie, like his former colleague Dumbell, was sceptical of airborne spread as the explanation for what happened in Meschede and instead thought indirect transmission via the night nurse or doctors more likely. Similarly, he thought indirect contact with microbiology staff was the most likely cause of Janet Parker's infection.

When pressed as to why he thought so, Downie described experiments he had performed in the early 1960s in Madras, where they found it difficult to recover any airborne smallpox virus from the wards inhabited by smallpox patients, even after sampling many litres of air using equipment invented at Porton Down. Downie also pointed out that had airborne spread been common, the WHO's attempts at eradication would have failed.

Escott-Cox asked Downie whether he would be happy to describe his former pupil Bedson as 'meticulously careful'. Downie agreed and cited, as evidence, the fact that Bedson had worked for two years in Liverpool on rabbitpox, which was a notoriously contagious infection, but had never experienced any unplanned escape of the virus from infected to uninfected rabbits. Similarly, there were no instances of cross-infection in Bedson's lab of smallpox between tissue cultures or chick embryos.

The QC returned to the specific issues of changing gowns between rooms and aspirating on the open bench. Downie agreed that taking a gown on and off between one room and the next created more risk of liberating infectious material than leaving it on. His colleague Kevin McCarthy had shown experimentally that aspiration did not liberate bacteria, so he did not think there was much chance of the procedure generating an aerosol.

Downie was then cross-examined by the Prosecution. He agreed that Janet Parker had almost certainly acquired her smallpox from the lab and that she had acquired 'smallpox proper', rather than, say, whitepox. Downie recalled a young man in Liverpool who had acquired smallpox out of the blue in 1958 or 1959, but agreed that acquisition from a hidden human case after what appeared to be a successful WHO eradication campaign was most unlikely.

Colston pressed Downie to admit that the virus could not have escaped from the lab had there been an adequate containment policy. Downie pointed out that infections had been acquired even in laboratories purpose-built to handle the most dangerous pathogens, such as at Porton Down, but Colston qualified this by pointing out that such infections had been restricted to those working in the labs, not outsiders like Janet Parker.

Discussion followed as to whether ignoring recommendations for lab safety that were official, though not legally binding, meant running a risk. Downie said 'no, not necessarily', stating that he had never worn gloves when handling smallpox, even though the rules now suggested this. He was questioned as to when he had last worked on smallpox and explained that he stopped work on variola in 1971 or 1972.

The court adjourned for lunch.

AFTER LUNCH, THE DISCUSSION turned back to Meschede. Colston quizzed Downie on the inadequacy of the 'night-nurse' explanation in explaining 'patient No. 8', who had visited the front of the hospital for only 15 minutes, and 'patient No. 15', a nursing sister who had never left the second floor cloister. Downie suggested that both patients could have come into contact with the doctor on night duty at the hospital, even though this possibility was not discussed in the write-up of the incident. He also suggested that there were alternative explanations for what appeared to be airborne spread during another German outbreak in Monschau. Colston asked Downie whether, after what had happened in Germany, that someone running a hospital or laboratory who discounted the airborne route would be a fool. Downie said that airborne transmission could not be proven or disproven, but seemed very unlikely.

The dialogue returned to Downie's experiments on forty-seven patients in Madras in the early sixties. Here, he was able to recover smallpox virus only from samples taken within a few inches of a patient's mouth and had never recovered the virus from the air, despite sampling ten litres a minute for up to half an hour. Colston pointed out the apparent discrepancy between conclusions from Downie's work and the investigation into the Meschede outbreak, which had included smoke tests. Colston asked Downie to explain how health care workers might spread smallpox from patient to patient. Downie suggested on the hands or on the clothes, citing examples of outbreaks in laundry workers.

Colston summed up that—leaving aside airborne infection—smallpox was most commonly spread via direct contact or indirectly via clothing or hands. Downie agreed but pointed out that cases of transmission through letters sent in the post had also been reported. The Prosecution asked the professor if there were any other routes of infection. He suggested that anything in the patient's room might get contaminated and pass on infection, including carpets, bedding and even books.

Colston revisited the Cox report's advice on changing gowns, which Downie said was impractical when several people were going in and out of the pox lab several times a day. Escott-Cox intervened to point out that the Cox report had taken a poor policy on gowns as indicative of a careless attitude, rather than as a key lapse in safety.

Downie was asked about the Cox Report recommendation that all open manipulations of the smallpox virus be carried out in a safety cabinet, rather than on the open bench. His response was it would have been almost impossible to grind up smallpox scabs with a pestle and mortar within the confines of a safety cabinet. Attention returned to keys and policies for locking doors. Downie explained that in his time all qualified researchers and some technicians had keys to the smallpox lab and that, although a night watchman locked the lab at the end of the day, there were no special locks on the doors.

Downie agreed that had Janet Parker been vaccinated within the last three years, she would not have caught smallpox. However, in Liverpool, as in Birmingham, it was not thought practicable to vaccinate everyone working in the same building as the smallpox lab. Colston pressed the witness on whether his earlier statement that there was 'not much chance' of creating an aerosol during aspiration implied that there was still 'some chance'—drawing the response 'very little risk, if any'.

Escott-Cox returned to question his witness, establishing that Downie did not see absence of vaccination of all Medical School staff as lack of a safety procedure. Downie pointed out that vaccination was not without risk, causing serious complications in one in 50-100,000 cases and killing 300 people over a ten-year period in the USA.

The elderly professor left the witness box.

57

THE UNIVERSITY MEN

NEXT ON THE STAND was Gordon Skinner, whose qualifications included a basic medical degree, a research degree and membership of the Royal College of Obstetricians and Gynaecologists. He had worked alongside Henry Bedson for a decade and was now a senior lecturer in medical microbiology in Birmingham and acting head of department. He explained that he worked in a lab next door to the pox lab and that his research focused on herpes viruses. He was one of two safety officers.

In the Q and A with Escott-Cox, Skinner made clear that it was certainly uncommon for any unauthorised personnel to enter the corridor outside the pox lab, that everyone in his department knew that vaccination was available to them and that Professor Bedson was the most safety conscious person he had ever encountered. He said that he always entered Bedson's lab with trepidation, as it was absolutely first class in terms of orderliness and he was worried about being hauled over the coals for some minor misdemeanour.

When asked if Bedson's interest in the lab had faltered as he took on departmental duties, Skinner's answer was blunt: 'Well, nonsense, would be my response to that'. He had never found the pox lab door unlocked or had any concerns about safety in that lab.

Just before the end of the day, Skinner was cross-examined by Colston, who tried to work out *who* took responsibility for *which* aspects of safety in the Medical School. After repeated questioning, Colston established that Skinner knew *for certain* that people in the Department of Medical Microbiology were offered vaccination, but was less certain about the rest of the Medical School.

The court adjourned overnight.

THE FOLLOWING MORNING, after Escott-Cox clarified that there was no written policy in the Medical School on vaccination outside the Department of Microbiology, Colston resumed his cross-examination of Gordon Skinner, establishing that Skinner did no research on smallpox and had handled only one diagnostic request in the last four years. Skinner used to visit the outer animal pox lab once a fortnight or so. He did not know how much time Bedson spent on teaching or administration. Colston pointed out that Skinner was now acting Head of Department and asked him to estimate how much time he himself spent on administrative tasks. Skinner prevaricated, before guessing a third-to-a-half of his time. However, he pointed out that Bedson probably spent less time on administrative tasks, as he was more experienced than Skinner.

After yet another meander through use of gowns and placement of safety codes, Colston attempted to raise the issue of mouth pipetting, only to be challenged by Escott-Cox, who pointed out that this had not been discussed with any previous witness. Colston asked whether Dr Skinner was 'shattered' when the WHO raised concerns over the practice. Skinner said 'no', but that Bedson was 'very concerned over this'.

The dialogue rambled on for an hour or so without establishing much, apart from that Skinner was not personally acquainted with Janet Parker and did not know precisely how vaccination had been offered to people outside his department or how the vaccine fridge was organised.

Skinner was re-examined by the Defence and revealed that perhaps a hundred people a year were vaccinated from outside Bedson's department. Skinner found it absurd that being head of department might have deprived Bedson of the chance to supervise his own lab.

NEXT IN THE WITNESS BOX was Reginald Farr, a Cambridge-educated medical physicist, employed as a Senior Lecturer at the University of Birmingham. Escott-Cox established that Farr had visited Bedson's pox lab on 11 October 1978, performing a thorough daylong inspection for radioactivity. Farr reported that he found no readings in excess of background levels of radioactivity and concluded that no spillages of radioactive material had taken place in the lab. When pressed, he qualified this to mean that no virus radiolabelled for electrophoresis could have been spilt on the benches or floors, but this did not exclude release via aerosol.

Farr was followed in the witness box by Sandy Buchan, the Scottish virologist who had worked for twelve years in the Department of Medical Microbiology in Birmingham and was now a Lecturer in the department. He had come to know Henry Bedson very well and could confirm that Bedson had a genuine interest and concern for safety 'which was part of the man'. Buchan explained that he had helped Bedson establish electrophoresis in the pox lab and often visited the animal pox room EG34, although not the smallpox room EG34b. He had never once found the door to the outer lab unlocked and he had found the animal pox room to be extremely neat and tidy at all times.

Buchan then described his own analyses of lab notebooks and of Bedson's timetables to determine whether there had been any changes in the run-up to the Janet Parker incident. He reported only a modest increase of 8% more tissue culture dishes being used in Bedson's lab in the first half of 1978 compared to a similar period in 1977. However, he made clear that Bedson's teaching load had dropped considerably a couple of years before, when a post-graduate course had been abandoned.

Escott-Cox quizzed Buchan about how the pox lab staff worked their lunch breaks, but drew a blank. The barrister then asked Buchan how often he had seen strangers on the pox lab corridor; the answer was 'infrequently'. When asked if he knew Janet Parker, Buchan said he knew her by sight, having encountered her on two occasions. The first was when she was, as a union member, picketing the entrance that Buchan used to enter the Medical School. The second was in July 1978, when Buchan was taken to meet her in the Department of Anatomy to share expertise in photography.

Next, Buchan was asked to interpret the results of a safety test carried out by Bedson and his staff in the smallpox room in November 1974, which established that no smallpox virus could be grown from swabs of the benches and safety cabinet. Two 'pocks' on chick membranes were recovered from the floor, but it was unclear whether these represented smallpox or some other virus or just random events.

On cross-examination, Buchan presented his estimate of how much of the Abid virus had been produced in the pox lab in Birmingham: this came to around five thousand million virus particles in a dessertspoon of liquid. The Prosecution badgered Buchan repeatedly over the interpretation of the results of the 1974 safety test, but Buchan made it clear that he could not help the court on this matter. Along the way, Escott-Cox joked about the spelling of 'pocks' versus 'pox' and pointed out that Colston was asking 'stop beating your wife' questions, in that Buchan had already said that the two pocks might have nothing to do with smallpox at all.

Colston attempted to clarify the circumstances in which Sandy Buchan met Janet Parker. Buchan explained that he had been in her studio for less than five minutes, had stood as close to her as he now was to the barrister and was not wearing a lab coat at the time. Colston then forced Buchan to agree that he sometimes went into the animal pox lab without a white coat on. Buchan admitted that he had written a note when in Parker's studio, but could not remember whether he had brought his own pen with him or borrowed one from Parker. He also could not accurately estimate how often he visited the pox lab—it was somewhere between once a day and once a week, but varied over time. Buchan had no fixed point in his memory to tie down when he visited Parker: he thought it was July 1978, but it could have been late June. He also had no memory of ever giving a cold room key to Mrs Millar.

The last fifteen minutes in court that day were spent trying, in vain, to establish whether Sandy Buchan knew anything about the minutes of a meeting of the University's Pathogenic Organisms Sub-Committee that took place on 22 February 1977. Colin Colston made it clear that he wanted to find the minutes of the meeting and present them in court and also to retain Buchan's services as a witness that could represent the University.

THE NEXT MORNING STARTED with a heated exchange of words between the two legal teams, with Escott-Cox accusing the Prosecution of launching a belated fishing expedition and making a deliberate tactical move to apply pressure on the Defence. If the Prosecution thought the minutes of that particular committee so important, why had they not attempted to obtain them in the many months leading up to the trial? The chief magistrate stepped in to limit the altercation, saying that the court had heard arguments from both sides on this matter—with the implicit assumption that they should move on.

Sandy Buchan was recalled as a witness and again cross-examined on his encounter with Janet Parker. When Buchan confirmed that he had visited Parker in her dark room, Colston threw out a snide question: 'You were going to give Mrs Parker some of your expertise...'

Buchan explained that he had been asked by Parker's colleague, Mr Fuller, to let Parker know what kind of photographic film, developer and fixer he used in his own photographic process. Buchan clarified that he did not enter the dark room, but stayed in the doorway around five to six feet away from Parker, who was inside the dark room. He told her that he used Agfa X-Ray film.

Buchan explained that he had not been introduced to Janet Parker by name, knowing her merely as the photographer who worked in Anatomy. It thus took a couple of days after Janet Parker was diagnosed with smallpox before Buchan mentioned his earlier encounter with the photographer to Henry Bedson.

Buchan left the stand and was replaced by Arthur Shakeshaft, chief engineer at the University of Birmingham. Under examination and cross-examination, Shakeshaft described the ducts in the animal pox room, making clear that the outer cover to the ducts had been unscrewed and taken off during a visit by the DHSS man Dr Robinson on 9 September 1978 and then screwed back in place, but not very tightly. He explained that the ducts were not ventilation ducts, but a cosmetic feature to hide pipework and that they had been blocked with bricks at floor level and sealed up in various ways to prevent leakage of steam from the basement of the building, but they were not likely to be airtight.

Next, the final witness was called to give evidence in court—a witness who would stay on the stand for the next day and a half.

58

THE KMcC CALCULATIONS

THE 57-YEAR-OLD PROFESSOR Kevin 'KMcC' McCarthy was sworn in and clarified that he was Professor of Medical Microbiology at the University of Liverpool and Consultant in charge of Medical Microbiology Services to the Royal Liverpool Hospital. He confirmed his general and specialist medical qualifications and his acquaintance with other relevant smallpox experts: Allan Downie (whose chair he had taken over in 1966), Henry Bedson and Keith Dumbell. He had worked on smallpox since 1946, in both research and diagnostic settings.

Escott-Cox and KMcC agreed that it was not possible to work on dangerous pathogens such as the smallpox virus with no risk whatsoever. McCarthy confirmed that the safety standards at Liverpool were no different from elsewhere in the country and that he had served on the Cox inquiry into the 1973 outbreak in London. He pointed out that the UK had been responsible for more lab work on smallpox than anywhere else in the world and, up to 1973, all this work (apart from at Porton Down) had taken place on the open bench, rather than in a safety cabinet.

McCarthy also noted that recommendations in the Cox report represented guidance rather than cast-iron rules, as evidenced by use of the verb form 'should' rather than 'must' and that, in a lab run by a smallpox expert, the head of the lab was best placed to decide on practice. He provided an example of the hazards of over-specified rules by pointing to the recently issued Howie code on lab work, which provided instructions on how to sterilise safety canisters that would have caused an explosion.

The discussion turned to Henry Bedson. KMcC let the court know that Bedson had, after the 1973 outbreak, called together all those working on smallpox to see if they could tighten up on lab safety. He had known Bedson for twenty or more years as a colleague and as a friend. He knew from personal observation that Bedson was a careful and meticulous operator and the most safety-conscious microbiologist that he knew.

McCarthy then explained the reasoning behind the smallpox eradication campaign, focusing on isolation of contacts, before moving on to the potential for an animal reservoir. He mentioned gerbilpox and whitepox and explained how Bedson, acting on a suggestion from Sandy Buchan, had adopted electrophoresis in the hope of finding fingerprints that differentiate smallpox from whitepox.

KMcC had visited Bedson's lab on numerous occasions and thought it was being run on very safe lines. He confirmed that his Liverpool lab was run on similar lines and fell short of the recommendations of the Godber report for similar reasons—and, like Bedson, he had received DPAG approval for his lab, despite these potential shortcomings. When pressed, he named seven UK smallpox labs that had passed muster with DPAG, but failed to meet all of Godber's recommendations.

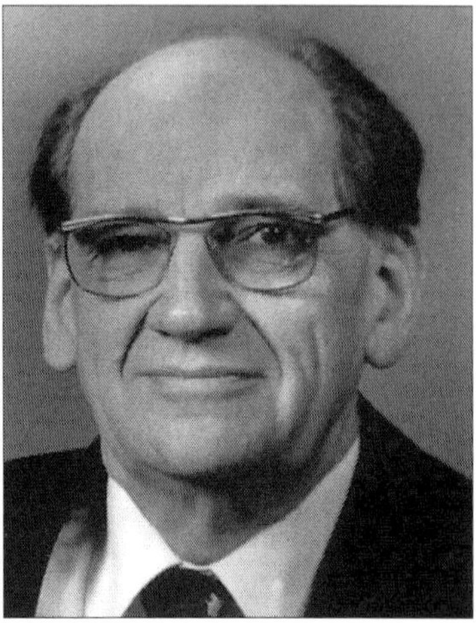

KEVIN MCCARTHY
'KMcC': Professor of Medical Microbiology at Liverpool whose calculations electrified the courtroom
{Source: Mary McCarthy}

Escott-Cox then asked about the risks of vaccination. McCarthy quoted the rate of severe complications of 1 in 50,000 to 1 in 100,000 and recounted from his own experience how a four-year-old girl with eczema had caught vaccinia infection from her older sister, who had been recently vaccinated, and had nearly lost a leg to amputation. Like Dumbell, he explained that the rationale for vaccinating everyone in a workplace had faded once smallpox had become uncommon, because there was no added benefit of protecting against smallpox caught in the community. The vaccine strain was infectious and potentially fatal in those with eczema or with weakened immune systems. McCarthy fully backed the approach used in Birmingham, where vaccinations were offered only after balancing risks of vaccination with the risks of acquiring smallpox.

They discussed airflow into the smallpox lab and storage of discarded pipettes and McCarthy made it clear that he had no concerns about safety on these counts. He described an experiment in which he had contaminated a piece of fabric from a lab coat with a million doses of smallpox virus and found that no virus was recoverable a day later. His verdict on long distance airborne spread of smallpox in Meschede was 'not proven' in Scottish legal parlance and KMcC confirmed that lack of cross-contamination between different viral preparations in the Bedson lab was evidence of a high standard of safety.

Escott-Cox probed his witness for an opinion on whether tissue culture dishes should be moved from one lab to another within a sealed container. McCarthy joked that this would be like trying to carry a tea tray around in a suitcase, thereby increasing the risk of spillage. Similar arguments applied to moving infected eggs within a rack or trying to transfer them to a sealed container. KMcC pointed that although he loved gadgets, in the lab, the finest instruments available were one's own fingers.

Questioning turned again to the issue of aspiration outside a safety cabinet. McCarthy made the point that this commonly used procedure would have been abandoned, had it had been associated with release of virus by aerosol, as any resultant cross-contamination would have ruined experiments. He described some experiments he had performed to quantify the risk, using a harmless lab strain of the bacterium *E. coli*.

He started off by placing a small dish containing four millilitres of liquid containing bacteria inside a larger dish containing solid agar culture medium. He then performed the aspiration step on the liquid and incubated the agar overnight. He calculated that there were 480 million bacteria in the liquid and he found only one colony grew on the agar, which may not have even originated from the aspiration itself.

McCarthy calculated how many litres of liquid containing a similar density of smallpox particles would be needed to get a single virus particle from the smallpox lab into the room upstairs, incorporating Lidwell's earlier calculation that only one in 1.1 million airborne particles in the lab would get through to the room. The figure he came up with was 53,000 litres—or fifty-three tonnes of liquid!

He then made use of Sandy Buchan's testimony on annual use of petri dishes to calculate that it would have taken between two thousand and twenty thousand years of lab work before a single virus particle would reach the room upstairs. He quipped that if one also took into account that the ducts may have been even less likely to transmit particles before being interfered with, then the time needed to transmit a single particle might stretch back to the dinosaurs!

McCarthy explained at length how performing the aspiration outside the safety cabinet was far less clumsy and, therefore, far safer than trying to do it with thick tubes threading through holes into the safety cabinet.

Next, the discussion turned to lab coats, which the professor pointed out did offer significant protection against gross splashes. He explained that in the USA, there had been use of what were effectively space suits to give total protection in the lab. Colin Colston provided reassurance that he would not be suggesting that people should have been wearing space suits in Birmingham.

Next, KMcC made clear that changing gowns between every manoeuvre in the labs was impractical in that it would have required a much larger autoclave than was available and DPAG must have known that gowns were not being changed that often from what they saw on their visit. Plus, he concurred that taking gowns on and off was a fiddly business likely to generate more aerosols than leaving them on for most of the day. He did another back-of-envelope calculation to suggest that the number of virus particles liberated from a coat contaminated from a tiny splash was likely to be in the tens, rather than in the hundreds of millions implicit in Lidwell's assumptions.

He found no problem with an eighteen-year-old Anita Dickerson working in a smallpox lab and saw no need to wipe down the outside of containers with disinfectant. He made clear that Dickerson had probably worked only with inactivated serum. Similarly, he concluded that the two pocks reported in Bedson's safety experiment were probably non-specific, because otherwise the ever-diligent Bedson would have followed them up.

As his initial examination of his last witness drew to an end, Brian Escott-Cox asked Professor McCarthy to speculate on how he thought Janet Parker might have contracted smallpox. The medical man started with a lawyerly response, outlining three possibilities. First, it could be the result of an unwished-for event, without obvious cause that happens despite the best practice, the best equipment and the best conscience. Second, it could be the result of a misjudgement, despite best efforts, as to the risk of an established procedure. Third, it could be the result of a conscious decision not to adopt the practice assessed as carrying the minimum risk.

KMcC said he heard nothing to support the third option, but that the first two remained possible. He discounted aerial spread. He speculated that there could have been indirect spread via a missed case or someone uninfected carrying virus on his or her person, say in the hair or in the nose. In the post-eradication era, smallpox labs were going to have to have a shower, but that in the past they were given approval without this.

THE DEFENCE BARRISTER RETURNED to his seat and cross-examination by Colin Colston began. McCarthy was quizzed about his lab in Liverpool and specifically about the relationship between labs, freezers, incubators corridors and air ducts. He explained that he did not grow smallpox in tissue cultures and pointed out that his lab was initially situated on an open corridor and then on a blind corridor with an electric lock. However, smallpox virus stocks were held in a lockable freezer out in the corridor.

Colston questioned the validity of KMcC's aspiration contamination experiment. Did not the results simply reflect the skill of a very great authority on smallpox, far more polished than those who had been working in Birmingham? McCarthy pointed out that, although he had had thirty-nine years experience of smallpox, he was on thirty-eight different committees at the moment and had very little time to polish his skills in the lab.

He accepted that his experiments did not show that aerosol production during aspiration was completely impossible, but that with the need for 20,000 years work to get smallpox into the upstairs room, there was a reasonable margin of safety. Colston pointed out that not everyone was as skilled as the professor in the lab. McCarthy responded by saying that Lidwell's experiments had only found airborne spread of particles when the lab door was open and the safety cabinet off, so things would have been even safer under normal working conditions, with the door closed and the cabinet on.

Colston grilled McCarthy about whether the two rooms in the Birmingham pox lab should be seen as one lab or two. McCarthy was adamant that they should be seen as two, as the smallpox lab was maintained under negative pressure by the safety cabinet. McCarthy accepted that infection was more likely to have arisen from the outer lab, but not through the air. And as escape via the air could be discounted, the fact that the windows did not close fully in the outer lab was irrelevant.

Next, Colston asked McCarthy the key question: 'How on earth did Mrs Parker get infected?' The professor responded, 'we do not know the answer to that and it may be we will never know the answer.'

In the last few minutes of that final Thursday of the trial, the conversation turned grouchy, with the Prosecution and the witness accusing each other of encouraging speculation over spread of the virus via the nose or hair. The court adjourned for the night—but they were not yet done with Professor McCarthy.

THE NEXT MORNING, COLSTON started by grilling McCarthy over his interpretation of Bedson's 1974 safety experiment; in particular, whether the lack of follow-up of the two pocks associated with the floor meant that they were necessarily non-specific and so not evidence of a spill involving smallpox virus. McCarthy stood his ground on this issue, but yielded on the point that repeating the test would have presented no practical difficulty.

McCarthy made clear his disagreement with the idea that written rules on safety should be slavishly obeyed without interpretation by the skilled worker, but accepted that one should do one's best to maintain an up-to-date set of rules. Colston pointed out that it would not be hard to keep the written rulebook updated with a team of just four people in the Bedson lab—McCarthy's response was that there was no need, with such a small expert team.

Next, the two men haggled over whether the statement in the local rules that vaccination was 'offered to those working elsewhere in the Medical School' implied that it was offered to *all* or just *some* of the workers in that category. Yet again, KMcC was forced to point out that the policy of vaccinating everyone in the work place was unevenly applied across the country, with the Central Public Health Lab in Colindale doing less vaccination of neighbouring departments than Birmingham had. The professor rammed the point home: 'the judgment must be a clinical judgement as you are assaulting a person in a sense in vaccinating them.'

Linguistic tussles followed over the meaning of 'open work' in the Birmingham lab rulebook, whether 'all' meant 'all' in the relevant line in the rulebook, whether the corridor outside the Birmingham pox lab could be described as 'communal' or why a non-specific phrase about offering vaccination to those outside the department had been left in the rule book, when there were detailed specifications as to which people were to be vaccinated.

The barrister pointed out that Linda Harper had accepted that aspiration on the open bench fell under the term 'open work', but McCarthy countered with the barbed comment, 'If that is considered open work by the senior person in Birmingham University, I would agree with you, but we have not had the opportunity of asking the senior person, because he is dead.'

The two men then considered the risks of something untoward happening during aspiration, like a sneeze or a heart attack. McCarthy accepted that falling off a stool might have an effect, but this would also be true for work done in a safety cabinet. Colston attacked the assumption that the speed of airflow into the pipette during aspiration was necessarily the same in Birmingham as in KMcC's experiment in Liverpool.

A short while later, the barrister asked again about who should be vaccinated, focusing, as an example, on Mrs Millar, who came down to the pox lab corridor to borrow the key to the cold room. McCarthy said he would not vaccinate such a person, pointing out that in Liverpool he had never vaccinated the milkman, but had vaccinated the window cleaners. The barrister and the professor wrangled over the calculation of the complication rate after vaccination.

Again, the issue of gowns was raised and attention refocused on the 1973 outbreak and the investigations that followed it, including Shooter's report into that outbreak (embedded within the Cox Report), in which Shooter claimed that Ann Algeo could have been infected from a pre-existing spill rather than during harvesting of smallpox virus from eggs. When asked if this made sense scientifically, McCarthy said 'no', so the barrister questioned whether Professor Shooter had got it wrong. In a series of responses, McCarthy made it clear that Shooter was a *bacteriologist*, not a *virologist* and could not be considered as 'a man of authority' in dealing with smallpox, as he had never worked with it.

The discussion ranged fruitlessly over the recommendations from various reports, which included the barrister trying to establish that it was generally accepted that all work on smallpox should be done in a safety cabinet and labs locked when not in use. McCarthy made it clear that in his opinion locking doors was not all that important, as the extent of smallpox contamination in the lab should be nil. However, he agreed he would have 'given his staff a rocket' for leaving the door to the smallpox lab open and that a malicious person who wanted to infect themselves could gain access to smallpox if lab doors and freezers were left unlocked.

McCarthy challenged the legitimacy of the Godber report, pointing out that it claimed that some UK polytechnics were holding the smallpox virus, which was plainly nonsense. He also found fault with the requirement that junior staff should be 'continuously' supervised by senior staff in the smallpox lab and he saw the availability of a shower in the lab as an additional help, but not a rigid requirement. Colston asked McCarthy to agree that it was hard to imagine a lab worse sited for smallpox work than the lab in Birmingham. McCarthy could not agree, pointing out that the situation was far worse in Colindale and much of a muchness in all the other UK smallpox labs.

After lunch, Colston pressed the witness on comparisons between the Birmingham lab and others, pointing out that only in Birmingham was diagnostic work combined with an active research programme. Later that afternoon, discussion turned to 'acts of God' and the need for, to use as a 'homely term', a 'belt and braces' approach to safety in the smallpox lab. McCarthy pointed out that perfection was impossible and that the WHO had had to close their own lab in Moscow on safety grounds. KMcC made it clear that he did not wish to say that, with regard to Birmingham, that 'there were matters in the system which could and should have been improved', particularly bearing in mind the leak of the Shooter Report and widespread public comment together with the passage of time and incompleteness of his knowledge. He also dismissed the suggestion that Sandy Buchan might have acted as a passive carrier of infection as an extremely remote possibility, no more likely than lots of other human activities in the Medical School building.

When Professor McCarthy was re-examined by Escott-Cox, he clarified that his smallpox lab in Liverpool had been relocated and upgraded, not so much in response to the Cox Report, but because smallpox labs were now being asked to take on responsibility for diagnosis of a more dangerous infection, Lassa fever. He pointed out that since the pox lab had been closed in Birmingham, suspected cases of Lassa fever were being transported in portable isolators to Liverpool and there had been at least one death that would have been avoided if the Birmingham lab were still functioning.

They explored the potential for a malevolent individual to gain access to pathogens in the lab and what would happen if there were a fire. McCarthy said a chief fire officer had reassured him that contents of freezers would be cooked before the building collapsed. He confirmed he had come across a vial of smallpox in a lab audit that had been overlooked because it was poorly labelled.

They discussed the WHO requirements for a smallpox lab in the post-eradication era, which McCarthy said had not been met even by Porton Down. Escott-Cox asked if eradication had seemed inevitable in 1977. The professor exclaimed 'Oh no!' and reminded the court that his colleague Keith Dumbell had just returned from a tiring and detailed survey looking for smallpox in Ethiopia and that eradication had been announced just one week before. Just before the interrogation came to an end, Escott-Cox asked whether the witness was surprised to hear of anything that he thought should not have been happening in Bedson's lab and he gave a one-word answer: 'no'.

THE PROSECUTION CALLED a now-visibly-nervous Sandy Buchan back to the witness box. Buchan confirmed that Bedson had made the policy decision not to vaccinate casual visitors, such as Mrs Millar, who came to borrow the key to the cold room and that the two of them had discussed this point 'long ago'. Colston leapt to his feet to challenge the witness, asking how he had now come to remember something from so long ago that he had not previously mentioned, and asking Buchan whether he could even remember what he had said five minutes before.

The overwrought Buchan was unable to give a straight answer, twice batting back the response 'If you say that is the sequence of events I agree with you'. Buchan was by now very tense, almost shaking and speaking in a quiet strangled voice.

When challenged on his memory, Buchan said he remembered some things and not others, like most people, and his recall responded to triggers. The Prosecuting barrister asked whether anything had triggered a better recollection of his encounter with Janet Parker.

Escott-Cox stepped in and established that Buchan's hesitancy was because he was very nervous and that his recall of the detail of the vaccination policy had been triggered by earlier discussion of the matter in court.

That week's proceedings ended when the two legal teams agreed to allow as admissible, Escott-Cox's observation that it was possible to make a phone call in the telephone room without doing so next to the air duct.

59

SUMMING UP

AS THE THIRD WEEK of the trial began, Colin Colston cracked a joke, saying that he was asking to speak for fifteen minutes and his learned friend Escott-Cox had agreed to start coughing at sixteen minutes.

Colston opened his summing up by focusing on the issue of 'reasonable practicability', as laid out in the *Health and Safety at Work Act* of 1974, which made it clear that the accused had to show that there were no better practicable means than those actually used to satisfy duties under the act. Colston pointed out that approval from DPAG for the Birmingham smallpox lab in 1976 did not give blanket approval for everything that was happening in 1978. He highlighted the discrepancies between the testimonies from Linda Harper and Kevin McCarthy as to whether the 'open work' on smallpox prohibited by Bedson's own rules included aspiration of spent tissue culture fluid on the bench. He claimed that Bedson as a great communicator must surely have made the issue clear to Linda Harper, who was a 'highly intelligent woman' and could not have 'got the wrong end of the stick'.

Colston highlighted an inconsistency in McCarthy's reasoning, who had, on the one hand, claimed that the Liverpool lab was special and warranted an upgrade because of a new requirement to handle Lassa fever samples, which apparently did not apply to the Birmingham lab, and then, on the other hand, to say lives were lost because the Birmingham lab was no longer open and able to handle Lassa samples. His point was that both labs should be upgraded.

Colston finished his summing up by railing against what he saw as an inadequate and poorly specified vaccination policy for staff in the Medical School, which in his view constituted 'an absolute offence' under the law.

Conspicuous by its absence in Colston's summing up was any mention of the pox-in-the-ducts hypothesis he had been so keen to champion early in the trial.

BY CONTRAST WITH the Prosecution's succinct summary, Brian Escott-Cox QC took well over an hour to present his conclusions. In so doing he rehearsed not only his own arguments, but also those that could be used by the Prosecution.

Escott-Cox started off by emphasising how this case was unique in that there was no simple chain of cause and effect, as there might be if, say, someone had put his hand into an unfenced press and injured himself. In addition, all the experts had agreed that it was impossible to do research work of this kind without some inevitable risk, but that did not mean that the accused could be judged guilty for simply doing the work. The Prosecution had to establish that the employees in the East Wing had been subjected to *unnecessary* risks, over and above those unavoidably inherent in the work. And the employer's duty of care extended only to employees, rather than, say, students, burglars or terrorists. Escott-Cox made it clear that all those working in the smallpox lab were solidly protected by vaccination, so the only people under consideration for any breach in duty were those working elsewhere in the Medical School.

Next, the barrister classified the potential charges against the University under three headings: *vaccination*, *pox-in-the-ducts* and *lab procedures*. He made it clear that the systems put in place had to be defective for the University to be found guilty, rather than a momentary lapse of judgment by an individual. He also made clear that the University was not saying that their system was 'unsafe, but they could not make it any safer on grounds of practicability or financial constraints'. Instead, the case for the University was and always had been 'Our system is safe, full stop' and the issue of 'so far as is reasonably practicable' does not apply.

Escott-Cox explained that the duty to protect against risks applied only to risks that were known or could reasonably be anticipated and not taken to ludicrous limits. As an example, he pointed out that it was well established that gas mains sometimes explode, but that no one was suggesting that the University should provide special curtains to prevent injury from glass that might be blown out of their windows in the East Wing.

Then he attempted to raise and neutralise four 'matters of prejudice' that should not be allowed to influence the outcome of the trial: the adverse publicity in the press; the highly charged emotions evoked by smallpox; the tragic deaths of Bedson and Parker; and the risk that the presumption of innocence be abandoned, so that the University has to justify its actions, rather than the Prosecution prove guilt.

Escott-Cox used gentle humour to mock the way in which Colston's detailed scrutiny of laboratory practice had made things seem a lot more dangerous than they actually were. He made the wistful claim that Colston could make the actions undertaken by a bishop standing up to give a sermon sound dangerous or could make cooking the Sunday dinner sound like a death trap.

The lawyer considered the vaccination issue, pointing out the absence of official guidance on this matter from any recent documents, the risks of vaccination and the careful approach to screening potential vaccinees adopted by the Medical School. He acknowledged that the Prosecution had repeatedly taunted the Defence about the University's house rules. However, he claimed that saying that vaccination was 'on offer' was no different from saying a product was 'on offer' in a supermarket, which did not imply that every householder in the district had been leafleted about it. If it was not obvious that vaccination was on offer, how was it that at least a hundred people were turning up for vaccination in the Medical School every year?

Escott-Cox showed a protective streak, pointing out how inappropriate it was for his learned friend to have interrogated Sandy Buchan as if he were a criminal charged with burglary, rather than accept him as a serious scientist, who was plainly nervous in court and reluctant to say anything unless obviously the truth.

He moved on to the pox-in-the-ducts issue. He dismissed Lidwell and his particle dispersal tests because the tests had been carried out only after the panels to the air ducts had been removed and damaged and hastily and incompletely put back in place, rather than testing the set-up as it would have been in the summer of 1978. In any case, Professor McCarthy's slightly sarcastic presentation of his calculations had shown that the astronomical quantities of particles released in Lidwell's tests were at odds with the effects of day-to-day work in the lab. Escott-Cox reminded the court how three eminent smallpox experts had all dismissed the possibility of long-range airborne infection with smallpox, whether in Meschede or Birmingham, and, so, to find the University guilty because it neglected this risk, would be to fly in the face of the greatest authorities in the world!

However, the barrister went further than just appealing to authority. He pointed out that if airborne spread had been a common and foreseeable problem, the eradication campaign would not have worked, Janet Parker would not have been the only person infected outside a lab and the relevant authorities would all have insisted that smallpox labs be hermetically sealed.

As Escott-Cox turned to the final issue of laboratory practice, he again turned to humour, suggesting that if anyone mentioned a white coat, it would be enough to make you scream, or at least turn off your hearing!

Next, he exploited the rhetorical device of *pathos*—an appeal to the listener's emotions—evoking the meticulous safety-obsessed personality of Henry Bedson and the sense of quiet orderly efficiency, safety and calm that prevailed in his lab. He provided haunting summaries of the witnesses who had spoken up for Bedson: the 'robust Scotsman' Gordon Skinner, Dr Linda Harper 'with her experience and great care', Jennifer Durham, 'the little blonde lady, with very little academic qualifications but years of careful laboratory experience'. He made it clear that there was no financial motive to cut corners on safety. Nor was there any evidence of inadequate training or supervision or of neglect of lab duties by Bedson or of any increase in workload or any need to rush things.

Escott-Cox highlighted the way the Prosecution had belittled Anita Bate as 'only a trainee', 'only nineteen years old', 'a school-leaver', who had never been given any safety rules or instruction by Bedson or Skinner, when in fact she gave evidence to the fact that she had been adequately trained and supervised. The barrister said this gave some indication of the 'shifting sands' of allegations that they had had to contend with in the case.

Escott-Cox summed up the evidence from expert witnesses that aspiration outside the safety cabinet was a perfectly safe procedure, no more complicated to a skilled lab worker than cooking scrambled eggs. In any case, it was not his job to show it was safe—the Prosecution had to prove that it was unsafe and they had no evidence for that. In fact, there were good reasons for believing that use of a shorter tube made possible by aspiration on the bench made things safer overall. And the only way any of this mattered was if viruses, like mosquitoes, could fly under the door and sting people elsewhere in the building, which was not true!

The QC next rounded on the 'key-and-corridor issue', stressing that the kind of people working in the East Wing of the Medical School were not common factory workers, but intelligent and sophisticated people, who would have no trouble understanding and complying with the *No Admittance* signs. He told an anecdote about a landowner in the Cotswolds who failed to deter trespassers from picnicking in his woods until he put up a sign saying 'Beware of the snakes'. For similar reasons, why on earth would any unprotected person visit the smallpox lab or corridor? In fact, they would be under a duty not to!

Escott-Cox dismissed the supposed problems with the use of gowns, saying that experts had agreed this was a non-issue, particularly if one discounts the potential for airborne transmission —and that repeatedly changing gowns was more hazardous than leaving them on.

The barrister marshalled three lines of evidence to show that contamination of the lab with smallpox was not a concern: the lack of radioactivity detected by Mr Farr; the lack of cross-contamination of viral cultures; and the evidence from Professor Dumbell that he could grow no smallpox from Bedson's containers.

Escott-Cox reminded the court that Bedson's lab had passed muster with DPAG, the DHSS and the WHO (albeit with reservations) and to convict the University would therefore be tantamount to over-ruling these august bodies. He poured scorn on one witness for the Prosecution, Dr Harris, who he claimed was neither independent nor an expert on smallpox, and he noted how another Prosecution witness, Professor Keith Dumbell, had given testimony that favoured the Defence.

In his last few minutes in the stand, Escott-Cox pointed out the flawed logic of the Prosecution case, whereby all three issues of vaccination, pox-in-the-ducts and lab techniques mattered only if long-range airborne transmission of smallpox were possible and that had not been proven. He noted the dreadfully regrettable death of Janet Parker, but made clear that the fact that she contracted smallpox and died did not in itself prove any breach of duty on the part of the University.

Escott-Cox's oration ended with a paean to Bedson guaranteed to stir the emotions, then and now:

'The work that Professor Bedson was doing was of great importance. We all know that. He was supported actively by the World Health Organization and the Medical Research Council. He was carrying out work with facilities provided for him by the University and I suppose in these days, and probably always, there is not the least reason in the world why we should not be very proud of the fact that these Britons have been in the forefront of this research, have been in the forefront of eradicating smallpox from the world, and men like Professor Bedson and his three colleagues are the men who were there, as it has been described in this case, pushing back the frontiers of scientific and medical knowledge to bring about these wonderful things, following in a fine tradition that this country can be proud of. I am not just saying that for emotional reasons, your worships. The university provided the facilities for Professor Bedson and in choosing him to use and run those facilities you may think that they might have been able to choose another man as good, they would have been hard pressed to choose a better man, a man of the greatest standing, a man of whom nobody has anything but respect and praise.

The procedures that he carried out, his great care, his great concern for the safety of others, all show that the University placed in him, in the right man, every confidence that their laboratory would be used in a safe and proper manner. No evidence which has been called in this case in my submission proves to the contrary. That university has a great reputation and rightly so, not merely in this city where we can be justly proud of it but elsewhere. It is not just a question of the burden of proof in this case, but I would ask your worships to say that the great reputation can go on unsullied by a finding of guilt on these summonses, allegations that have been made and which are far from proven.

I do not wish to repeat myself and I am not going over any of this ground again, but I ask you to look at all those matters and to look and see if I am right, and if you agree I am right on that one central issue that in the absence of long-range airborne infection no known or reasonably anticipated danger can exist, to say, and be happy to say, as I am sure you would be, without fear of recrimination that this summons is not made out and bring in a finding of not guilty.'

It was, by now, late morning. The senior magistrate thanked Mr Escott-Cox and announced that the court would adjourn until ten o'clock the next morning.

60

VERDICT

MR JAMES BAILEY, CHAIRMAN of the court and the senior of the three magistrates, began Day Twelve of the case by thanking Mr Colston and Mr. Escott-Cox for their presentation of evidence and the assistance they had given the magistrates in hearing the case. He then returned the court's verdict: 'It is our unanimous decision that the information laid against the University of Birmingham is dismissed'.

The chairman agreed that the costs of the case could be met from central funds. Both lead barristers thanked the magistrates for agreeing to hear the case themselves, rather than insist it go to the Crown Court.

The 'Not Guilty' verdict in a court of law meant that the University and Professor Bedson were now exonerated. However, the HSE was not the only agency to bring a case over the smallpox incident—in May, the ASTMS issued sixteen writs against the University on behalf of Janet Parker's husband and mother and fourteen members of the union who had suffered 'personal injury and/or physical harm'. As a result Janet Parker's husband, Joseph, was awarded £25,000 in compensation for her death.[1]

ON 9 DECEMBER 1979 a commission of experts signed a parchment declaring that infection with smallpox had been eradicated from the face of the planet.[2] The following year, the World Health Assembly ratified the eradication of smallpox, declaring 'solemnly that the world and its peoples have won freedom from smallpox, which was a most devastating disease sweeping in epidemic form through many countries since earliest time, leaving death, blindness and disfigurement in its wake…'[3]

In 1999, a paper entitled *A variant of variola virus, characterized by changes in polypeptide and endonuclease profiles* was published in the journal *Epidemiology and Infection*.[4] The authors included Keith Dumbell, Linda Harper, Sandy Buchan and Henry Bedson. A poignant footnote states: 'Henry Bedson died in 1978 but was closely involved in the planning and execution of the polypeptide work.'

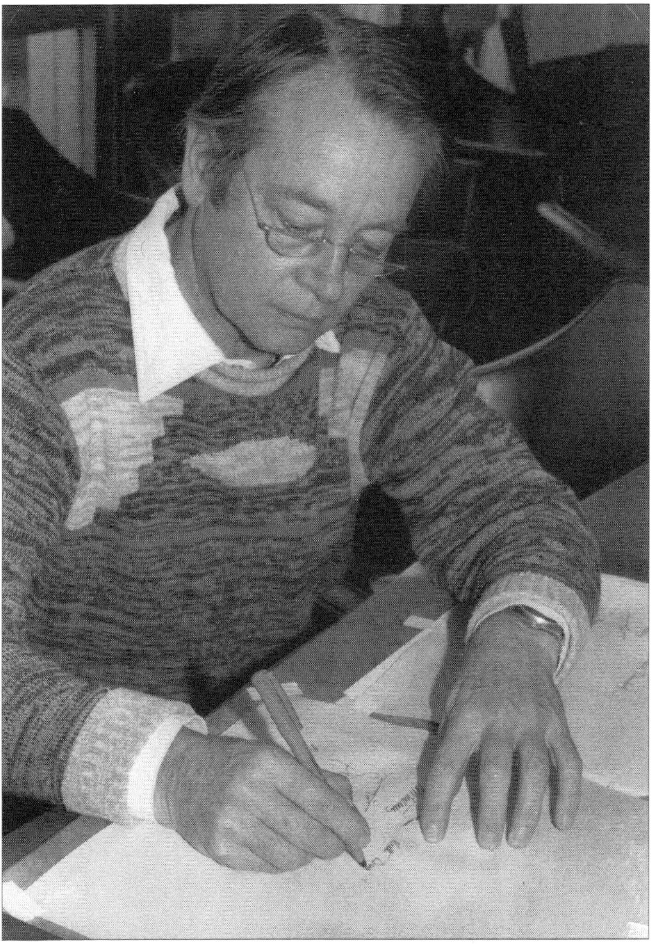

BRITISH SMALLPOX EXPERT, KEITH DUMBELL
In 1979, signing the WHO parchment certifying the eradication of smallpox
{Source: K. Dumbell}

61

PERSONAL INTERLUDE

HARRY'S HUMOUR

I first met Harry Smith through a colleague Brendan Wren in the early 1990s. Brimming with the prejudice of youth, I found it odd that my colleague should show such deference to a short old man with a strong regional accent. However, I soon developed a sense of deference myself when I learned that it was Harry who had discovered anthrax toxin and that he had worked at Porton Down and in Birmingham.

Harry celebrated his eightieth birthday shortly after I arrived in Birmingham. Over the next ten years, I often saw Harry out and about on the University campus, on his way to seminars. I asked him if he remembered the smallpox incident. He said, 'yes, he did' and expressed great sadness as he recalled being told that Bedson had cut his throat.

Several years later, as I started work on this book, my thoughts returned to Harry, particularly as another long-standing Birmingham academic, Jeff Cole, suggested to me that the Shooter Report was a cover-up and that Harry, who had signed the Official Secrets Act, might know what really happened.

Through another colleague, Steve Busby, I learned that Harry, now in his nineties, often came to the University for a lunchtime drink in the Staff House bar. We hatched up a plan—and one day, as Harry was leaving the bar, I confronted him, asking what he could tell me about the real story of the 1978 incident. He saw off the intrusion with a terse response: 'I know more than I can say', before shuffling off into a car.

Harry died a few weeks later and we gathered to pay our last respects at a local crematorium. The heavily religious ceremony was largely lost on a bunch of hard-headed academics. Afterwards, I asked Steve Busby whether Harry was religious and was told 'no, he was just an atheist with a strange sense of humour'. That put Harry's remarks on the smallpox incident in a new light—perhaps his 'mock-007' response was just another example of Harry's sense of humour—and rather than sitting on some hidden truth, he was just stringing me along. So, I learned to be comfortable with the idea that smallpox in Birmingham was neither conspiracy nor cock-up—just a mystery that will outlive us all.

But then new evidence turned up...

PART SEVEN

AFTERMATH

62

BIRMINGHAM 2013

BERYL OPPENHEIM GREW UP in Johannesburg[1] and graduated in medicine from the University of the Witwatersrand in 1977. She completed her specialist training in Medical Microbiology in South Africa before moving to the UK in 1985. She spent most of the next fifteen years working in Manchester, before moving to Heartlands Hospital (the new name for the East Birmingham Hospital) in 2001.

A decade later, Beryl moved to a consultant job at the Queen Elizabeth Hospital, which shares a campus with the University of Birmingham Medical School. A short while later, she took on the role of Director of Infection Prevention and Control within the local NHS Trust.

However, little in Beryl's distinguished career prepared her for what happened when a patient with a new deadly and contagious viral infection arrived in her hospital—right in the heart of Birmingham and just a few hundred yards from where Janet Parker had caught smallpox more than three decades before.

On 20 September 2012, Dr Ali Mohamed Zaki, an Egyptian virologist working in Saudi Arabia, announces the existence of a frightening new infection in an email to the emerging diseases network ProMED. In his posting, he describes the first case, a fatal lung infection in a 60-year-old Saudi man, and announces culture of a new coronavirus.[2] This prompt disclosure quickly leads to a diagnostic test; unfortunately, it also leads to Dr Zaki losing his job.[3]

The story then shifts to the UK.[4] Late in 2012, a 38-year-old man of Pakistani heritage, Khalid Hussain, is diagnosed with a brain tumour. Khalid works as a travel agent in Rotherham, but, after the diagnosis, moves to Birmingham to receive chemotherapy at the Queen Elizabeth Hospital. In the closing weeks of 2012, Khalid's father, Abid Hussain, who has lived in Birmingham for many years, travels to Pakistan with his daughter to let his relatives know of his son's diagnosis.

In late January, on his way back from Pakistan, Abid visits the Muslim holy cities of Mecca and Medina in Saudi Arabia, to pray for Khalid. While in Arabia, he develops a fever and a cough.

On 28 January, Khalid meets his father at Heathrow Airport and drives him home. Abid's symptoms worsen and he is admitted to Birmingham's City Hospital on 5 February. Initial investigations show that Abid is carrying influenza virus. However, when anti-flu drugs fail to make an impact, a sample is tested for the new coronavirus and found to be positive.

Just as in 1978, the recognition that a patient is carrying a deadly viral infection prompts an immediate search for contacts and an exhaustive public health response. Contacts are tracked down from Abid's plane journey, from his family and among health care workers. Over one hundred close contacts are identified in the UK, including Abid's son Khalid and Abid's sister Zaida, who both test positive for the new coronavirus.

Abid is transferred to Manchester for specialist care, where he spends many weeks in a coma before the damage to his lungs leads to his death. Zaida recovers quickly. However, Khalid's cancer treatment has suppressed his immune system and made him highly susceptible to infection. He is admitted, seriously ill, to the Queen Elizabeth Hospital in Birmingham on Saturday 9 February.

Over the next ten days, as head of infection control, Beryl Oppenheim juggles demands from many quarters simultaneously. She ensures that Khalid is placed under stringent isolation in a negative-pressure room in the hospital's Intensive Care Unit. She makes difficult decisions about the family's access to the potentially infectious patient. She weighs up the risk to hospital staff from the new infection and advises health care workers on infection control She liaises with external organisations and interacts with experts on emerging viral infections, while also briefing the hospital's communications team, who keep the media informed.

Ten days after admission, despite the best efforts of the doctors on the Intensive Care Unit and the Medical Microbiology team, Khalid Hussein loses his battle with the virus, leaving behind a grief-stricken wife, Azima, and three-year-old twin boys, Danyal and Zain.

THE NEW INFECTION is named *Middle Eastern Respiratory Syndrome* (or *MERS*) shortly after the Birmingham outbreak and at the time of writing just under 2000 cases have been reported worldwide.[5] Transmission of MERS in hospitals remains a risk, as evidenced by outbreaks in Saudi Arabia and South Korea. The fact that in 2013, just as in 1978, Birmingham saw off the threat of a deadly viral epidemic stands testament to the professionalism of the city's health care professionals—then and now.

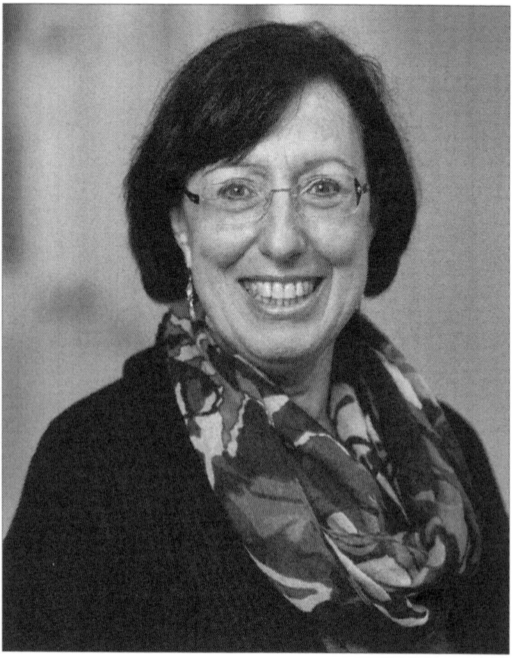

BERYL OPPENHEIM
Infection control doctor in Birmingham during the 2013 MERS incident
{Source: B. Oppenheim}

63

WORST-CASE SCENARIOS

...these dead shall not have died in vain.
Lincoln at Gettysburg, under the influence of smallpox.

THE TRAGIC DEATHS of Janet Parker and Henry Bedson represent the worst-case scenario for health and safety at work. In an ideal world, Parker's death from laboratory-acquired infection and Bedson's suicide triggered by work-related stress would be 'never-events'—like a maternal death in childbirth or surgery on the wrong patient—that should never be allowed to happen.[1] However, in the real world, laboratory-acquired infection and stress in the workplace sadly remain an enduring problem.

Accidents or near-misses still occur in microbiology laboratories, despite ever-tighter regulation and the efforts of organisations like the UK's Health and Safety Executive.[2] The *Guardian* reported in early 2018 that the HSE investigated over forty mishaps at specialist laboratories over a two-year period.[3] *USA Today* paints a similar picture in the USA, with over eleven hundred incidents involving 'select agents' reported by labs from 2008 to 2012, most requiring medical attention.[4]

Perhaps the most worrying recent near-miss in the UK occurred in May 2012, when staff at the Animal Health and Veterinary Laboratories Agency in Weybridge, Surrey, posted mislabelled tubes containing live anthrax bacteria to labs across the UK, some of which were then handled on the open bench.[5] The timing was ironic, as the UK government was just then preparing for a potential bioterrorist release of anthrax at the London Olympics. Two years later, a high-security lab at the US Centers for Disease Control and Prevention also sent samples of live anthrax bacteria to low-security labs, thinking they had been inactivated.[6]

The Amerithrax incident—the deliberate release of anthrax into the American postal system by biodefense scientist Bruce Ivins—highlights the need to take malicious behaviour into account in risk assessments on dangerous pathogens.[7] Aside from five deaths through deliberate release, this incident also resulted in one case of lab-acquired infection, caught by handling vials contaminated on the outside with *Bacillus anthracis*.

A few years later, in the wake of the outbreak of *Severe Acute Respiratory Syndrome* (*SARS*) in 2002-3, there were four separate lab accidents that resulted in infections with the SARS virus; in one case, an infected lab worker spread the virus to other people.[8] More recently, multistate outbreaks of laboratory-associated *Salmonella* infection, linked to clinical and teaching labs in the US and associated with at least one death, have prompted a call for a centralised registry of laboratory-acquired infections.[9]

What of the worst-case scenario: death from an infection caught in a lab? Sadly, over 170 deaths from lab-acquired infection have been documented in the medical literature, although most occurred before 1978.[10] In recent years, such deaths have become rare, but there is no room for complacency. In 2014, Simon Silver reviewed recent deaths associated with research labs,[11] including the death of Malcolm Casadaban from plague at a University of Chicago lab; the death of Richard Din in California from laboratory-acquired meningococcal meningitis and the deaths of six African researchers from Ebola virus infection—Mohamed Fullah, Mbalu Fonnie, Alex Moigboi, Sidiki Saffa, Alice Kovoma, S. Humarr Khan—poignantly named as posthumous authors on an Ebola genome-sequencing paper.[12]

Aside from death, lab-acquired infection can lead to serious life-changing injury. In 2005, a former colleague of the author, Jeannette Abu-Bobie, caught meningococcal septicaemia while working at an Environment Science and Research laboratory in New Zealand. As a result, she lost both legs, her left arm and the fingers on her right hand. After initially denying responsibility, the New Zealand authorities eventually paid compensation.[13]

These worst-case scenario outcomes have informed debate on research on potentially pandemic viruses, particularly research involving gain-of-function mutations, which might increase virulence or transmissibility in humans. In 2014, the US authorities instituted a moratorium on gain-of-function research on influenza, MERS and SARS. However, the moratorium was lifted in late 2017, with the chairman of the National Science Advisory Board for Biosecurity providing the bullish justification: 'nature is the ultimate bio-terrorist and we need to do all we can to stay one step ahead'.[14]

Laboratory-acquired infection with poxviruses remains a concern. From 2005 to 2008 in the USA alone, there were sixteen reported laboratory exposures to vaccinia and six laboratory-acquired infections, four resulting in hospitalisation.[15] Infections with genetically engineered vaccinia strains have been reported.[16] Laboratory infection has also been described with buffalopox virus, a close relative of vaccinia.[17]

Poxviruses still sometimes play the trickster. In July 2010, a laboratory researcher working on a pox virus harmless to humans developed a painful, ulcerated lesion on the ring finger of his right hand, which was subsequently associated with flu-like symptoms.[18] A subsequent investigation revealed that he had been infected with a strain of cowpox virus, which was being stored in a freezer in the lab, even though no one was currently working on it. It turned out that the cowpox virus had contaminated six virus or cell culture stocks in the lab and poxvirus DNA was detected in three environmental swabs taken from laboratory surfaces, including a freezer handle and the outside and inside of a box, where only poxviruses harmless to humans were stored.

Although Janet Parker's case remains unusual in affecting an outsider rather than a lab worker, it is not unique in that regard. Just a few months after Parker's death, accidental release of anthrax spores from a Russian bioweapons lab in Sverdlovsk led to at least sixty-six deaths among bystanders downwind from the site.[19]

Janet Parker's case also illustrates a persistent problem with laboratory-acquired infection: often, no obvious breach of protocol or mishap in the lab can be identified that might account for the infection. Back in the 1970s, 80% of laboratory-acquired infections fell into the *unexplained* category, with no obvious route of infection.[20] Recent studies suggest this percentage has fallen,[21] but hard-to-explain infections still occur and coming up with a neat chain of causality often remains impossible. For example, there is no doubt that Malcolm Casadaban's infection with a weakened version of the plague bacillus was acquired from the lab.[22] He was suffering from an unsuspected condition, haemochromatosis, that made him more susceptible than usual to infection with this pathogen. However, it remains unclear how enough of the bacterium got into his tissues to cause infection, when to establish a similar infection in susceptible mice requires administration of half a billion bacterial cells.

It may be argued that we could avoid the risk of laboratory-acquired infection if we simply stopped working on pathogens. However, handling potentially dangerous pathogens in the clinical diagnostic lab is unavoidable and the only way to be sure that no infections are ever acquired in the research lab would be to ban all research on pathogens—which would mean no new anti-microbial drugs or vaccines. Instead, as we press on with work on dangerous pathogens, the Birmingham smallpox incident reminds us how badly things can go wrong and should force us to recognise that risk assessments and training in health and safety are not simply paper exercises, but vital tools in the prevention of harm.

STRESS IN THE WORKPLACE remains an enduring problem, afflicting over half a million workers per year in the UK and accounting for over twelve million working days lost.[23] Stress, burn-out, bullying and related mental health problems among academics are on the rise.[24] Henry Bedson's suicide reminds us of the worst-case scenario here and the duty of care that employers have to their staff and that we all have to our colleagues.[25] Sadly, contemporary cases echo what happened to Bedson. In 2003, the British microbiologist David Kelly committed suicide after political and press harassment in relation to the UK Government's dossier on weapons of mass destruction in Iraq.[26] In 2012, Stefan Grimm, who held a Chair in Toxicology at Imperial College London, took his own life, after being told that he was 'struggling to fulfil the metrics' of his professorial post.[27]

The kind of intrusive harassment by the news media that contributed to Henry Bedson's suicide remains all too common, as revealed by the News International phone hacking scandal and the subsequent Leveson Inquiry.[28] In 2013, British primary school teacher Lucy Meadows killed herself after her gender reassignment became national news.[29] At her inquest, the coroner adopted a stance chillingly similar to that adopted by his predecessor at Bedson's inquest: in closing the inquest, he turned to the reporters present and said, 'And to you the press, I say shame, shame on all of you.'

An unwelcome development is that the Internet makes persecution of vulnerable individuals much easier. British journalist Jon Ronson's exploration of public shaming *So You've Been Publicly Shamed* shows how lives can be destroyed by the online herd mentality.[30] Sadly, social media have also fuelled the alternative facts agenda pioneered by Clive Jenkins and Sheila McKechnie in the 1970s—but the fake news is now often propagated by those in government.[31]

64

AFTERLIFE OF THE POX

As a psycholinguist who once wrote an entire book on the past tense, I can single out my favourite example in the history of the English language:

> *'Smallpox was an infectious disease caused by one of two virus variants, Variola major and Variola minor.'*

Yes, "smallpox was".
Steven Pinker (2018) *Enlightenment Now*

WHAT OF SMALLPOX THESE last forty years? Here, the news is good. Eradication stands firm—in Pinker's words, smallpox still *was* rather than *is*. There have been no cases of smallpox in humans or wild animals, whitepox proved to be a contaminant[1] and there has been no spillover of taterapox from gerbils to humans.

Other poxviruses present variable threats to humans. Variola's close relative, camelpox, is a worldwide problem in camels, but, despite its close evolutionary relationship to smallpox, there has been only a handful of human infections, with no human-to-human transmission [2] Among camel handlers in Rajasthan, the rash took a similar course to smallpox, with papules, vesicles, ulceration and finally scabs, but was restricted to the fingers and hands.[3] Buffalopox has also proven a problem, with recurrent reports of human infections in India and elsewhere, but again infection is mostly limited to the hands with no well-documented human-to-human transmission.[4]

Monkeypox represents a more significant threat, closely mimicking smallpox clinically and sometimes proving fatal, even though the virus responsible is only distantly related to variola virus.[5] Despite its name, monkeypox most commonly spills over into humans from rodents. Several hundred human infections have now been documented and outbreaks have proven a recurrent problem in remote villages of Central and West Africa close to tropical rainforests. Although human-to-human transmission seems to be less efficient than for smallpox, the longest chain of human-to-human spread has involved seven transmission events.[6]

In 2003, the United States experienced a monkeypox outbreak among humans and captive prairie dogs, but fortunately with no deaths or human-to-human spread. Epidemiological investigations traced the source back to a shipment of wild Gambian pouched rats (*Cricetomys gambianus*) from Ghana.[7] Fortunately, vaccination with vaccinia is protective against monkeypox, which limits the potential for pandemic spread.

Cowpox continues to cause sporadic infections in humans, often caught from domestic cats.[8] However, the viruses given the name 'cowpox' appear to be a heterogeneous group that represents at least five distinct species.[9]

The vaccinia virus used in vaccine formulations is quite distinct from the cowpox viruses and the history and origins of vaccine strains remain unclear.[10] Genomic analysis of an early twentieth century vaccine formulation using ancient-DNA approaches revealed that at least some historical vaccine preparations contained the horsepox virus rather than vaccinia.[11]

Interestingly, the vaccinia virus has acquired a curious troublesome afterlife in the post-eradication era, not just spreading from human to human after vaccination (often through sex[12]), but also going wild in the cattle population in Brazil, causing infections in humans and livestock with appreciable economic impact.[13]

ALTHOUGH SMALLPOX AS a human disease has been eradicated, stocks of the smallpox virus still exist. In the years following eradication, the world's stocks of variola virus were destroyed or transferred to two WHO-designated laboratories with the highest containment facilities (*BSL-4 labs* in the jargon)—one in the USA, at CDC, Atlanta, Georgia, the other within Russia's State Research Centre of Virology and Biotechnology, also known as VECTOR.[14]

The WHO initially recommended destruction of all stocks of variola virus in 1986, but on several occasions since then, the virus has experienced a stay of execution.[15] Authorities have argued that the virus stocks are needed for continuing research on smallpox, while critics argue that the stocks present a continuing unnecessary risk of lab-acquired infection or escape of the virus from the lab.[16] In defence of the policy of retaining stocks of variola virus, the US Institute of Medicine produced reports in 1999 and 2009 evaluating research needs and achievements.[17]

So what has been achieved in the science of smallpox since eradication? Genome sequencing has elucidated the relationships between more than forty variola virus strains and confirmed the close relationships with camelpox and taterapox.[18] Most recently, recovery of a seventeenth century variola genome from a Lithuanian mummy and recovery of variola genomes from Czech museum specimens have suggested that all extant strains of the smallpox virus have a relatively recent common ancestor—no longer ago than the fourteenth or fifteenth century CE—and that the smallpox virus lineage diverged from the ancestor of taterapox and camelpox as recently as the third century CE, i.e. long after Ramesses V.[19] These findings cast doubt on the widely-held view that smallpox is an ancient disease and refocus interest on an old observation that virulent smallpox was unknown in the UK and Europe before the sixteenth century.[20]

Genome sequencing has also primed the development of novel DNA-based diagnostic assays allowing rapid recognition of smallpox and smallpox-like illnesses.[21] In the scariest post-eradication excursion of live variola virus, a new animal model of smallpox has been established in cynomolgus macaques and used to test new drugs and explore the remarkable way in which the smallpox virus manipulates the host immune response.[22]

Biodefence-driven concerns about the re-emergence of smallpox have delivered a productive research programme yielding new tools for preventing and treating the infection. New drugs active against smallpox include tecovirimat, which works by preventing the virus from leaving infected cells, and brincidofovir, a new more active version of an old drug cidofovir, which works by inhibiting viral DNA synthesis.[23] Neither are yet licenced for use against smallpox, but the US has created a stockpile of tecovirimat, for use in the event of an outbreak. Safer derivatives of vaccinia virus have been developed, including Imvanex, a vaccine strain unable to replicate in human cells, and Lc16m8, an attenuated, replicating smallpox vaccine developed in Japan.[24]

Various scenarios for the return of smallpox have been entertained. An obvious risk is accidental infection from an overlooked laboratory source. Smallpox DNA was found in a South African laboratory in 2013, but soon destroyed in the presence of WHO officials.

More worryingly, in July 2014 sixteen sealed glass vials of variola virus were discovered in cardboard boxes found in an unused part of a storeroom in a Food and Drug Administration lab at the National Institutes of Health in Bethesda, Maryland.[25] The vials appeared to date back to the 1950s. They were immediately transferred to the CDC's high-containment facility in Atlanta, which confirmed the presence of variola virus DNA. Luckily, none of the vials broke before reaching the high-containment facility. However, after arrival there, they remained in limbo for several months as international protocols require that the WHO witnesses the destruction of the samples, but no WHO staff had the necessary clearance to enter the CDC's facility. They were finally destroyed in February 2015.[26]

Concerns have been raised—but then downplayed—about the potential release of smallpox virus from long-dead human material, for example museum samples, archaeological remains or bodies thawing out from permafrost.[27]

A more pressing concern is that smallpox might be revived for malevolent purposes, such as biowarfare or bioterrorism. Mindful of such risks, in June 2001, US authorities simulated a covert smallpox attack on the United States in an exercise entitled 'Dark Winter'. After a fictional deliberate release of illegally held laboratory stocks of the smallpox virus, they contemplated how an initial infection of three thousand individuals could lead to a million deaths after four rounds of infection.

In recent years, an alternative doomwatch scenario has emerged: re-creation of smallpox virus using genetic engineering. This worrying possibility has been rendered all the more credible by publication in early 2018 of a study in which horsepox virus (a close relative of the smallpox virus) was synthesised from scratch in a Canadian lab, providing would-be terrorists with a recipe for construction of the variola virus.[28] However, one has to question why a bioterrorist would go to all the bother of building a smallpox virus, which has a large and complex genome, when obtaining more dangerous alternatives, such as Ebola virus, or creating a small genetically engineered virus carrying a lethal toxin, would require far less effort.[29]

Nonetheless, there are plans and guidelines in place for coping with a smallpox outbreak[30] and in the unlikely case that smallpox returns—and this book requires a new title—we will be better prepared than we were in the pre-eradication era, as we now have new drugs and vaccines, plus a global stockpile of 600-700 million vaccine doses. We beat smallpox once and can be confident that we will do so again—*if* it ever returns.

65

PERSONAL INTERLUDE

CDC & MLK

It is 31 May 2015 and thanks to a thunderstorm, I am stuck in New York. I am en route to an American Society of Microbiology meeting in New Orleans, but have stopped off for a couple of days in the Big Apple. Yesterday, I visited Ellis Island and the Statue of Liberty. Today, I grabbed some lunch in downtown Harlem. It has been an unbearably hot sultry day, so I arrived early at the airport to benefit from the air conditioning.

The heat and humidity have now culminated in a thunderstorm. I am supposed to be flying out this afternoon on to New Orleans, but a lightning strike has grounded all planes. No one can say when we will be able to fly. As we reach early evening, my jet-lagged brain, stuck five hours ahead, is telling me I desperately need to sleep. It looks as if we are going to arrive in New Orleans very late that evening.

After struggling with fatigue and the uncertain wait for news for several hours, I finally pluck up courage to ask the man at the desk how easy it would be for me to re-book on a flight the next morning. He seems positively pleased that I am volunteering to abandon the delayed flight. I search for a nearby hotel and as I take a brief taxi ride across a multi-lane highway, the heavens open, there is a roar of thunder and lightning illuminates the sky.

I sleep well and the next morning's flight is uneventful. I arrive just in time to meet my hosts for lunch, stepping straight out of the taxi from the airport into the diner. My trip has been hosted by former microbiology colleague from Birmingham, Lars Westblade, who now works at Emory University in Atlanta, Georgia. After lunch, I participate in a conference session on the use of genomics in clinical microbiology and then grab a couple of late afternoon beers with the American science writer Carl Zimmer and one of the big names in microbiome studies, Julie Segre. I go to bed early and fly out the next day to Atlanta, Georgia.

Lars has persuaded me to stop by at his workplace, Emory University in Atlanta, to give a seminar and meet local medics and academics. It was meant at first to be a one-night stop, but once news of my visit gets out, Lars tells me I have an invite to stay a second night, hosted by the Centers for Disease Control and Prevention (CDC). I am flattered to be asked and snap up the offer.

As soon as we arrive in Atlanta, Lars takes me to a local bar, Leon's Full Service, in the university suburb of Decatur, where, clearly well known to the bar staff, he orders us both a cocktail called Penicillin—a heady concoction of scotch, honey-ginger syrup and lemon juice. Alcohol helps me re-tune my body clock.

Over drinks, Lars explains that the Southern states are still different from the North, pointing out that here Lincoln's war is sometimes ironically styled the War of Northern Aggression. Later that evening, I check into the tranquil, quietly atmospheric Emory Conference Center Hotel, designed by the eminent American architect Frank Lloyd Wright.

After a fruitful day at Emory discussing microbial genome sequencing, the following evening I switch over to becoming a guest of CDC, where my host is an agreeable bioinformatician called Scott Sammons. We dine with other CDC staff, then visit a local bar, which sports an impressive array of microbrewery-produced beers. During our conversation, I mention that I used to work in Birmingham, know the doctor who diagnosed the last case of smallpox and have started writing this book. Scott says he hadn't any inkling of my interest in smallpox, but would see what he could do to integrate it into my itinerary.

First thing next morning, Scott picks me up from the hotel and takes me to a New York-style deli, the General Muir, just across the road from CDC. There we meet Dr Inger Damon, who is dressed in a navy-style uniform that reflects her role as an officer in the United States Public Health Service Commissioned Corps. We discuss the Birmingham 1978 incident and I ask if she is worried that someone might recreate smallpox from scratch using DNA synthesis. She nods in agreement.

At the time we meet, my interests in smallpox are still limited to uncovering what happened in Birmingham in 1978 and I have not familiarised myself with recent research. Only later do I realise that I have had an audience with the world's foremost smallpox expert, who still works with live variola virus.

As Scott takes me into CDC, he explains how much they have boosted their security after the 9-11 attacks, with a perimeter wall with such deep foundations that it could withstand a car bomb. He drops me off at the CDC Museum, where I come face to face not just with exhibits from the smallpox eradication campaign, but a range of material illustrating CDC's enduring frontline role in disease control, including AIDS, swine flu, the deliberate release of anthrax and efforts to eradicate guinea worm and polio.

One eye-catching poster reminds me that CDC doesn't just work on infection. Under the faces of Martin Luther King, James Chaney and Malcolm X sits a banner proclaiming they were 'great men who fought for a great cause and who died for their beliefs. Their deaths were a tragedy, but not a waste.' The poster reaches the rather ungainly conclusion that African Americans who believe they cannot quit smoking are also likely to die for their beliefs.

We walk across to another building on the CDC campus, to grab a buffet lunch before my seminar. I look out of the window across the campus and experience a frisson of excitement, as I realise that I am just a few hundred yards away from the last vestiges of one of mankind's most fearful microbial adversaries.

After the seminar, and having just twigged that Atlanta was the home of one of my heroes, Martin Luther King, I ask Scott if he minds breaking the journey to the airport at the city's Martin Luther King Jr. National Historic Site, which includes King's birthplace, his church and his final resting place. Scott is more than happy to oblige and seems mildly embarrassed to admit that, although the site is only twenty minutes away from CDC by car, he has never been there. I ask him if he remembers segregation, to which he replies 'yes, I grew up in South Georgia and my school was segregated until I started fifth grade. I also remember our local doctor's surgery having segregated waiting rooms'.

We park up and more or less stumble into the Ebenezer Baptist Church. We are quickly directed downstairs into the church's main auditorium, where we are given a talk by the African American orator, Stephon Ferguson, on the King family's links to the church and the tragic history of their lives cut short by violence.

What starts off as a routine lecture soon turns into something altogether grander, as Ferguson asks us to cast our minds back to August 1963, as Martin Luther King Jr addresses the crowd from the Great March on Washington. Suddenly, Ferguson, the only speaker licenced by the King family to recite MLK's speeches, is transformed into the great civil rights leader, his baritone voice projecting the 'I have a dream' speech across the auditorium.

As the speech draws to a close, the line about 'Let freedom ring from Stone Mountain of Georgia' catches my attention. Scott has clearly noticed it too because, as the soaring rhetoric ends, he lets out a quiet 'Wow, that was quite something—I live just near Stone Mountain, it's just half an hour's drive away!'

With the speech's climactic final words 'free at last, free at last, thank God Almighty, we are free at last' echoing through my head, my thoughts turn to a world free of smallpox, thanks to the same idealism that permeated King's speech. Sadly, it's a world that King died too soon to see, but it is one inherited by his children and his children's children, while ironically the great orator and the great trickster slumber a few miles apart.

66

EMERGENCE OR ERADICATION?

ALTHOUGH THE THREAT OF resurgent smallpox may be small, other viruses have emerged since eradication as real or potential threats to global health. As documented in David Quammen's excellent book, *Spillover*,[1] these emerging diseases are usually the result of viruses jumping from animals to humans.

In 1981, just a year after smallpox was declared gone, AIDS was first recognised in the United States[2] and the causative virus, HIV—a spillover from chimps—went on to infect more than 76 million people, killing over half of them.[3] However, as a testament to human ingenuity, within a few years of recognising the new disease, highly active anti-retroviral therapy was developed to treat the infection.[4]

Between November 2002 and July 2003, an outbreak of SARS that started in southern China spread to 37 countries and went on to cause eight thousand cases and over seven hundred deaths.[5] As we have seen, another emerging viral infection, MERS, was first recognised in Saudi Arabia in 2012, but was soon seen more widely in humans and in camels, with over two thousand human infections reported to date.[6]

From 2013 to 2016, Ebola virus disease caused devastating loss of life and societal disruption in Guinea, Liberia, and Sierra Leone, killing over 11,000 people, and striking with a case fatality rate of around 70% in the worst hit areas.[7] There was limited overspill into Nigeria, Mali, Senegal, the UK, Italy, the USA and Spain.

In 2015, Zika virus hit the headlines as the cause of an epidemic spreading across Brazil and to other parts of the world, bringing the risk of microcephaly when acquired during pregnancy.[8]

On top of all this, the threat of pandemic flu hangs in the air—as does the spectre of antimicrobial resistance.[9]

AND YET, THE EXAMPLE of smallpox provides a powerful signal that the battle against infection can be won. In 2011, the United Nations Food and Agriculture Organization announced that rinderpest, a disease of cattle, had been eradicated from the planet[10]—the second disease after smallpox to be wiped out completely.

By the time most of you are reading this, the decades-long battle against dracunculiasis (also called Guinea worm), spear-headed by former US president Jimmy Carter, will almost certainly have been won—a countdown to zero that began in 1986, when there were around 3.5 million cases in over twenty countries in Africa and Asia.[11] Polio will not be far behind, with just 22 cases in 2017, with transmission limited to just three countries: Nigeria, Pakistan, and Afghanistan.[12]

On the horizon sit several more diseases ripe for eradication, including once-global viral infections like measles, rubella, mumps or tropical parasitic diseases like onchocerciasis, cysticercosis, lymphatic filariasis.[13] The global goliath is malaria[14], which Bill Gates believes can be eradicated by 2040. Given that the number of children who die from the disease has been halved in just fifteen years, he is probably right— after all, eradication of smallpox was just the start!

67

SO, WHAT ACTUALLY HAPPENED?

When you are puzzled by how somebody got infected with smallpox, the first question, probably the only question, you need to ask, is:
'Who has been naughty?'
Keith Dumbell (2018), quoting D. A. Henderson or Alan Downie[1]

FOUR DECADES ON, two questions remain: how did Janet Parker become infected with smallpox and why did she die from the infection?

When it comes to the source of infection, the arguments rehearsed during the trial of *Cook versus the University of Birmingham* still hold firm today: nothing that was being done in Bedson's smallpox lab can be linked in a tidy chain of causality—let alone culpability—to Janet Parker's illness. This absolves Bedson and the University of Birmingham of any blame for what happened.

Nonetheless, Shooter and his men were right in pointing out that lightning struck twice in that East Wing—it is hard to dismiss smallpox in two photographers working near a smallpox lab as mere coincidence. However, Shooter's pox-in-the-ducts explanation remains untenable, as none of the procedures underway in the smallpox lab could have generated an aerosol of viral particles of sufficient density for infection to drift upstairs.[2]

So what *did* happen? Even forty years ago, the odds were stacked against establishing a full account of events, with both protagonists in this tragic incident dead before serious inquiries could get underway. One might reasonably argue that nothing new can be added now, after the passage of so much time. However, conversations with two now-elderly participants in the 1979 trial have convinced me otherwise—as they have provided potential explanations for the *means*, the *motive* and the *opportunity* behind these tragic events.

PROFESSOR KEITH DUMBELL was a friend and colleague of Henry Bedson and is now one of the very few surviving experts with hands-on experience of smallpox in the pre-eradication era. Disgusted by the hysteria generated by the 1978 incident, Dumbell moved to

South Africa in the early 1980s. When I spoke and corresponded with him in 2017, he had reached the grand old age of 95, but was still intellectually as bright as a button, using Skype to ask me questions I could not easily answer on the genomics of variola virus.

Dumbell is convinced that those involved in the 1978 incident did not reveal the whole truth during Shooter's inquiry and the court case. He recalls that shortly after the incident, on a trip to Birmingham in Desmond Robinson's car, he asked the DHSS man 'off the record' whether he had any idea what had happened. Robinson replied that *he* did not have any idea, but that *somebody* did. He went on to say that he had interviewed lots of people and that when interviewing one particular individual at Birmingham, he had the strong feeling that something was being held back; that not all was being told. However, he mentioned no names.

In pursuit of this hidden truth, Dumbell has formulated a theory that provides the *means* and a previously unrecognised *opportunity* for infection. He begins his argument by positing that, given that the virus could not leave the pox lab to meet the photographer, the photographer must have gone to the pox lab to meet the virus.

Dumbell is also keen to explain why Janet and her predecessor Tony McLennan were singled out as photographers in their susceptibility to laboratory-acquired smallpox. His interest in an occupational explanation was kindled when the Shooter panel asked him if there was any hazard specific to photographers. He told them that he did not know of any, but the question has stayed with him.

After much thought, Keith's suggestion is—now that dermatitis caused by contact with developing fluid or other photographic reagents is recognised as an occupational hazard[3]—occupationally-acquired contact dermatitis, or even just dried out, defatted skin might have made it easier for the smallpox virus to breach the usual solid barrier of the skin and reach living cells. Assuming that work surfaces in the lab were contaminated with even a minute amount of variola virus, simply touching them in the presence of damaged skin without gloves on would provide a *means* for Janet (and Tony) to become infected.

What about *opportunity*? Keith notes that Janet Parker's smallpox followed an unusual course, in that it evolved slowly, even though it did eventually result in her death. Given this unusual time course once smallpox was established—together with the fact that Janet did not acquire infection in the normal way from another infectious human—Keith suggests that the incubation period in Janet Parker might have been much shorter than the usual twelve days. This argument is strengthened by the fact that similar shortening of the incubation period has been reported after direct inoculation of the variola virus into the skin.[4] This means that Janet might have been infected even after 3 August, the last date smallpox virus was handled in the lab according to Shooter's report.

According to Dumbell, this creates a previously unrecognised *opportunity* for her to acquire the infection, because Bedson left for a holiday in Wales shortly afterwards—and with the boss away, attitudes to safety might have been relaxed, even if only unconsciously, and someone might have granted Janet access to the pox lab after Bedson had left. Or perhaps the cleaners were in and out of the lab doing an end of term clean and left the door open or unlocked?

However, Dumbell's theory lacks a crucial component: *motive*. What on earth would have motivated Janet Parker to visit the pox lab? To answer this question, we must turn to testimony from another sagacious elder.

BRIAN ESCOTT-COX QC was the barrister who defended the University of Birmingham in the 1979 case. When I met him at his home in early 2018, despite his eighty-five years of age, he was astute, articulate and keen to share his understanding of what happened.[5]

Escott-Cox explained that during the 1979 court case, as a defence barrister, he met up several times each day with his instructing solicitor, Adrian Davis—typically for an hour first thing before each day's proceedings, then again during the two-hour lunch break and at the end of each day's session in court.

During one of these meetings, two or three days into the trial, Escott-Cox recalls that he turned to Davis to ask him, 'Adrian, you have got your ear very close to the ground on this. Do you know what actually happened?.' The solicitor said 'Well, all I can tell you is this. There is a very strong rumour going around...'

Before sharing the rumour, Escott-Cox reminded me that Janet had been infected towards the end of July, after the students had left for the summer. However, he noted that the University did not really shut down until the beginning of August, when most staff disappeared to take their summer holidays. He reminded me that, back in those pre-digital days, people who wanted to take photographs had to use cameras with films in them, with flash bulbs and other accessories—and, as a professional photographer, Janet could get these things very quickly and at an advantageous price.

Then, Brian shared the rumour that best explains what happened in 1978. According to the rumour, in the run-up to the summer holidays, Janet visited all the departments of the Medical School, knocking on doors, asking people before they went off on their holidays whether they wanted any photographic film or other materials—letting people know that she could get these things at a reduced price. Perhaps, she made a small mark-up on the film she supplied—Shooter reported that she did private work for her colleagues—or, perhaps, she just did all these favours from the goodness of her heart? Perhaps, some of the film she ordered was used for work purposes , but some for taking holiday snaps?

Crucially, the rumour went, one of Janet's visits was to the pox laboratory—and that was how she caught smallpox.

Certainly, an end-of-year trip up and down stairs and along corridors would have provided a clear *motive* for her to visit the pox lab. If she knocked on the outer door and found no answer, she might have been tempted to enter the outer lab. Maybe, Janet then put her hands down on a work surface contaminated with variola virus? Or maybe she knocked on the door of the inner smallpox lab and someone handling smallpox came out to greet her? After all, if this had become a familiar annual ritual—and given that Janet was known around the place—no one would have challenged her. In any case, she had been vaccinated, just not all that recently.

Although back in 1979, Davis qualified his assertion with the caveat: 'I am bound to say that there is not a shred of evidence to support it.', when Escott-Cox and I discussed this potential explanation, four additional pieces of evidence fell into place and, in Brian's words, provided *prima facie* evidence that the rumour was true.

First, the Shooter Report makes much of the fact that during the last two weeks in July and the first week in August, Janet Parker was on the phone several times a day, every day, busily contacting suppliers to order photographic materials. The Report stresses that Parker placed an unusually large number of orders on 25 July. Shooter's explanation for this behaviour was that the Department's accounting year ended on 31 July.

However, Shooter's photographer-on-the-phone explanation seems incomplete on two counts. Why did only Janet become infected, when her unvaccinated coffee mates also used the telephone room? And what on earth was Parker intending to do with all the photographic material she was ordering? Janet's strenuous efforts on the phone make a lot more sense if they were twinned with an exhaustive trek around the Medical School to take orders for photographic materials, just in time for the summer holidays.

Second, the photographer-doing-the-rounds rumour is strengthened by—and explains—Sandy Buchan's fleeting encounter with Janet Parker, mentioned in the Shooter Report and in the court case. In itself, Buchan's visit to the photographic studio probably presents too indirect a link to the pox lab to account for Parker's infection. But remember why it took place: because Buchan had been asked by a colleague to let Janet know what kind of photographic film, developer and fixer Buchan used in his own photographic process. Why did she want to know this, when they did not even know each other? Presumably, because she was aiming to order stock for all her colleagues—including those, like Buchan, that she did not even know.

Third, if Sandy Buchan knew or merely suspected that Parker's trips around the building taking orders meant that she might have visited the pox lab, this could explain why he was quite so nervous when questioned in court about his encounter with her. He was not asked directly whether he knew of any reason why Janet should visit the pox lab, but he was perhaps anxious that he might have to share his suspicions. It is worth noting that during the trial, one of the witnesses, Edgar Morris, claimed that Bedson had told him that one of the staff in the Bedson lab had discussed work with Janet Parker. However, it remains unclear whether this contact between the pox lab and Parker included just Sandy Buchan or whether it involved another of Bedson's staff.

Fourth, if this custom of photographers offering colleagues discounts on photographic material was a well-established practice in the Medical School, stretching back several years, it might have given Tony McLennan a reason to visit the pox lab in 1966 and so explain why the two photographers were singled out by smallpox. In support of this explanation, Escott-Cox points out that McLennan must have caught smallpox in the run up to the UK's half-term holiday in February, when colleagues might have been keen to get hold of some film to take photographs on their skiing holidays.

It is worth stressing that Dumbell's ideas and Escott-Scott's explanation are not mutually exclusive—Janet Parker could have visited the pox lab, taking orders, while Bedson was away and also have experienced a shorter-than-usual incubation period because of a peculiarity in the way she got infected.

ALTHOUGH THE PHOTOGRAPHER-on-the-rounds hypothesis provides a cogent explanation of how and why Janet Parker acquired smallpox, why has it taken until now for these details to surface? Why did Shooter miss it and why did it not come to light during the trial?

One potential explanation stems from the personality of Reggie Shooter, whom Dumbell describes as a perfect English gentleman, with an otherworldly faith in the essential goodness of humanity. For a man like Shooter, it seemed far easier to believe in a physical explanation for Parker's acquisition of smallpox—virus travelling up a duct—rather than accept that his fellow humans might be holding something back.

Escott-Cox on the other hand, after a lifetime cross-examining criminals, has a much clearer understanding of what Kant dubbed the 'crooked timber of humanity'. When I asked him why none of those working in the pox lab volunteered information about Parker's itinerant habits during the inquiry or during the trial, he shot back a response worthy of Mandy Rice-Davis: 'Well, they wouldn't, would they?!'[6]

He went on to explain that had anyone from the pox lab met Janet Parker in this way and not followed all the University's rules, they would have been in breach of the *Health and Safety at Work Act* and as a result would probably lose their job. In addition, assuming Parker had ignored warnings in the corridor and on the door and nonetheless entered the pox lab, she would have fallen foul of the Health and Safety at Work Act, which stresses that 'It shall be the duty of every employee while at work to take reasonable care for the health and safety of himself and of other persons who may be affected by his acts or omissions at work.' These two factors—fuelling the desire not to incriminate themselves or their colleague Janet—would have provided a clear motivation to stay silent.

Of course, if we accept that the most probable explanation is that Janet Parker visited the smallpox lab, this does not make her recklessly culpable and obviously to blame for her own fate. All it required was a fleeting encounter—and if Parker had knocked on doors year on year and never come to any harm, perhaps she had fallen under an anaesthetic of familiarity and just never considered that she might be at risk. If she did think about it, Janet Parker knew that she had been vaccinated against smallpox just twelve years before and it was not unreasonable to believe that was probably protection enough.

THIS LEADS US ON to the question of why Janet Parker's illness took the course that it did. The fact that she had been vaccinated many years before would not be expected to provide complete protection,[7] but some residual immunity might explain why Janet Parker did not suffer from the most acute fulminant form of smallpox, nor the haemorrhagic variety. Instead, she survived for an entire month with her illness, before dying.

However, even with a copy of medical notes to hand, it is impossible to explain precisely why her illness took such a protracted and ultimately fatal course. This problem is exacerbated by the fact that, within the isolation hospital, her doctors could not perform many of the usual investigations crucial to the management of the critically ill, such as advanced imaging, or advanced biochemical, haematological or immunological tests.

We know that Janet Parker was in renal failure when admitted to hospital, but it is not clear why. Was her renal failure entirely due to her smallpox or due to an underlying disease of the kidneys, particularly as she reported urinary symptoms. Keith Dumbell reports that he and a nephrologist colleague took a needle biopsy of the kidney from Janet six hours after she died and the resulting pathologist's report documented the condition *acute tubular necrosis*, 'with some evidence of cellular recovery'.[8] It is unclear what caused the tubular necrosis: perhaps poor blood flow to the kidney or a direct toxic effect of the smallpox virus. Perhaps, she had a hidden generalised illness—e.g. systemic lupus erythematosis—that might make her more vulnerable to organ failure. Or might an unrecognised immune deficiency account for the unusual course of her illness? However, this remains pure speculation. Unfortunately, we have to accept that we are never going to be able to provide a comprehensive clinical explanation of why Janet Parker was destined to die from her infection.

68

LAB IN A SUITCASE

IT IS APRIL 2015 and an Ebola epidemic has exploded across West Africa, with deaths mounting and the virus spreading from Guinea to neighbouring Sierra Leone and Liberia.[1]

Josh is in a state of extreme psychological stress. His tissues are awash with adrenaline and his blood pressure is sky high. Over the past few days, he has had six vaccinations, a full medical examination and a mad rush to London and back to get a visa stamped in his passport. He has also been down to the UK defence research labs in Porton Down to test out the protocols he has been throwing together. He has had to fill in umpteen forms for the WHO, but thanks to a bounced email they are now saying they still don't have a contract for him. He has spent hours and hours packing and re-packing his bags, trying to cope on his own while his supervisor is laid up with flu and communicating only sporadically via *WhatsApp*.

Josh's mission-impossible is to fit a virology lab into just two suitcases. In Henry Bedson's day, this would have included an electron microscope the size of a room. At the heart of Josh's set-up is a tiny DNA sequencer the size of a USB stick, developed by the British company Oxford Nanopore and called the MinION.

The stressed-out scientist is in a lab at the University of Birmingham, the day before he is due to travel, trying to cram three sequencers, four laptops, a bunch of chemicals, a miniature centrifuge, a PCR machine and a heating block into a pair of suitcases, one of them an ultra-tough Pelican case bought from eBay for the fragile equipment. He knows he has to take everything he could possibly need with him, but keep the weight down. He has to maintain a cold chain for some reagents, so he is leaving it to the last minute to add in cooling packs and insulation. He is sick with worry that he is going to arrive in Africa with a crucial piece missing and be unable to do anything useful. After packing and repacking, his baggage now weighs less than 50 kilograms. He finally leaves the lab at midnight, shuffling home to grab some sleep.

JOSH QUICK IS A PhD student at the University of Birmingham, working in the Institute of Microbiology and Infection under the supervision of microbial bioinformatics guru Nick Loman (@pathogenomenick to his loyal Twitter fans). Thanks to his own PhD apprenticeship with the author, Nick is used to tracking the spread of pathogens through changes in their genomes. Watching the Ebola outbreak from a distance, he is frustrated at how few viral genome sequences are being generated, when genome sequencing should be a core part of any modern surveillance programme. Without this information, how can you expect to work out who is infecting whom and how strains are evolving and spreading?

The problem is that, until now, the only way to sequence Ebola genomes has been to ship samples across international borders to specialist labs thousands of miles away, with export delays and expensive shipping costs, only for samples to arrive at their destination in poor shape. As a MinION 'fan boy', Nick knows we can do better—he is convinced he can get the sequencing done out in the field, as close to the patients as possible.

Nick initially plans to use his connections with the UK military to get on-site genome sequencing underway in Sierra Leone—but it's a slow process. However, thanks to a chance encounter at a conference in Birmingham, Nick hooks up with a charismatic British poxvirus-expert-turned-Ebola-hunter, Miles Caroll and seizes the opportunity to launch his plans more quickly and easily in Guinea. Miles is already doing Ebola genome sequencing, but, like Nick, he is frustrated at the slow pace of progress using established sequencing approaches. He tells Nick he is off to Guinea on WHO business in two weeks time and suggests Nick gets ready to fly out with him on the very same flight.

Nick briefly considers going out to Africa himself, but his lab experience is no match for Josh's—and, besides, now he's a dad, he has family responsibilities. Josh's girlfriend isn't too keen on him rushing off into a danger zone, just as she is helping a close friend through a crisis, but a sense of duty and adventure prevails. Nick injects his quirky sense of humour and love of barbecuing into the project by naming their three MinION sequencers Ribz, Chicken, and Brisket.

AFTER SOME RESTLESS sleep, Josh sets off by car at 3.00am for an early morning flight from Heathrow airport. British airlines have suspended all flights to the Ebola-stricken countries in West Africa, so Josh is forced to fly with Air France via Paris Charles-de-Gaulle. As he checks in, the airline demands that he pays a €60 surcharge for the excess weight of his baggage, but Josh is not resentful, just pleased to be on his way.

This is Josh's first trip to sub-Saharan Africa and, despite the lack of sleep, he is wide awake with excitement as, late that afternoon, he flies into Conakry, a bustling capital city that sprawls across a small island and narrow peninsula jutting into the Atlantic Ocean. As he travels with Miles Caroll in a WHO Land Rover from the airport to the city's Donka Hospital, the young scientist comes face to face with the heat, the noise and the crowded streets of an African city.

Thanks to Miles' involvement in a project entitled the European Mobile Laboratory (co-ordinated by German virologist Stephan Günther), Josh is granted workspace in Donka Hospital. He unpacks his suitcases on to two wooden tables and within minutes he has turned an empty room into a state-of-the-art sequencing laboratory.

Josh starts work that very afternoon, generating some pilot data from samples left over from the diagnostic lab. He works with basic personal protective clothing (gloves, gown and goggles), relying on the Ebola treatment centre run by *Médecins Sans Frontières* and diagnostic lab run by the European Mobile Laboratory project to carry out a decontamination process with chemicals and heat to rid samples of live virus. The only problem is that no one has ever tested the decontamination process on samples as heavily laden with virus as those coming from this epidemic. Josh just has to trust that the WHO's assessment of the risks is adequate. Under the contract he has signed with them, he is paid just a single dollar, but is given the promise that he will be evacuated for treatment in Geneva, should he fall ill.

Later that evening, Josh checks into the country's premier hotel, the Hotel Palm Camayenne, especially approved for WHO workers on account of its five-star facilities and security. Josh uses the hotel Wi-Fi to send data back to Birmingham. His supervisor Nick Loman is astonished to find a data file waiting for him on Google Drive when he gets up the next day.

Josh's nerves calm, once he realises that what had been bothering him most was fear of the unknown. It doesn't help that political tensions are running high, with riots on the streets, as the President, Alpha Condé, is trying to delay elections on account of the Ebola outbreak. As a result, Josh is issued with a WHO gilet that makes his role clear. However, Josh is reassured by the stringent infection control measures in place across the whole city, with hand-washing checkpoints kitted out with chlorine almost everywhere. Every ten minutes, he is confronted with a Thermoflash check, where an electronic, infrared thermometer measures body temperature, when pointed at the head for less than a second. Ebola patients are confined to highly secure Ebola treatment centres.

Josh is excited to find the hotel and city bustling with ex-pat doctors and foreign aid workers associated with a wide range of non-governmental organisations. Many seem to show a fearless adventurer disposition, free of any ties back home and drawn to the thrill of working in a risky environment. WHO rules mean that Josh cannot travel by foot at night, but he manages to eke out a social life at the hotel. He also makes daytime trips on foot to a local Lebanese restaurant and forays by car to restaurants after dark. On one such journey, a vehicle carrying local gendarmes crashes into the side of their Land Rover, only to speed away from the scene. Luckily, no one is hurt.

Over the next twelve days, despite frequent power outages, Josh sequences Ebola virus genomes from fourteen patients. He has to send all his data back to Birmingham before the genomes can be analysed. By comparing viral genomes, Josh and Nick are quickly able to work out that there are two distinct lineages of Ebola virus circulating in Guinea. The genome sequences also provide valuable information on how the disease is travelling along and across the border between Guinea and Sierra Leone. Early on, Josh and Nick start to generate daily reports with latest findings, which Miles presents to the local Ministry of Health and WHO contacts, who quickly get hooked on the new data.

After a month in Africa, as Josh prepares to fly home, he makes plans to leave the portable lab behind in the hands of his colleague Sophie Duraffour. They have decided to move the lab out of the capital thirty miles away to the town of Coyah, closer to most of the Ebola patients. However, this means that they can no longer use the Palm Camayenne's Wi-Fi to upload data. Instead, they are going to have to rely on a local 3G network.

Josh spends his final days in Africa getting his driver to hand over huge wads of Guinean Francs to market traders in exchange for local SIM cards, so Josh can evaluate network options. In his attempts to get a 10 Gigabyte top-up bundle, he has to buy seventeen top-up cards. Fortunately, he soon settles on a South African provider, MTN, which gives speeds that are acceptable, even if not quite as good as the hotel Wi-Fi.

Shortly after Josh leaves, Sophie and her colleagues move the mobile Ebola genomics lab to Coyah, where , with only intermittent running water, it's a lot less comfortable than the Palm Camayenne. A team of volunteers from the UK and Europe, as well as Guinean clinical scientists Raymond Koundouno and Joseph Bore continue to sequence genomes until the epidemic finally ends in May 2016.

As Josh gets back to the UK, his girlfriend puts him into temporary quarantine. A year later, they are engaged to be married. In February 2016, Josh, Nick, and colleagues describe their findings in a paper[2] in the prestigious journal *Nature*, which in turn leads to Nick gaining a professorship and Josh a PhD. Both soon throw themselves into the new challenge of diagnosing and tracking the newly emerging Zika virus in South America.

IT IS NOW TIME to leave Birmingham and its university. As we do so, it is worth reflecting how the legacy of Henry Bedson lives on in his workplace. In the 1970s, Bedson, Buchan and their colleagues were pioneers in exploiting molecular biological techniques to track the emergence, evolution and spread of deadly viruses.[3] Forty years on, their legacy endures through the work of Josh Quick and Nick Loman. Thanks to all their efforts—and similar efforts around the world[4]—we can be sure that should smallpox (or something like it) re-emerge, we will be ready to detect and track it with unparalleled speed and accuracy, using mobile genomics labs to pinpoint minute changes in any virus's genetic make-up .

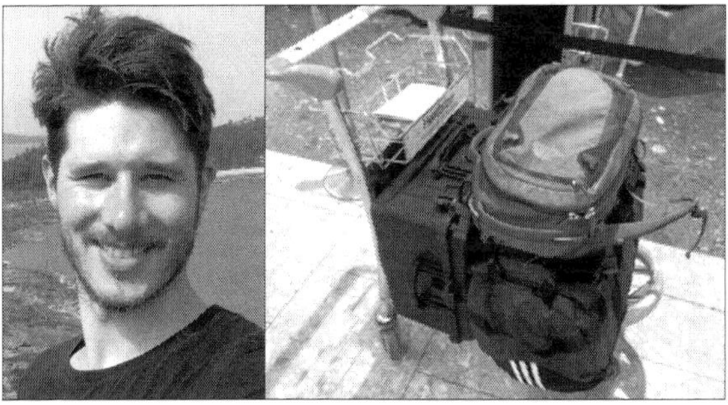

JOSHUA QUICK AND HIS LAB IN A SUITCASE
Suitcases on a trolley at Heathrow Airport;
the light bag on top was for Josh's clothes and personal items
{Source: J. Quick}

69

LAST WORDS

Reason is the capacity for consciously making sense of things, establishing and verifying facts, applying logic, and changing or justifying practices, institutions, and beliefs based on new or existing information.
Wikipedia

'RAGE' REMAINS AN appropriate response to what smallpox did to Janet Parker in 1978 and to people around the world for many centuries. But it was *Reason* that brought smallpox to an end in Bangladesh and Birmingham—a chain of reason that stretches back to the Edward Jenner and to the Enlightenment.[1]

It is easy to look back at the years leading up to 1978—the seventies and the tail end of the sixties—as a decrepit decade, a time of dreary deadlock and a world divided. The USA experienced the assassination of Martin Luther King, the Vietnam War, the Cold War and the Oil Crisis. In the UK we saw industrial discord, frequent power cuts, the three-day week and the IRA's mainland bombing campaign.

But let's not forget that this was a time when Americans sent men to the moon 'in peace for all mankind' and celebrated their bicentenary with photos from the surface of Mars. This was a time when cold war adversaries shook hands in space and the first space station orbited our planet. This was a time when humankind sent Voyager probes off on a grand tour of the solar system to turn half-glimpsed smudges in the night sky into newly mapped worlds. This was a time when we could fly from London to New York in three hours, faster than the speed of sound, and arrive before we set off. This was a time, before the mind virus of neoliberalism took hold, when British society stood at a peak of equality.[2]

Let's not forget that these were *the last days of smallpox*. This was a time when we put aside petty differences of country, creed or colour and worked together on the basis of our common humanity to drive a vicious virus out of every ounce of human flesh. A time when we took on a microbial adversary that killed millions—and won!

GLOSSARY

Aerosol: a suspension of fine solid particles or liquid droplets in air.

Alastrim: a mild form of smallpox, also called variola minor, caused by a less virulent form of the variola virus.

Anti-vaccinial immunoglobulin: an antibody preparation raised against the vaccinia virus that provides protection to those exposed to smallpox.

Aspiration: withdrawal by suction of fluid from a vessel, such as a petri dish.

Area Health Authority (AHA): a body responsible for planning and delivering health care within an area of England and Wales, established by the National Health Service Reorganisation Act 1973.

ASTMS: Association of Scientific, Technical and Managerial Staff; a white-collar union representing laboratory and technical workers in universities, headed by Clive Jenkins.

Autoclave: a sealed vessel using superheated steam under pressure to sterilise laboratory equipment and laboratory waste; similar in principle to a pressure cooker.

Barrister: a type of British lawyer specialising in courtroom advocacy.

Bifurcated needle: a narrow two-inch-long steel rod, with two prongs at one end with a gap designed to hold a single dose of smallpox vaccine.

Camelpox: a disease of camels caused by a virus closely related to the smallpox virus, characterised by a rash and generalised infection.

CDC: leading national public health institute of the United States, with special responsibility for infection; located in Atlanta, Georgia; home to last remaining stocks of smallpox virus. Over the years variably called *Communicable Disease Center*, *Centers for Disease Control* and now *Centers for Disease Control and Prevention* but with the acronym *CDC* used throughout.

Centrifugal: when applied to the rash of smallpox, indicating that the eruption is most severe on the face and extremities, as opposed to the *centripetal rash* of chickenpox, which is most severe on the trunk.

Centrifuge: an instrument with a rapidly rotating container that applies centrifugal force to its contents, typically to separate liquids from solid material.

Chorioallantoic membrane (or CAM): a membrane rich in blood vessels found within fertilised eggs: The CAM of hen's eggs can be used to grow and identify poxviruses.
Confluent smallpox: a rare, severe form of smallpox in which the pustules ran into each other leading to the sloughing off of large sheets of skin.
Consultant: a senior hospital-based physician or surgeon in the UK who has completed specialist training.
Coronaviruses: a group of viruses that cause a variety of diseases in humans and other animals, including SARS and MERS.
Cowpox: an infection of cattle that sometimes spreads to humans; caused by a poxvirus.
Culture medium: a nutritious substance capable of sustaining cultured cells in the laboratory.
Cytopathic effect (CPE): the structural changes that can be seen under the microscope when cells are damaged by viral infection.
Department of Health and Social Security (DHSS): a ministry of the British government from 1968 until 1988 responsible for healthcare and social services.
Dangerous Pathogens Advisory Group (DPAG): a body set up in the wake of the 1973 London outbreak and the Cox Report to advise on laboratory work in the UK on dangerous pathogens.
EF26 (or the telephone room): a room used for storage and containing a phone that could be used to make external calls.
EG34 (or the animal pox lab): the large outer room within Bedson's pox lab in which work on viruses other than smallpox took place.
EG34b (or the smallpox lab): the small inner room within Bedson's pox lab in which the smallpox virus was handled.
Electrophoresis: see *Polyacrylamide gel electrophoresis.*
Endogenous viruses: viruses or viral fragments that have integrated into the genome of their host.
Fumigation: a method for killing pests, including viruses and bacteria, that uses a toxic gas to treat an enclosed space, such as a laboratory, a house or a car.
General Practitioner (GP): in the UK, a doctor who provides frontline healthcare outside hospitals.
Grammar School: (in the UK) a publicly funded secondary school to which pupils are admitted on the basis of ability; now largely subsumed into the comprehensive school system.
Haemorrhagic smallpox: a rare severe form of smallpox, usually fatal, characterised by bleeding from the mouth and other orifices.

Health and Safety Executive (HSE): an organisation created by the UK's Health and Safety at Work Act 1974; responsible for safety in the workplace.

House officer: in the UK, a recently qualified doctor practising under supervision in hospital during the first three years after graduation.

Lesion: a localised change in a tissue indicative of disease.

Macule: a flat patch of skin altered in colour (typically red in smallpox).

Malignant smallpox: a rare severe form of smallpox, usually fatal, characterised by skin lesions that do not progress to the pustular stage, but instead remain soft and flat.

Medical Officer of Health: from the 1850s to early 1970s, a community physician in the UK responsible for public health within a local municipality.

MERS: Middle East respiratory syndrome: a life-threatening viral infection of humans affecting the lungs, first described in Saudi Arabia in 2012.

Methisazone: an antiviral drug used in the past to treat smallpox.

Mimivirus: a giant virus of amoebae, comparable in size and complexity to some bacteria, distantly related to the smallpox virus.

Petechiae: red or purple round pinpoint spots caused by bleeding into the skin, typically appearing in clusters forming a rash.

Petri dish: a shallow, circular, transparent dish with a loose-fitting flat lid used for the culture of microorganisms.

Pipette: a slender tube relying on suction to transfer or measure defined quantities of liquid in the laboratory.

Polyacrylamide gel electrophoresis: an analytical method to resolve protein components in a mixture based on the size of the molecules: adapted by Henry Bedson and Sandy Buchan to fingerprint poxviruses.

Porton Down: a scientific campus in Wiltshire, England that has been home to military and civilian microbiology research labs working on dangerous pathogens.

Poxviruses: a family of large complex DNA viruses with a propensity to cause skin lesions: Includes the vaccinia and variola viruses, along with camelpox, taterapox and many others.

Pustule: a raised skin lesion filled with pus.

QC (Queen's Counsel): an eminent barrister appointed by the Queen and enjoying certain privileges including wearing a silk gown.

Safety cabinet: an enclosed, ventilated workspace for working safely with pathogenic microorganisms.

Severe acute respiratory syndrome (SARS): a viral infection of animal origin that caused an outbreak in 2002-3 that spread from China to 36 countries.

Syncytium: a collection of cultured cells that have fused together: a rare side effect of infection with some strains of the smallpox virus.

Taterapox: a poxvirus isolated from a gerbil captured in West Africa in 1968; very closely related to the variola virus.

Tissue culture: the growth of cells from animal or plant tissues separate from the organism, typically stuck to a solid surface while bathed in culture medium. The cultured cells can be used to grow virus particles.

Umbilicated: when applied to a smallpox spot, having a small central depression so that the spot resembles the umbilicus.

Vaccinia virus: a poxvirus used as a live vaccine against smallpox; related to but distinct from the virus that causes cowpox.

Vaccine: a preparation capable of producing immunity against a specific disease without causing symptoms comparable in scale or type to that seen during natural infection.

Vaccination: administration of a vaccine to produce immunity against a disease.

Variola: the Latin term for smallpox.

Variola major: the classical, more severe form of smallpox, with a death rate of 15-30%.

Variola minor: see alastrim.

Variola virus: the virus that causes smallpox; also called *the smallpox virus.*

Vesicle: a raised skin lesion filled with clear fluid; a variety of blister.

Viraemia: the presence of virus particles circulating and reproducing in the bloodstream.

Whitepox virus: a virus isolated from monkey tissue, originally believed to be a new poxvirus but later recognised to be variola virus present as a laboratory contaminant.

WHO (the World Health Organization): an agency of the United Nations with responsibility for global public health; established in 1948, with headquarters in Geneva.

PEOPLE

Henry Bedson: British microbiologist; Professor of virology and head of the smallpox lab in Birmingham in 1978.

Pat (Ann) Bedson: Wife of Henry Bedson. Later remarried as Pat Fisher.

Rahima Banu Begum: Last person to be naturally infected with variola major.

Alexander (Sandy) Buchan: virologist at the University of Birmingham.

Leslie Collier: British virologist who developed a method for creating a freeze-dried vaccine.

Colin Colston: Barrister who acted for the Health and Safety Executive in the 1979 court case.

Adrian Davis: solicitor and senior partner in the firm of Johnson and Co., who instructed the Prosecution in the 1979 court case.

Keith Dumbell: English smallpox expert, Professor of Virology at St Mary's Hospital Paddington in 1978; Bedson's collaborator and friend, subsequently moved to South Africa.

David Ennals: Secretary of State for Health and Social Services, i.e. head of the DHSS in Callaghan's Labour government 1976-9.

Brian Escott-Cox QC: Senior barrister who defended the University of Birmingham in the 1979 court case brought by the Health and Safety Executive.

Alasdair Geddes: Infectious disease physician who made the clinical diagnosis of smallpox in the Birmingham 1978 outbreak.

Donald Ainslie (D.A.) Henderson: American physician who directed the smallpox eradication campaign.

Brodie Hughes: Dean of Medicine at the University of Birmingham at the start of the 1978 outbreak.

Clive Jenkins: Flamboyant trade union leader who led the ASTMS and leaked the Shooter Report to the press.

Edward Jenner: English physician who kick-started the process of vaccination.

Tony McLennan: photographer who worked at the Medical School in Birmingham and first case in the 1966 smallpox outbreak.

Sheila McKechnie: Trade unionist who made exaggerated claims against the University of Birmingham.

Hugh Morgan: Professor of Tropical Medicine at the East Birmingham Hospital who took responsibility for Janet

Parker.

Willie Nicol: Medical Officer for the Birmingham Area Health Authority who led the public health response to smallpox in 1978.

Janet Parker: Medical photographer at the University of Birmingham; victim of smallpox.

Desmond Robinson: representative of the DHSS who directed control measures at the University of Birmingham during the 1978 incident.

Reginald Shooter: English bacteriologist who led the government inquiry into the 1978 smallpox incident.

Deborah Symmons: Senior House Officer who cared for Janet Parker in 1978, subsequently Professor of Rheumatology and Musculoskeletal Epidemiology in Manchester.

Colman Treacy: Junior barrister who defended the University of Birmingham in the 1979 court case.

Owen Wade: Dean of Medicine at the University of Birmingham during the height of the 1978 smallpox outbreak.

Fred Witcomb: Father of Janet Parker.

Hilda Witcomb: Mother of Janet Parker. Last case of smallpox.

Viktor Zhdanov: Soviet virologist who proposed the eradication of smallpox.

ACKNOWLEDGEMENTS

I am grateful to many people for their help with this endeavour, particularly Alasdair Geddes, whose vivid reminiscences sparked the whole thing off; Deborah Symmons, who kindly provided access to her notes from the time; and Roberta Bivins, who helped me obtain a copy of the transcript of the 1979 court case. I thank Jas Bains for scanning, copying and organising the transcript of *Cook v University of Birmingham*. This book would not have been possible without the interviews generously given by Alasdair Geddes, Deborah Symmons, Surinder Bakhshi, Keith Dumbell, David Veale, Joel Bremen, Brian Escott-Cox and Josh Quick.

I thank all those who have commented on drafts of the text, including Graham Beards, Roberta Bivins, Steve Busby, Philip Butcher, Inger Damon, Keith Dumbell, Brian Escott-Cox, Stanley Falkow, John Heath, Anne-Marie Krachler, Nick Loman, Robin May, Conall McCaughey, Johnjoe McFadden, Charles Penn, Josh Quick, Josh Rappoport, Andy Richards, Branko Rihtman, Lucy Ryan, Simon Silver, Soad Tabaqchali, Mark Webber and Lars Westblade. I am very grateful to Georgina Lloyd for her diligent proof reading and copy editing.

I thank Emma Denham, Andy Richards, Lucy Ryan and Lawrence Young for support and encouragement. I am grateful to Nick Loman for putting me in touch with Steve Rivo and Nicki Carrico at TDG and to Steve and Nicki for including coverage of the Birmingham incident in the international version of their documentary, *Invisible Killers: Smallpox*. I am especially grateful to Andy Richards for providing news cuttings and for granting permission to use photos from the *Birmingham Mail* archive, as well as publishing excerpts from this book in the newspaper. I am grateful to Nick Caya and his colleagues at word-2-kindle.com for their help in formatting the Kindle version of the book. Finally, I thank my wife and children for putting up with my smallpox obsession for the best part of a decade.

Responsibility for any errors or any opinions remains my own.

NOTES

1. FROM BERKELEY TO BIRMINGHAM

1. Jefferson (1806).
2. Jenner's home in Berkeley is now a museum: https://jennermuseum.com
3. Jenner's experiments are in described in Jenner (1798). Jenner was not the first to use vaccination with cowpox to induce immunity to smallpox: those with prior claims include Dorset famer Benjamin Jesty: https://en.wikipedia.org/wiki/Benjamin_Jesty However, it was Jenner's efforts to publicise and proselytise that led to the widespread adoption of vaccination.
4. For a full account of the global eradication campaign, see Fenner, Henderson, Arita, Jezek, & Ladnyi (1988).

2. A CHILD IS BORN

1. The record of Janet Parker's birth: https://www.freebmd.org.uk/cgi/information.pl?cite=LQukJUKXUJOu8IRYMy6PmQ&scan=1 Janet's maiden name and the surname of her parents was *Witcomb*, although some sources use the erroneous spelling *Whitcomb*.
2. Information on the global state of smallpox between the world wars from Fenner, Henderson, Arita, Jezek, & Ladnyi (1988).
3. Detailed descriptions of the clinical features of smallpox can be found in Fenner, Henderson, Arita, Jezek, & Ladnyi (1988) and Dixon (1962).
4. Estimate of world total of smallpox virus particles based on reports from infection in cynomolgus monkeys (Jahrling *et al.*, 2004), where there were 100,000 viruses per gram in the brain and a thousand million virus particles per gram in the adrenals, kidneys, spleen and liver:. If one assumes a similar viral load in the average human of say 30,000 grams, this would mean a total viral load per viraemic case of at least 3 thousand million virus particles. According to Fenner, Henderson, Arita, Jezek, & Ladnyi (1988) p.175, there were probably 50 million cases of smallpox worldwide in the early 1950s. Assuming a similar disease burden in 1938 of 50 million cases, each viraemic for one week, then there would have been a point prevalence of around a million viraemic

cases at the time of Janet Parker's birth, carrying a total of 3 thousand million million (or 3 x 10^{15}) virus particles. According to Wikipedia, there are 100-400 thousand million stars in the Milky Way. Even if the smallpox estimates are wrong by a factor of ten or even a hundred, the number of variola virus particles remains 'astronomical'.

4. VIRUS WORLD

1. Pasteur's tomb is part of a museum dedicated to his life: https://www.pasteurfoundation.org/about/pasteur-museum.
2. Waller (2002).
3. Jupille's struggle against the rabid dog is also commemorated in a bronze statue in the garden of the Institut Pasteur, Paris.
4. For accessible introductory guides to the history and nature of viruses, see Zimmer (2015), Rybicki (2015).
5. Negri (1906); Mervyn (1925).
6. For preparedness against real zombies, rather than their viral analogues, see https://www.cdc.gov/phpr/zombie/index.htm
7. Forterre (2006).
8. Clokie, Millard, Letarov, & Heaphy (2011); Steward *et al.* (2013).
9. https://www.ncbi.nlm.nih.gov/gene?LinkName=nuccore_gene&from_uid=10313991 Esposito *et al* (2006)
10. Forterre (2006).
11. Bugert & Darai (2000).
12. La Scola *et al.* (2003); Raoult *et al.* (2004).
13. Colson, de Lamballerie, Fournous, & Raoult (2012); but for a challenge to this view, see Yutin, Wolf, & Koonin (2014).

5. OUT OF AFRICA

1. https://en.wikipedia.org/wiki/Ramesses_V
2. Ruffer & Ferguson (1911).
3. Hopkins (1980).
4. Reed, Light, Allen, & Kirchman (2007); Wertheim, Smith, Smith, Scheffler, & Kosakovsky Pond (2014). But note that in each case, a close relative of the ancient parasite was also acquired by inter-species transmission.
5. Wolfe, Dunavan, & Diamond (2007); Quammen (2012).
6. Sharp & Hahn (2011).
7. Kemp, Causey, Setzer, & Moore (1974); Kemp (1975).
8. Lourie, Nakano, Kemp, & Setzer (1975).
9. Buist (1887).

10. Paschen (1906).
11. Nagler & Rake (1948).
12. pp.20-21 in Fenner, Henderson, Arita, Jezek, & Ladnyi (1988); Steinhardt, Israeli & Lambert (1913).
13. Goodpasture, Woodruff, & Buddingh (1932).
14. Nelson (1943).
15. Baxby (1972). Subsequent studies did show subtle differences between camelpox and smallpox in tissue culture: Bedson (1972); Baxby (1974).
16. Baxby, Hessami, Ghaboosi, & Ramyar (1975).
17. Duraffour, Meyer, Andrei, & Snoeck (2011).
18. Camels have never naturally caught smallpox and even when injected with a large dose of the virus, produce just a few transitory vesicles.
19. Afonso *et al.* (2002); Esposito *et al.* (2006).
20. Li *et al.* (2007).
21. Hughes, Irausquin, & Friedman (2010); Shchelkunov (2009); Firth *et al.* (2010); Babkin & Babkina (2012): but see discussion in *Afterlife of the Pox* below for more recent estimates.
22. Babkin & Babkina (2015).

5. FROM THE OLD WORLD TO THE NEW

1. Razi (1848).
2. Benedictow (2004).
3. Diamond (1997).
4. Motolinía (1914). Motolinía was the nickname of Toribio de Benavente (1482–1568).
5. Patterson & Runge (2002).
6. d'Errico (2017).
7. Baron (1827).
8. Fenner, Henderson, Arita, Jezek, & Ladnyi (1988); Glynn & Glynn (2005); Hopkins (2002); Williams (2010); Henderson (2009); Kotar & Gessler (2013).

7. GETTYSBURG 1863

1. Assuming Lincoln first fell ill on 18 November and given the usual incubation period of 10-14 days, Lincoln must have acquired smallpox between 4 November and 8 November, with this most likely to have happened on 6 November.
2. Helm (1928).
3. The following account is taken from Goldman & Schmalstieg (2007).

4. Basler (1972).
5. Witcover (2014);
https://www.alternatehistory.com/forum/threads/wi-president-hannibal-hamlin.367834
https://groups.google.com/forum/#!msg/soc.history.what-if/S-6J3pGO1fg/vKNGd26EjjAJ

8. INTO THE TWENTIETH CENTURY

1. Chapter 8 in Fenner, Henderson, Arita, Jezek, & Ladnyi (1988).
2. Mack (1972); Bhatnagar, Stoto, Morton, Boer, & Bozzette (2006).
3. https://en.wikipedia.org/wiki/Trickster
4. Chapter 17 in Dixon (1962).
5. Millard (1943).
6. Hogben, McKendrick, & Nicol (1958).
7. p. 312 in Dixon (1962).
8. Wanklyn (1913), cited in Dixon (1962).
9. p. 328, p. 419, p. 429 *et seq*. in Dixon (1962).
10. Gordon & Lewis (1969).
11. Millard (1945); Clark *et al.* (1944).
12. Bradley, Davies, & Durante (1946).
13. Weinstein (1947).
14. Clark *et al.* (1944).
15. Bradley (1948).
16. Irons (1953).
17. Mack (1972); Bhatnagar, Stoto, Morton, Boer, & Bozzette (2006).

9. BRIGHTON 1950

1. Breen (1956).
2. "Monthly Weather Report of the Meteorological Office: December 1950" (1950).
3. Information on the Brighton outbreak drawn from Breen (1956); Cramb (1951); Hounsome (2007); Gaston (2013); Collis (2013). A Pathé news reel covering the outbreak is available from: https://www.britishpathe.com/video/town-tackles-smallpox-scare
4. 13 Kemp Street, Brighton BN1 4EF
5. "Obituary G. E. Breen" (1981).
6. Clark & Grasty (1999).
7. Price (2003).
8. According to

http://www.nlcaonline.org.uk/page_id__253.aspx the business was named Tivoli Laundry with its main site at 28A Crescent Road, in the Round Hill suburb of Brighton and receiving depots at 5 Kemp Street (a few doors down from the Bath family home) and in Southover Street.

9. According to Hounsome (2007), the greengrocer's was in Down Terrace, Brighton, BN2 9ZH, which was the scene of a 2009 film of the same name.

10. BRADFORD 1962

1. Information on the Bradford outbreak drawn from: *Smallpox 1961-2, Reports on Public health and Medical Subjects* (1963); Tovey (2004); Tainsh (1962); Douglas & Edgar (1962); Bradley (1963).
2. "Death not due to smallpox" (1962).
3. Tovey (2004).
4. For a full analysis of the political ramifications and press coverage associated with this outbreak and other UK outbreaks in 1962, see Butterworth (1966); Gordon (1983); Bivins (2007); Bivins (2015).
5. "Pakistanis' windows broken" (1962).
6. Corina (1962).
7. "Pakistanis' windows broken" (1962).
8. *Hansard*, January 23 1961, col 32-7.
9. "Smallpox and race relations" (1962).

11. SOUTH WALES 1962

1. Information on the South Wales outbreak is drawn from: *Smallpox 1961-2, Reports on Public health and Medical Subjects* (1963); Stewart "Smallpox1962"; Bivins (2015); Culley (1963).
2. In 1962, the now-abandoned term *toxaemia of pregnancy* was used to describe what we now call *pre-eclampsia*.
3. Patient names and patterns of spread can be found here: https://smallpox1962.wordpress.com/6-rhondda/0-8-4-how-smallpox-spread-in-rhondda/
4. For the boy to acquire infection from Mansfield, he must have experienced a very short incubation period of 5-7 days, which could perhaps be explained if he came into intimate contact with large amounts of virus shed from Mansfield contaminating the room or instruments. p. 27 in *Smallpox 1961-2, Reports on Public health and Medical Subjects* (1963).
5. Albert Cook was in the ward above the boy and there is no other plausible source of his infection. However, for him to

acquire infection, variola virus must have travelled through two open windows, or have been spread by fleeting contact with the boy's mother or hitched a ride on some newspapers. p. 28 in *Smallpox 1961-2, Reports on Public health and Medical Subjects* (1963).

6. According to https://smallpox1962.wordpress.com/5-documents/5-008-the-case-of-trevor-thomas/ the most likely link was a GP shared with Marion Jones; according to p. 28 in *Smallpox 1961-2, Reports on Public health and Medical Subjects* (1963) a social visitor might have passively conveyed the virus.
7. Over the course of less than a month—from mid-Dec 1961 to mid-Jan12 1962—there were five importations of smallpox from Pakistan: the 9-year-old girl mentioned in the previous chapter; Shuka Mia, a 27-year-old Pakistani man, Mohammed Siddique, who infected a doctor in the West Midlands; Imrat Khan, a 24-year-old, who died in the Long Reach Smallpox Hospital and a 30-year Pakistani man who travelled to Birmingham, where he recovered and failed to infect anyone.
8. Mentioned in a memo from Dr A. R. Culley in the Board of Health to Dr W. H. Bradley, Ministry of Health, London https://smallpox1962.wordpress.com/5-documents/5-001/ and identified as a potential missing link by James Stewart: https://smallpox1962.wordpress.com/4-cardiff-jan-1962/
9. According to p. 26 in *Smallpox 1961-2, Reports on Public health and Medical Subjects* (1963) there were three other unexplained cases of smallpox that year sharing the common factor of proximity to smallpox hospitals, including Sophia Evans (see below) and two men who passed close to Long Reach Hospital in Dartford, London when Imrat Khan was a patient there.
10. By this time, Sophia Evans had not left the ward for over a year. However, six infectious smallpox patients were being cared for in the Smallpox Hospital at Heddfan, three quarters of a mile away from Glanrhyd Hospital and were perhaps the most likely source of her infection according to p. 26 in *Smallpox 1961-2, Reports on Public health and Medical Subjects* (1963).
11. Manworth (2002).

13. STAFFORDSHIRE 1966

1. Chief, Smallpox Eradication Program (1967) *Variola Minor—in England and Wales, 1966*, reproduced in Shooter (1980).

Events described in this chapter draw on this report from the Smallpox Eradication program.

2. The White Cock Inn, which was located at Uttoxeter Road, ST11 9JG, was subsequently turned into an Indian restaurant before being demolished and the site redeveloped for housing. http://closedpubs.blogspot.co.uk/2012/04/white-cock.html
3. McLennan has been named in the press, e.g. Docherty & Foulkes (2003).
4. A young mother, Vivienne Jean Yates, who died during the outbreak from an acute exacerbation of long-standing asthma, was found on laboratory testing to have had smallpox at the time of her death, but the infection is not recorded as contributing to her death. "Smallpox case inquiry" (1966).

14. BIRMINGHAM 1967

1. https://en.wikipedia.org/wiki/Operation_Cedar_Falls
2. https://en.wikipedia.org/wiki/Torrey_Canyon_oil_spill
3. https://en.wikipedia.org/wiki/1967
4. Biographical details on Alasdair Geddes are drawn from interviews with the author and from Geddes' unpublished autobiography, *My Story*.
5. *Hansard*, 12 May 1967, col 1961-74; Chapter 15 in Dixon (1962).
6. https://en.wikipedia.org/wiki/Witton_Isolation_Hospital
7. "A thief risks smallpox" (1966).
8. *Hansard*, 12 May 1967, col 1961-74.
9. https://www.youtube.com/watch?v=XV1zRG14fCg ; https://www.britishpathe.com/video/hospital-burnt-down ; http://www.macearchive.org/films/midlands-news-03051967-witton-isolation-hospital-fire ; http://www.macearchive.org/films/midlands-news-03051967-witton-isolation-hospital-burned-down
10. It is worth noting that several other smallpox hospitals were burnt down at the end of their working life—a similar fate befell Laceby Hospital, near Grimsby, in September 1970, Penrhys Hospital in 1971, Ainsley Isolation Hospital in 1972 and Long Reach Hospital in 1977.
11. *Hansard*, 12 May 1967, col 1961-74.

15. WEST GERMANY 1970

1. Information on the Meschede outbreak is drawn from Wehrle, Posch, Richter, & Henderson (1970); Gelfand & Posch (1971) "Smallpox Outbreak - Meschede, Federal Republic of Germany,

1970" (1970); Preston (2002).

16. LONDON 1973

1. Information on the 1973 outbreak is drawn from: Cox, McCarthy & Millar (1974); Pennington (2002).
2. The inference that Ann Algeo was brought up as a Catholic is based on the choice of a university in Dublin and a shared interest in the Irish Catholic magazine.
3. https://en.wikipedia.org/wiki/The_Troubles
4. Hay, Odds, & Campbell (2017).
5. Keith Dumbell attests to Algeo's animated personality and the lively nature of the relationship between her and Mr Bruno, claiming that investigators at the time held in mind an image of Bruno chasing Algeo around the lab with smallpox-infected eggs in hand. Dumbell, K. Interview with the author. 13 November 2017.
6 Rondle was an extreme nighthawk in terms of his body clock, working late into the night, but seldom appearing in the work place before midday: Dumbell, K. Interview with the author. 13 November 2017.
7. "Philip Cox, radar operator – obituary" (2015).
8. Keith Dumbell in an interview with the author highlighted another human cost of the outbreak, making it clear that Charles Rondle never really recovered from this incident, which resulted in a serious increase in alcohol consumption followed by repeated bouts of ill health resulting in early death in his late fifties or early sixties.

17. LOOK BACK IN ANGER

1. Darwin (1856).
2. Miele (1995).
3. Beer (2000).
4. Darwin (1860).
5. Dawkins (1976).

18. THE EXPANDING CIRCLE

1. pp 100-101 in Darwin (1871).
2. https://en.wikipedia.org/wiki/List_of_wars_by_death_toll
3. https://en.wikipedia.org/wiki/Common_Sense_(pamphlet); http://www.gutenberg.org/ebooks/147
4. https://en.wikipedia.org/wiki/Idealism_in_international_relations
5. https://en.wikipedia.org/wiki/World_Health_Organization

6. https://en.wikipedia.org/wiki/Brock_Chisholm
7. https://en.wikipedia.org/wiki/Palace_of_Nations; the WHO moved to a new headquarters building in Geneva in 1966: http://www.who.int/archives/exhibits/galleries/building/en/
8. Chapter 9 in Fenner, Henderson, Arita, Jezek, & Ladnyi (1988).
9. Manela (2010).

19. ZHDANOV

1. Bentham (1907).
2. https://en.wikipedia.org/wiki/Felicific_calculus
3. MacAskill (2015).
4. This account of Zhdanov's life is drawn from: Bukrinskaya (1991); Uryvaev (2011); Chapter 9 in Fenner, Henderson, Arita, Jezek, & Ladnyi (1988).

20. D. A.

1. https://en.wikipedia.org/wiki/Citizenship_in_a_Republic
2. This account of DA's life and work and of the eradication campaign is drawn from Henderson (2009); Henderson (2011); Fenner, Henderson, Arita, Jezek, & Ladnyi (1988); Manela (2010); Behbehani (1983); "Donald Henderson, epidemiologist who helped to eradicate smallpox – obituary" (2016); Geddes (2016).
3. Rubin (1980).
4. See also Roy (2010).

21. PERSONAL INTERLUDE: WMD

1. Clark *et al.* (1944).

22. WHITEPOX

1. Dumbell & Kapsenberg (1982).
2. Arita & Henderson (1976).
3. Gispen & Brand-Saathof (1972).
4. Noble (1970); Arita, I. *et al.* (1972); Breman, Bernadou & Nakano (1977).
5. Arita & Henderson (1976).
6. In fact, concerns about an animal reservoir proved unfounded and the whitepox strains were later dismissed as contaminants: Dumbell (1982); Esposito (1985).
7. Bedson & Dumbell (1961); Dumbell, Bedson & Rossier (1961).

23. BEDSON

1. Account of Henry Bedson's early life is drawn from: http://munksroll.rcplondon.ac.uk/Biography/Details/334; "Obituary: Henry Samuel Bedson" (1978) and interviews with Keith Dumbell.
2. Biographical details on Samuel Bedson from http://munksroll.rcplondon.ac.uk/Biography/Details/335; note that *Bedsonia* was later reclassified by taxonomists as a form of *Chlamydia*.
3. The author, like Bedson, is an alumnus of this august institution, which is now part of Barts and The London School of Medicine and Dentistry.
4. Wade (1978a).

24. BANGLADESH 1973

1. Chapter 16 in Fenner, Henderson, Arita, Jezek, & Ladnyi (1988).
2. Biographical details on Alasdair Geddes are drawn from interviews with the author and from Geddes' unpublished autobiography, *My Story*.
3. Foster, Hughes, Tarantola, & Glasser (2011).

25. BANGLADESH 1975

1. www.zero-pox.info/targetzero/Staff_1975-10-27.pdf
2. Bangladesh Smallpox Eradication Programme (1976) Joarder, Tarantola, & Tulloch (1980).
3. https://phil.cdc.gov/details.aspx?pid=7720
4. https://phil.cdc.gov/Details.aspx?pid=7765; Voice of America (2009).
5. Massung *et al.* (1994).

26. SOMALIA 1977

1. Chapter 21 and Chapter 22 in Fenner, Henderson, Arita, Jezek, & Ladnyi (1988).
2. Chapter 31 in Fenner, Henderson, Arita, Jezek, & Ladnyi (1988).
3. The Apollo program is estimated to have cost $25.4 billion: https://en.wikipedia.org/wiki/Apollo_program

28. PAKISTAN 1970

1. https://en.wikipedia.org/wiki/A_Psalm_of_Life
2. https://en.wikipedia.org/wiki/Great_man_theory; for an alternative view, see Tolstoy (1922).
3. The provenance and characteristics of the Abid strain and

related strains are described by Dumbell in Appendix 3 in Shooter (1980) and in Dumbell, Harper, Buchan, Douglass, & Bedson (1999). Whole-genome sequencing places isolates from Pakistan, Kuwait, Vellore and Yugoslavia in a single clade, which is probably also home to Abid, on the basis of a shared protein polymorphism. However, it is worth stressing that Dumbell, Harper, Buchan, Douglass, & Bedson (1999) suggest that the Abid strain may not have the reported provenance as it appears highly adapted to culture in the laboratory. For simplicity, I have stuck with the narrative from Shooter (1980), but the metaphor that variola strains achieve a kind of nirvana in the lab remains equally forceful if the Abid strain in fact represents a highly passaged strain of uncertain pedigree.

29. THE PHONEY WAR

1. This estimated date range is derived by subtracting the range of incubation periods for smallpox (7-17 days) from the date of onset of Parker's symptoms (August 11). However, as Dumbell points outs (personal communication), it is possible that the incubation period could have been even shorter if infection occurred through an unorthodox route.
2. Rubins, Hensley, Relman, & Brown (2011).
3. Bidgood & Mercer (2015).
4. This account of the pathogenesis of smallpox is drawn from: Wahl-Jensen *et al.* (2011) and Chapter 3 in Fenner, Henderson, Arita, Jezek, & Ladnyi (1988).

30. BIRMINGHAM 1978

1. This chapter is largely drawn from https://en.wikipedia.org/wiki/Birmingham; https://en.wikipedia.org/wiki/History_of_Birmingham
2. Uglow (2002).
3. Darwin & Harris (2004). See also: http://www.gutenberg.org/ebooks/author/3099.
4. https://www.youtube.com/watch?v=GxZ1xn2ml10; http://www.imdb.com/title/tt1230174/
5. https://en.wikipedia.org/wiki/Smethwick_in_the_1964_general_election
6. https://en.wikipedia.org/wiki/Rivers_of_Blood_speech
7. https://en.wikipedia.org/wiki/Birmingham_Six
8. Laws (2017).
9. Cashmore (1979).

10. Stubbs (2016).
11. Campbell & Campbell (2006).
12. Adeney (2017).
13. Baker (2003).
14. https://en.wikipedia.org/wiki/Mormon_sex_in_chains_case
15. https://en.wikipedia.org/wiki/Labour_Isn%27t_Working
16. https://en.wikipedia.org/wiki/Winter_of_Discontent
17. https://en.wikipedia.org/wiki/University_of_Birmingham; https://en.wikipedia.org/wiki/Red_brick_university
18 Lodge (1975).
19. https://en.wikipedia.org/wiki/University_(Birmingham)_railway_station

31. THE FLUEY PHOTOGRAPHER

1. This chapter is drawn from Shooter (1980), "Janet Parker" (1978), the transcript of Cook v The University of Birmingham (1979); Janet Parker's medical records, provided by Deborah Symmons; and an interview with Brian Escott-Cox QC in February 2018.
2. https://www.freebmd.org.uk/cgi/information.pl ?r=232145463:9533&d=bmd_1513933595
3. "Husband tells of life without Janet" (1979).
4. "PO engineers hold out for 35-hour week" (1978).
5. https://en.wikipedia.org/wiki/Kings_Norton
6. https://en.wikipedia.org/wiki/Crossroads_(UK_TV_series)
7. "Danger germs 12-year mystery" (1978).
8. "Midnight knock starts parents' ordeal" (1978).
9. Sandy Buchan's testimony in Cook v. University of Birmingham (1979); discussed in Chapter 57.

32. THE VIRAL OFFENSIVE

1. https://en.wikipedia.org/wiki/Tet_Offensive
2. This account of the clinical features and pathogenesis of smallpox is drawn from: Ricketts (1908); Dixon (1962); in Fenner, Henderson, Arita, Jezek, & Ladnyi (1988); Wahl-Jensen, V. *et al.* (2011).

33. A UNICORN ON THE LAWN

1. Biographical details for Deborah Symmons come from an interview with the author in October 2016. Except where indicated, the account of Parker's illness is drawn from Shooter (1980) together with Janet Parker's medical notes and contemporary notes on events made by Deborah

Symmons.

2. "Shops clear shelves of tinned salmon" (1978); Ball *et al.* (1979).
3. http://www.britishempire.co.uk/article/littlebromwich.htm
4. https://en.wikipedia.org/wiki/SOAP_note
5. Parker's haemoglobin level was 9.4g/dl, while the lower limit of normal for an adult female is 12.1g/dl. The white cell count was 15 x 10^9 cells per litre, where the upper limit of normal is 11. Parker had a lower than usual proportion of lymphocytes (17%, with a lower limit of normal of 33%) and a slightly higher than usual proportion of eosinophils (9% when normal is <7%). Her neutrophils were described as "right-shifted", meaning that the ratio of mature to immature cells was increased, suggesting that the bone marrow was not churning out as many blood cells as usual. The level of sodium ions in her blood was much lower than usual (120 mmol/L when normal is >135), while the level of potassium ions was normal. She had a raised level of urea (26.9 mmol/L, when normal is <7).
6. Daughter of Ron Fothergill, who had been a consultant on the unit, but was forced to retire earlier that year after a heart attack.
7. Geddes (1995).
8. https://en.wikipedia.org/wiki/Zebra_(medicine)

34. THE DIAGNOSIS

1. This and the subsequent chapter are drawn from interviews with Alasdair Geddes and Deborah Symmons, together with notes on events made at the time by Geddes, as recorded in Shooter (1980), and contemporary notes made by Symmons and shared with the author in 2017. According to Graham Beard (personal communication), Thomas Henry Flewett claimed to have played a role in the clinical diagnosis of Parker's smallpox. However, neither Geddess, nor Symmons have any recollection of this. Samples from Parker were sent to Flewett's virology lab at the East Birmingham Hospital, but not processed once the diagnosis had been made at the Medical School. However, this meant the lab had to be fumigated and staff put into quarantine.

35. MEETINGS AND CONTACTS

1. Mack (1972).
2. Probably from the affluent area of Kelvinside, according to

fellow Scot Geddes. Nicol can be seen in the Pathé newsreel of the burning of Witton hospital: https://www.britishpathe.com/video/hospital-burnt-down
3. Interview with Surinder Bakhshi, 21 September 2016.
4. Details of Nicol's life from "Dr William Nicol, MBChB, FFCM, DPH" (1981). Details of events are drawn from contemporary notes on events made by Deborah Symmons and from her interview with the author.

36. SAVING A CITY FROM SMALLPOX

1. https://en.wikipedia.org/wiki/Alpha_Tower
2. Biographical details from an interview with Surinder Bakhshi, 21 September 2016.
3. https://en.wikipedia.org/wiki/Kuomboka
4. The timeline of events here is drawn from notes on events made at the time by Geddes, as recorded in Shooter (1980),
5. "Doomwatch wife smallpox alert" (1978).
6. Department of Health and Social Security and the Welsh Office (1975).
7. Details of the management of the outbreak drawn from Nicol & Bakhshi (1980).
8. https://en.wikipedia.org/wiki/Bank_Holidays_Act_1871
9. Interview with Surinder Bakhshi, 21 September 2016.
10. "Ennals orders inquiry into smallpox case" (1978); "Tories press for laboratory code" (1978).
11. "Smallpox chief drama" (1978).
12. "Smallpox warning from worried countries"(1978).
13. Nicol & Bakhshi (1980).
14. "Lonely vigil of prisoner at No. 9 "(1978).
15 Docherty & Foulkes (2003).
16. Cummings (1978); there are obvious parallels between Callaghan's failure to call an autumn election in 1978 and Gordon Brown's failure to do so in 2007.
17. https://en.wikipedia.org/wiki/Pope_John_Paul_I
18. Nicol & Bakhshi (1980).

37. THE MEDICAL SCHOOL

1. https://en.wikipedia.org/wiki/University_of_Birmingham_Medical_School; https://www.birmingham.ac.uk/university/colleges/mds/about/history.aspx
2. https://en.wikipedia.org/wiki/Thomas_Arthur_Lodge
3. http://manchesterhistory.net/architecture/

1930/medicalschool.html
4. https://en.wikipedia.org/wiki/Olympiastadion_(Berlin).
5. Biographical details on Brodie Hughes from: http://livesonline.rcseng.ac.uk/biogs/E007346b.htm "Obituary EBC Hughes" (1989); "Obituary Brodie Hughes. Neurosurgeon in sight and sound" (1989).
6. Details of events taken Hughes (1978) and Wade (1978c).

38. PERSONAL INTERLUDE: THE GHOSTS OF BIRMINGHAM PAST
1. Relman, Schmidt, MacDermott, & Falkow (1992).
2. Bentley *et al.* (2003).
3. Jahrling *et al.* (2004).

39. THE CHRISTIE COMMITTEE
1. Biographical details from "Obituary A. B. Christie" (1992).
2. Christie (1965).
3. Details of the Christie Committee from Appendix 1 in Shooter (1980).

40. BACK TO WORK
1. Details of events taken Hughes (1978) and Wade (1978c).

41. THE LAST SUPPER
1. Details of events taken from Wade (1978c); McCarthy (n.d.); Wade (1996); "Ennals orders inquiry into smallpox case" (1978).

42. THE NEW DEAN
1. Biographical details from Kendall (2009); Wade (1996).

43. THE MOST UNKINDEST CUT OF ALL
1. "The Weather" (1978).
2. The following account of events is derived from: Wade (1978c); McCarthy (n.d.); Wade (1996); Osman (1978); "Smallpox expert is critical" (1978); "Press harried smallpox professor, says coroner" (1978); "Suicide plea of smallpox chief" (1978).
3. Observation made by Keith Dumbell during interview on 15 January 2018.
4. Personal Communication, Alasdair Geddes.
5. "Suicide man 'not hounded'" (1980).

44. AT THE HELM

1. Wade (1978c); Wade (1996).
2. p. 36 in Shooter (1980).
3. McKechnie later became director of the homelessness charity Shelter and then of the Consumers' Association. In 2001, she admitted "I am a fully paid-up member of the awkward squad and will remain so for the rest of my life." She died in 2004. https://en.wikipedia.org/wiki/Sheila_McKechnie
4. "Genetic manipulation: the birth of a myth" (1978); "Was the Birmingham Outbreak Really Smallpox?" (1978).

45. CATHERINE-DE-BARNES

1. https://en.wikipedia.org/wiki/Catherine-de-Barnes; http://www.solihull.gov.uk/Resident/Libraries/Local-family-history/localhistory/catherinedebarneshistory
2. Docherty & Foulkes (2003); https://en.wikipedia.org/wiki/Catherine-de-Barnes_Isolation_Hospital; the former hospital site is located here: https://goo.gl/maps/jd1zP4t3uqs
3. Details of the course of Janet Parker's illness are taken from an interview with Deborah Symmons, 24 October 2017 and from a copy of Janet Parker's medical notes made available to the author by Professor Symmons. Justification for the release of Parker's medical details forty years after her death stems from continuing medical interest in the course of illness in the last fatal case of smallpox plus an interest in informing the public of the true nature of this hideous vaccine-preventable disease, lest we forget what can be achieved through vaccination. Although the UK's General Medical Council advises that patient confidentiality continues after the death of a patient, they recognise that "the potential for disclosing information about, or causing distress to, surviving relatives or damaging the public's trust will diminish over time". https://www.gmc-uk.org/guidance/ethical_guidance/30625.asp
4. This photograph has already been released into the public domain by Alasdair Geddes in Geddes (2006).
5. "'I'm still amazed more weren't infected'" (2011).
6. "Smallpox case death 'due to heart attack'" (1978); "Smallpox father dies" (1978).
7. "Smallpox: 2 new suspects" (1978); "Smallpox 'beaten' and 260 cleared" (1978).

46. NINE ELEVEN
1. "Tight security at smallpox inquest" (1978); "Medical officer halts work on smallpox laboratory project" (1978).
2. "Husband may miss smallpox wife's funeral" (1978).
3. Gibbons (2011).
4. p. 5 in Shooter (1980).
5. "Mother of dead woman has smallpox" (1978); "Smallpox family in new tragedy" (1978).
6. p. 2 in Shooter (1980).

47. A POX IN THE DUCTS
1. Biographical details on Shooter from Roe & Roe (2013).
2. Cox, McCarthy & Millar (1974).
3. Wade (1978c).
4. This chapter draws heavily on Shooter (1980).
5. Lock (2012); "Sir Christopher Booth obituary" (2012).
6. Chris's wife Soad Tabaqchali recruited me to Barts in 1988 and mentored me for the following decade.
7. It was perhaps naïve to dismiss deliberate removal of the smallpox virus from the pox lab with intention to do harm, given subsequent history, i.e. the deliberate release of anthrax spores from a lab in 2001.

48. POXY POLITICS
1. Biographical details on Clive Jenkins from https://en.wikipedia.org/wiki/Clive_Jenkins; Pattinson (1999).
2. "Union leader blames 'new' virus for smallpox death" (1978).
3. Details except where indicated from Wade (1996).
4. "Clive the Leak" (1979).
5. "UNSAFE!" (1979).
6. McGinty (1979).
7. "Smallpox case is delayed" (1979).
8. *Hansard* (24 January 1979) col 434-48.

50. CASE FOR THE PROSECUTION
1. https://en.wikipedia.org/wiki/Aston_Webb
2. https://en.wikipedia.org/wiki/Victoria_Law_Courts
3. This account of the Cook v. University of Birmingham trial is based on a transcript of the case compiled by Cater, Walsh and Company and Meredith and Company and lodged by Owen Wade in the University of Birmingham's Special Collections, and an on interview with Brian Escott-Cox on 8 February

2018.
4. "Colston, His Honour Colin Charles (born 2 Oct. 1937), QC 1980; a Circuit Judge, 1983–2003." WHO'S WHO & WHO WAS WHO. 22 Feb. 2018.
5. "Cox, Brian (Robert) Escott (born 30 Sept. 1932), QC 1974; a Recorder of the Crown Court, 1972–98." WHO'S WHO & WHO WAS WHO. 22 Feb. 2018.
6. "Treacy, Rt Hon. Sir Colman Maurice (born 28 July 1949), a Lord Justice of Appeal, since 2012." WHO'S WHO & WHO WAS WHO. 22 Feb. 2018.

52. COMMON SENSE?

1. *Bacillus subtilis* var *globiggi* (also called BG; now reclassified as *Bacillus atrophaeus*): https://en.wikipedia.org/wiki/Bacillus_atrophaeus

60. VERDICT

1. “Union sues on smallpox” (1979); Docherty & Foulkes (2003).
2. Opposite the title page in Fenner, Henderson, Arita, Jezek, & Ladnyi (1988).
3. World Health Organization (1980).
4. Dumbell, Harper, Buchan, Douglass, & Bedson. (1999).

62. BIRMINGHAM 2013

1. Interview with Beryl Oppenheim 6 April 2017.
2. http://www.promedmail.org/direct.php?id=20120920.1302733
3. Hussain (2103); Zaki, van Boheemen, Bestebroer, Osterhaus & Fouchier (2012).
4. The Health Protection Agency (HPA) UK Novel Coronavirus Investigation Team Collective (2013); Varma (2013); Smith & Sample (2013).
5. https://en.wikipedia.org/wiki/Middle_East_respiratory_syndrome

63. WORST-CASE SCENARIOS

1. https://en.wikipedia.org/wiki/Never_events
2. http://www.hse.gov.uk; details of how to report a workplace health and safety problem to the HSE can be found here: http://www.hse.gov.uk/contact/concerns.htm
3. Sample (2018): for balance, see also: https://www.ibms.org/resources/news/ibms-response-to-the-guardian/

4. Young (2014).
5. Sample (2014).
6. https://www.cdc.gov/anthrax/news-multimedia/lab-incident/index.html
7. https://en.wikipedia.org/wiki/2001_anthrax_attacks; https://www.justice.gov/archive/amerithrax/docs/amx-investigative-summary2.pdf; http://www.johnstonsarchive.net/terrorism/anthrax.html
8. Normile (2004); Orellana (2004); Lim et al (2004).
9. Singh (2011); https://www.cdc.gov/salmonella/2011/lab-exposure-1-17-2012.html; https://www.cdc.gov/salmonella/typhimurium-labs-06-14/index.html https://www.cdc.gov/salmonella/typhimurium-07-17/index.html;
10. Singh (2009).
11. Silver (2015).
12. Gire *et al.* (2014); the paper is dedicated to five dead co-authors, but Sidiki Saffa is also highlighted as "deceased" on the author information.
13. http://www.stuff.co.nz/national/562741/Amputee-scientist-infected-at-lab-I-can-move-on-now
14. Kaiser & Malakoff (2014); https://www.rt.com/usa/413692-pandemic-pathogen-research-moratorium/
15. MacNeil, Reynolds & Damon (2009).
16. Jones, Ristow, Yilma, & Moss (1986); Openshaw, Alwan, Cherrie, & Record (1991); Mempel, *et al.* (2003); Lewis *et al.* (2006).
17. Riyesh et al (2014).
18. McCollum *et al.* (2012).
19. Meselson *et al.* (1994).
20. Pike (1976).
21. Wurtz *et al.* (2016).
22. Silver (2015).
23. http://www.hse.gov.uk/statistics/causdis/stress/
24. https://www.ucu.org.uk/article/7514/Constant-change-and-heavy-workloads-behind-rising-stress-levels-of-college-staff; https://en.wikipedia.org/wiki/Workplace_bullying_in_academia
25. The HSE provides advice for employers on what to do about stress in the workplace: http://www.hse.gov.uk/stress/what-to-do.htm The UK's NHS offers advice on how to deal with suicidal

thoughts and how to support someone with suicidal thoughts: https://www.nhs.uk/conditions/suicide/getting-help/ https://www.nhs.uk/conditions/suicide/helping-others/ Samaritans in the UK can be contacted on the phone at 116123 or by email at jo@samaritans.org Wikipedia provides an international list of suicide crisis lines: https://en.wikipedia.org/wiki/List_of_suicide_crisis_lines
26 https://en.wikipedia.org/wiki/David_Kelly_(weapons_expert) https://en.wikipedia.org/wiki/Hutton_Inquiry
27. https://en.wikipedia.org/wiki/Stefan_Grimm
28. https://en.wikipedia.org/wiki/News_International_phone_hacking_scandal https://en.wikipedia.org/wiki/Leveson_Inquiry
29. Pidd (2013).
30. Ronson (2016).
31. https://en.wikipedia.org/wiki/Fake_news; https://en.wikipedia.org/wiki/Alternative_facts

64. AFTERLIFE OF THE POX

1. Esposito, Nakano & Obijeski (1985).
2. Dahiya *et al.* (2016).
3. Bera *et al.* (2011).
4. Singh *et al.* (2007).
5. McCollum & Damon (2014).
6. Nolen *et al.* (2016).
7. Ligon (2004).
8. Vorou, Papavassiliou & Pierroutsakos. (2008).
9. Mauldin *et al.* (2017).
10. Qin, Favis, Famulski & Evans (2015).
11. Schrick *et al.* (2017).
12. Centers for Disease Control and Prevention (2007); Muzny, C.A. *et al.* (2009); Centers for Disease Control and Prevention, C.D.C. (2010).
13. Oliveira *et al.* (2017).
14. Chapter 28 in Fenner, Henderson, Arita, Jezek, & Ladnyi (1988).
15. Khalakdina, Costa & Briand (2016).
16. Arita & Francis (2014); Agwunobi (2007); Hammond (2007); Damon, Damaso & McFadden (2014); Lane & Poland (2011).
17. Arvin & Patel (2009).
18. Esposito JJ *et al.* (2006); Massung *et al.* (1994); Shchelkunov *et al.* (2000); Shchelkunov, Massung &Esposito (1995).
19. Duggan *et al.* (2016); Smithson, Imbery & Upton (2017).

20. Carmichael & Silverstein (1987).
21. Reviewed by Shchelkunova & Shchelkunov (2017); Damon, Damaso & McFadden (2014); Olson & Shchelkunov (2017).
22. Jahrling *et al.* (2004); Rubins (2004); Wahl-Jensen (2011); Valdivia-Granda, Kann & Malaga (2007).
23. Reviewed by Shchelkunova & Shchelkunov (2017); Damon, Damaso & McFadden (2014); Olson & Shchelkunov (2017).
24. Reviewed by Shchelkunova & Shchelkunov (2017); Damon, Damaso & McFadden (2014); Olson & Shchelkunov (2017).
25. Reardon (2014b).
26. Director of Laboratory Science and Safety, FDA (2016).
27. McCollum *et al.* (2014); Reardon (2014).
28. Noyce, Lederman &Evans (2018); Kupferschmidt (2018).
29. Thiessen (2014).
30. https://www.cdc.gov/smallpox/bioterrorism-response-planning/index.html; https://stacks.cdc.gov/view/cdc/27723; http://www.gov.scot/Publications/2002/12/15905/14661.

66. EMERGENCE OR ERADICATION?

1. Quammen (2012).
2. Centers for Disease Control (1981).
3. http://www.unaids.org/en/resources/fact-sheet
4. Delaney (2006).
5. Peiris, Yuen, Osterhaus & Stöhr (2003).
6. http://www.who.int/emergencies/mers-cov/en/
7. https://en.wikipedia.org/wiki/West_African_Ebola_virus_epidemic
8. https://en.wikipedia.org/wiki/Zika_virus
9. https://en.wikipedia.org/wiki/Influenza_pandemic; https://amr-review.org
10. http://www.fao.org/ag/againfo/programmes/documents/grep/A_RESO_18_FMD_Eradication.pdf
11. https://en.wikipedia.org/wiki/Eradication_of_dracunculiasis; https://www.cartercenter.org/health/guinea_worm/
12. https://en.wikipedia.org/wiki/Poliomyelitis_eradication
13. https://en.wikipedia.org/wiki/Eradication_of_infectious_diseases
14. http://endmalaria2040.org

67. SO, WHAT ACTUALLY HAPPENED?

1. Keith Dumbell, Interview, 9 March 2018. Keith remembers that this was a common saying , but cannot remember the precise source.

2. Silver (2014) reports an equally implausible scenario—that the smallpox virus was carried by ants that moved from room to room along electric wiring tracts. It seems he got the idea from my former colleague Jeff Cole and this says more about Jeff's sense of humour than about what really happened in 1978.
3. Lidén & Brehmer-Andersson, (1988); Aguirre, Landa, González, & Díaz-Pérez (1992); Brancaccio, Cockerell, Belsito, & Ostreicher (1993); Galindo, Garcia, Garrido, Feo, & Fernández (1994); Rustemeyer & Frosch (1995); Hansson, Ahlfors, & Bergendorff (1997); Marconi, Campagna, Fabri, & Schiavino (1999); Chen & Pratt (2015).
4. Chapter 6 in Dixon (1962).
5. Interview with Escott-Cox, 8 February, 2018
6. https://en.wikipedia.org/wiki/MRDA_(slang)
7. Dixon (1962) estimates that, relative to the unvaccinated, the risk of infection in the vaccinated after to exposure to variola major is reduced by a thousand to one in the first year after vaccination but falls to only one in eight after ten years and down to just 50% after twenty years.
8. Interview with Keith Dumbell, 9 March 2018.

68. LAB IN A SUITCASE

1. The events in this chapter are drawn from an interview with Josh Quick on15 March 2018 and from Loman (2016). Information on the Ebola outbreak: https://en.wikipedia.org/wiki/West_African_Ebola_virus_epidemic
2. Quick *et al.* (2016).
3. Harper, Bedson & Buchan (1979); Dumbell, Harper, Buchan, Douglass, & Bedson (1999).
4. On 16 March 2018 at the Nanopore Day Paris meeting, Jean-Luc Guérin and Guillaume Croville announced that they can obtain full length poxvirus genome assemblies directly from clinical lesions on the nanopore platform: https://twitter.com/pathogenomenick/status/974302851387351045 https://twitter.com/slecrom/status/974296751518646277

69. LAST WORDS

1. Pinker (2018).
2. Peck & Tickell (2002); https://www.equalitytrust.org.uk/how-has-inequality-changed

REFERENCES

"A thief risks smallpox" (1966, May 2). *The Guardian*, p. 1.

Adeney, M. "Derek Robinson obituary" (2017, November 1). *The Guardian*. Retrieved from https://www.theguardian.com/politics/2017/nov/01/derek-robinson-obituary

Afonso, C. L., Tulman, E. R., Lu, Z., Zsak, L., Sandybaev, N. T., Kerembekova, U. Z. *et al.* (2002). The genome of camelpox virus. *Virology, 295*, 1-9.

Aguirre, A., Landa, N., González, M., & Díaz-Pérez, J. L. (1992). Allergic contact dermatitis in a photographer. *Contact Dermatitis, 27*, 340-341.

Agwunobi, J. O. (2007). Should the US and Russia destroy their stocks of smallpox virus. *BMJ, 334*, 775.

Arita, I., & Francis, D. (2014). Is it time to destroy the smallpox virus. *Science, 345*, 1010.

Arita, I., Gispen, R., Kalter, S. S., Wah, L. T., Marennikova, S. S., Netter, R. *et al.* (1972). Outbreaks of monkeypox and serological surveys in nonhuman primates. *Bull World Health Organ, 46*, 625-631.

Arita, I., & Henderson, D. (1976). Monkeypox and whitepox viruses in West and Central Africa. *Bull World Health Organ, 53*, 347-353.

Arvin, A. M & Patel, D. M. (2009). *Live Variola Virus: Considerations for Continuing Research.* Washington (D.C.): National Academies Press; Institute of Medicine.

Babkin, I. V., & Babkina, I. N. (2012). A retrospective study of the orthopoxvirus molecular evolution. *Infect Genet Evol, 12*, 1597-1604.

Babkin, I. V., & Babkina, I. N. (2015). The origin of the variola virus. *Viruses, 7*, 1100-1112.

Baker, J. P. (2003). The pertussis vaccine controversy in Great Britain, 1974-1986. *Vaccine, 21*, 4003-4010.

Ball, A. P., Hopkinson, R. B., Farrell, I. D., Hutchison, J. G., Paul, R., Watson, R. D. *et al.* (1979). Human botulism caused by *Clostridium botulinum* type E: the Birmingham outbreak. *Q J Med, 48*, 473-491.

Bangladesh Smallpox Eradication Programme. (1976). Documentation for International Assessment Commission. Status Report June 1, 1976. Retrieved from http://www.zero-pox.info/other_docs/bangla_comm.pdf

Baron, J. (1838). *The life of Edward Jenner, with illustrations of his doctrines, and selections from his correspondence*. London: Henry Colburn. Retrieved from https://archive.org/details/lifeofedwardjenn02barouoft

Basler, R. P. (1972). Did President Lincoln Give the Smallpox to William H. Johnson? *The Huntington Library Quarterly*, 279-284.

Baxby, D. (1972). Smallpox-like viruses from camels in Iran. *Lancet*, *300*, 1063-1065.

Baxby, D. (1974). Differentiation of smallpox and camelpox viruses in cultures of human and monkey cells. *J Hyg (Lond)*, *72*, 251-254.

Baxby, D., Hessami, M., Ghaboosi, B., & Ramyar, H. (1975). Response of camels to intradermal inoculation with smallpox and camelpox viruses. *Infection and Immunity*, *11*, 617-621.

Bedson, H. S. (1972). Camelpox and smallpox. *Lancet*, *2*, 1253.

Bedson, H. S., & Dumbell, K. R. (1961). The effect of temperature on the growth of pox viruses in the chick embryo. *Journal of Hygiene*, *59*, 457-470.

Beer, G. (2000). Darwin's Plots. Cambridge University Press.

Behbehani, A. M. (1983). The smallpox story: life and death of an old disease. *Microbiol Rev*, *47*, 455-509.

Benedictow, O. J. (2004). *The Black Death 1346–1353: The Complete History*. Woodridge: Boydell & Brewer.

Bentham, J. (1907). An Introduction to the Principles of Morals and Legislation. Retrieved from http://oll.libertyfund.org/titles/bentham-an-introduction-to-the-principles-of-morals-and-legislation

Bentley, S. D., Maiwald, M., Murphy, L. D., Pallen, M. J., Yeats, C. A., Dover, L. G. *et al.* (2003). Sequencing and analysis of the genome of the Whipple's disease bacterium *Tropheryma whipplei*. *Lancet*, *361*, 637-644.

Bera, B. C., Shanmugasundaram, K., Barua, S., Venkatesan, G., Virmani, N., Riyesh, T. *et al.* (2011). Zoonotic cases of camelpox infection in India. *Vet Microbiol*, *152*, 29-38.

Bhatnagar, V., Stoto, M., Morton, S., Boer, R., & Bozzette, S. (2006). Transmission patterns of smallpox: systematic review of natural outbreaks in Europe and North America since World War II. *BMC Public Health*, *6*, 126.

Bidgood, S. R., & Mercer, J. (2015). Cloak and Dagger: Alternative Immune Evasion and Modulation Strategies of Poxviruses. *Viruses*, *7*, 4800-4825.

Bivins, R. (2007). "The People Have No More Love Left for the Commonwealth": Media, Migration and Identity in the 1961–62 British Smallpox Outbreak. *Immigrants & Minorities, 25*, 263-289.

Bivins, R. (2015). *Contagious Communities: Medicine, Migration, and the NHS in Post War Britain*. Oxford: OUP.

Bradley, W. H. (1948). Smallpox 1947. *Proc R Soc Med, 41*, 497-500.

Bradley, W. H. (1963). Smallpox in England and Wales 1962. *Proc R Soc Med, 56*, 335-338.

Bradley, W. H., Davies, J. O., & Durante, J. A. (1946). The outbreak of smallpox in Middlesex, 1944. *Br Med J, 2*, 194-196.

Brancaccio, R. R., Cockerell, C. J., Belsito, D., & Ostreicher, R. (1993). Allergic contact dermatitis from color film developers: clinical and histologic features. *J Am Acad Dermatol, 28*, 827-830.

Breen, G. E. (1956). The management of an outbreak of smallpox. I. Clinical aspects. *Public Health, 69*, 98-103.

Breman, J. G., Bernadou, J., & Nakano, J. H. (1977). Poxvirus in West African nonhuman primates: serological survey results. *Bull World Health Organ, 55*, 605-612.

Bugert, J. J., & Darai, G. (2000). Poxvirus homologues of cellular genes. *Virus Genes, 21*, 111-133.

Buist, J. B. (1887). *Vaccinia and variola: a study of their life history*. London: Churchill. Retrieved from https://archive.org/details/vacciniavariolas00buisuoft

Bukrinskaya, A. (1991). In memory of Victor Zhdanov. *Arch Virol, 121*, 237-240.

Butterworth, E. (1966). The 1962 Smallpox Outbreak and the British Press. *Race & Class, 7*, 347-364.

Campbell, A., & Campbell, R. (2006). *Blood and Fire*. Random House.

Carmichael, A. G., & Silverstein, A. M. (1987). Smallpox in Europe before the seventeenth century: virulent killer or benign disease. *J Hist Med Allied Sci, 42*, 147-168.

Cashmore, E. (1979). *Rastaman. The Rastafarian Movement in England*. London: Allen & Unwin.

Centers for Disease Control (CDC) (1981). *Pneumocystis* pneumonia--Los Angeles. *MMWR Morb Mortal Wkly Rep, 30*, 250-252.

Centers for Disease Control and Prevention (CDC) (2007). Vulvar vaccinia infection after sexual contact with a military smallpox vaccinee--Alaska, 2006. *MMWR Morb Mortal Wkly Rep, 56*, 417-419.

Centers for Disease Control and Prevention (CDC) (2010). Vaccinia virus infection after sexual contact with a military smallpox vaccinee -Washington, 2010. *MMWR Morb Mortal Wkly Rep, 59*, 773-775.

Chen, T., & Pratt, M. D. (2015). Photo developer allergic contact dermatitis in a photographer following paraphenylenediamine sensitization from a temporary henna tattoo. *J Cutan Med Surg, 19*, 73-76.

Christie, A. B. (1965). Motoring and Camping in Greece.

Clark, G., Seiler, H. E., Joe, A., Gammie, J. L., Tait, H. P., & Jack, R. P. (1944). *The Edinburgh Outbreak of Smallpox 1942*. Edinburgh: City of Edinburgh Public Health Department.

Clark, T., & Grasty, P. (1999). Obituary Liselotte (Lilo) Lennhoff. *Br Med J, 318*, 813.

"Clive the Leak" (1979, January 4). *Daily Express*, p. 1.

Clokie, M. R., Millard, A. D., Letarov, A. V., & Heaphy, S. (2011). Phages in nature. *Bacteriophage, 1*, 31-45.

Colangelo, P., Corti, M., Verheyen, E., Annesi, F., Oguge, N., Makundi, R. *et al.* (2005). Mitochondrial phylogeny reveals differential modes of chromosomal evolution in the genus Tatera (Rodentia: Gerbillinae) in Africa. *Mol Phylogenet Evol, 35*, 556-568.

Collis, R. (2013). *Death and the City: The nation's experience, told through Brighton's history*. Hanover Press.

Colson, P., de Lamballerie, X., Fournous, G., & Raoult, D. (2012). Reclassification of giant viruses composing a fourth domain of life in the new order Megavirales. *Intervirology, 55*, 321-332.

Colston, His Honour Colin Charles (born 2 October 1937), QC 1980; a Circuit Judge, 1983–2003. (2018). *WHO'S WHO & WHO WAS WHO* Retrieved from http://www.ukwhoswho.com/view/10.1093/ww/9780199540884.001.0001/ww-9780199540884-e-11586

Cook v The University of Birmingham. (1979, October 22 – November 6). Birmingham Magistrates Court.

Cooper, B. (2006). Poxy models and rash decisions. *Proc Natl Acad Sci U S A, 103*, 12221-12222.

Corina, F. J. (1962, January 18). More readers' views *Telegraph and Argus*, p. 6.

Cox, Brian (Robert) Escott (born 30 September 1932), QC 1974; a Recorder of the Crown Court, 1972–98. (2018). *WHO'S WHO & WHO WAS WHO* Retrieved from http://www.ukwhoswho.com/view/10.1093/ww/9780199540884.001.0001/ww-9780199540884-e-12125

Cox, P. J., McCarthy, K., & Millar, E. L. (1974). *Report of the Committee of Inquiry into the Smallpox Outbreak in London in March and April 1973*. London: HMSO.

Cramb, R. (1951). Smallpox outbreak in Brighton, 1950-51. *Public Health, 64*, 123-128.

Cruickshank, J., Bedson, H., & Watson, D. (1966). Electron microscopy in the rapid diagnosis of smallpox. *Lancet, 2*, 527.

Culley, A. R. (1963). The Smallpox Outbreak in South Wales. In Bradley, W.H. et al (1963) Smallpox in England and Wales 1962. *Proc R Soc Med, 56*, 335–346.

Cummings (1978, September 1). I am not worried about smallpox. I'M worried about an outbreak of Socialism in the Labour Party between now and Election Day... *Daily Express*, p. 11.

d'Errico, P. (2017). Jeffery Amherst and Smallpox Blankets. Lord Jeffery Amherst's letters discussing germ warfare against American Indians. http://people.umass.edu/derrico/amherst/lord_jeff.html

Dahiya, S. S., Kumar, S., Mehta, S. C., Narnaware, S. D., Singh, R., & Tuteja, F. C. (2016). Camelpox: A brief review on its epidemiology, current status and challenges. *Acta Trop, 158*, 32-38.

Damle, A. S., Gaikwad, A. A., Patwardhan, N. S., Duthade, M. M., Sheikh, N. S., & Deshmukh, D. G. (2011). Outbreak of human buffalopox infection. *J Glob Infect Dis, 3*, 187-188.

Damon, I. K., Damaso, C. R., & McFadden, G. (2014). Are we there yet? The smallpox research agenda using variola virus. *PLoS Pathog, 10*, e1004108.

"Danger germs 12-year mystery" (1978, August 26). *Birmingham Evening Mail*, p. 10.

Darwin, C. (1860). Letter to Asa Gray. Darwin Correspondence Project, "Letter no. 2814. *Darwin Correspondence Project* http://www.darwinproject.ac.uk/DCP-LETT-2814

Darwin, C. (1856). Letter to Joseph Hooker. Darwin Correspondence Project, "Letter no. 1924". *Darwin Correspondence Project* http://www.darwinproject.ac.uk/DCP-LETT-1924

Darwin, C. (1871). *The Descent of Man, and Selection in Relation to Sex*. London: John Murray. Retrieved from http://darwin-online.org.uk/content/frameset?pageseq=113&itemID=F937.1&viewtype=text

Darwin, E., & Harris, S. (2004). *Cosmologia: A Sequence of Epic Poems in Three Parts.*

Dawkins, R. (1976). *The Selfish Gene*. Oxford: Oxford University

Press.
"Death not due to smallpox. Queues for vaccination." (1962, January 30). *The Guardian*, p. 1.
Delaney, M. (2006). History of HAART – the true story of how effective multi-drug therapy was developed for treatment of HIV disease. *Retrovirology, 3*, S6.
Department of Health and Social Security and the Welsh Office. (1975). Memorandum on the Control of Outbreaks of Smallpox. HMSO.
Diamond, J. M. (1997). *Guns, germs, and steel : the fates of human societies*. New York: W.W. Norton & Co.
Director of Laboratory Science and Safety, F. D. A. (2016). FDA Review of the 2014 Discovery of Vials Labeled "Variola" and Other Vials Discovered in an FDA-Occupied Building on the NIH Campus. https://www.fda.gov/downloads/AboutFDA/ReportsManualsForms/Reports/UCM532877.pdf
Dixon, C. W. (1962). *Smallpox*. London: Churchill. Retrieved from https://www.nlm.nih.gov/nichsr/esmallpox/smallpox_dixon.pdf
Docherty, C., & Foulkes, C. (2003, October 4). Toxic SHOCK; Twenty five years ago a disease that many thought was dead and gone reared its head in Birmingham: smallpox. *The Birmingham Post*. Retrieved from https://www.thefreelibrary.com/Toxic+SHOCK%3b+Twenty+five+years+ago+a+disease+that+many+thought+was.-a0108504745
"Donald Henderson, epidemiologist who helped to eradicate smallpox – obituary" (2016, August 21). *The Telegraph*. Retrieved from http://www.telegraph.co.uk/obituaries/2016/08/21/donald-henderson-epidemiologist-who-helped-to-eradicate-smallpox/
"Doomwatch wife smallpox alert" (1978, 26 August). *Daily Express*, p. 2.
Douglas, J., & Edgar, W. (1962). Smallpox in Bradford, 1962. *Br Med J, 1*, 612-614.
"Dr William Nicol, MBChB, FFCM, DPH" (1981). *Community Medicine*, *3*, 365.
Duggan, A. T., Perdomo, M. F., Piombino-Mascali, D., Marciniak, S., Poinar, D., Emery, M. V. *et al.* (2016). 17th century variola virus reveals the recent history of smallpox. *Curr Biol*, *26*, 3407-3412.
Dumbell, K. R., & Bedson, H. S. (1964). The use of ceiling

temperature and reactivation in the isolation of pox virus hybrids. *J Hyg (Lond)*, *62*, 133-140.

Dumbell, K. R., Bedson, H. S., & Rossier, E. (1961). The laboratory differentiation between variola major and variola minor. *Bull World Health Organ*, *25*, 73-78.

Dumbell, K. R., Harper, L., Buchan, A., Douglass, N. J., & Bedson, H. S. (1999). A variant of variola virus, characterized by changes in polypeptide and endonuclease profiles. *Epidemiol Infect*, *122*, 287-290.

Dumbell, K. R., & Kapsenberg, J. G. (1982). Laboratory investigation of two "whitepox" viruses and comparison with two variola strains from southern India. *Bull World Health Organ*, *60*, 381.

Duraffour, S., Meyer, H., Andrei, G., & Snoeck, R. (2011). Camelpox virus. *Antiviral Res*, *92*, 167-186.

"Ennals orders inquiry into smallpox case" (1978, August 31). *The Guardian*, p. 1.

Esposito, J. J., Nakano, J. H., & Obijeski, J. F. (1985). Can variola-like viruses be derived from monkeypox virus? An investigation based on DNA mapping. *Bull World Health Organ*, *63*, 695-703.

Esposito, J. J., Sammons, S. A., Frace, A. M., Osborne, J. D., Olsen-Rasmussen, M., Zhang, M. *et al.* (2006). Genome sequence diversity and clues to the evolution of variola (smallpox) virus. *Science*, *313*, 807-812.

Fenner, F., Henderson, D. A., Arita, I., Jezek, Z., & Ladnyi, I. D. (1988). *Smallpox and its eradication*. Geneva: World Health Organization. Retrieved from http://whqlibdoc.who.int/smallpox/9241561106.pdf

Fenner, F., Wittek, R., & Dumbell, K. R. (1989). *The orthopoxviruses*. San Diego: Academic Press. Retrieved from https://www.nlm.nih.gov/nichsr/esmallpox/orthopoxviruses.pdf

Firth, C., Kitchen, A., Shapiro, B., Suchard, M. A., Holmes, E. C., & Rambaut, A. (2010). Using time-structured data to estimate evolutionary rates of double-stranded DNA viruses. *Mol Biol Evol*, *27*, 2038-2051.

Forterre, P. (2006). The origin of viruses and their possible roles in major evolutionary transitions. *Virus Res*, *117*, 5-16.

Foster, S. O., Hughes, K., Tarantola, D., & Glasser, J. W. (2011). Smallpox eradication in Bangladesh, 1972-1976. *Vaccine*, *29 Suppl 4*, D22-9.

Galindo, P. A., Garcia, R., Garrido, J. A., Feo, F., & Fernández, F.

(1994). Allergic contact dermatitis from colour developers: absence of cross-sensitivity to para-amino compounds. *Contact Dermatitis*, *30*, 301.

Gaston, H. (2013). *Lost Hospitals of Brighton and Hove*. Southern Editorial Services.

Geddes, A. (1995). Obituary HV Morgan. *Br Med J*, *311*, 1086.

Geddes, A. M. (2006). The history of smallpox. *Clin Dermatol*, *24*, 152-157.

Geddes, L. (2016, September 6). Donald Henderson obituary. *The Guardian*. Retrieved from https://www.theguardian.com/world/2016/sep/07/donald-henderson-obituary

Gelfand, H. M., & Posch, J. (1971). The recent outbreak of smallpox in Meschede, West Germany. *Am J Epidemiol*, *93*, 234-237.

"Genetic manipulation: the birth of a myth" (1978). *University of Birmingham Bulletin*, *333*, 2.

Gibbons, B. (2011, June 21). Haunting memories of smallpox drama *Birmingham Mail*. Retrieved from http://www.birminghammail.co.uk/news/local-news/haunting-memories-of-smallpox-drama-156484

Gire, S. K., Goba, A., Andersen, K. G., Sealfon, R. S., Park, D. J., Kanneh, L. *et al.* (2014). Genomic surveillance elucidates Ebola virus origin and transmission during the 2014 outbreak. *Science*, *345*, 1369-1372.

Gispen, R., & Brand-Saathof, B. (1972). "White" poxvirus strains from monkeys. *Bull World Health Organ*, *46*, 585-592.

Glynn, I., & Glynn, J. (2005). *Life and Death of Smallpox*. Cambridge: Cambridge University Press.

Goldman, A. S., & Schmalstieg, F. C. (2007). Abraham Lincoln's Gettysburg illness. *J Med Biogr*, *15*, 104-110.

Goodpasture, E. W., Woodruff, A. M., & Buddingh, G. J. (1932). Vaccinal Infection of the Chorio-Allantoic Membrane of the Chick Embryo. *Am J Pathol*, *8*, 271-282.7.

Gordon, C. W., Donnelly, J. D., Fothergill, R., Ker, F. L., Millar, E. L., Flewett, T. H. *et al.* (1966). Variola minor. A preliminary report from the Birmingham Hospital region. *Lancet*, *1*, 1311-1313.

Gordon, P. (1983). Medicine, racism and immigration control. *Critical Social Policy*, *3*, 6-20.

Greenough, P. (1995). Intimidation, coercion and resistance in the final stages of the South Asian smallpox eradication campaign, 1973–1975. *Social Science & Medicine*, *41*, 633-645.

Gubser, C., & Smith, G. (2002). The sequence of camelpox virus shows it is most closely related to variola virus, the cause of smallpox. *J Gen Virol*, *83*, 855-872.

Hammond, E. (2007). Should the US and Russia destroy their stocks of smallpox virus. *BMJ*, *334*, 774.

Hansson, C., Ahlfors, S., & Bergendorff, O. (1997). Concomitant contact dermatitis due to textile dyes and to colour film developers can be explained by the formation of the same hapten. *Contact Dermatitis*, *37*, 27-31.

Harper, L., Bedson, H., & Buchan, A. (1979). Identification of orthopoxviruses by polyacrylamide gel electrophoresis of intracellular polypeptides. I. Four major groupings. *Virology*, *93*, 435-444.

Hawkes, N. (1979). Science in Europe/smallpox death in Britain challenges presumption of laboratory safety. *Science*, *203*, 855-856.

Hay, R., Odds, F., & Campbell, C. (2017). Obituary Donald MacKenzie 1929-2017. http://www.bsmm.org/2017/08/31/obituary/

Health Protection Agency (HPA) UK Novel Coronavirus Investigation team (2013). Evidence of person-to-person transmission within a family cluster of novel coronavirus infections, United Kingdom, February 2013. *Euro Surveill*, *18*, 20427.

Helm, K. (1928). *The true story of Mary, wife of Lincoln*. New York and London: Harper & brothers. Retrieved from https://archive.org/details/truestoryofmaryw00helm

Henderson, D. A. (2009). *Smallpox: The Death of a Disease* (1 ed.). Prometheus Books.

Henderson, D. A. (2011). The eradication of smallpox--an overview of the past, present, and future. *Vaccine*, *29 Suppl 4*, D7-9.

Hogben, G. H., McKendrick, G. D., & Nicol, C. G. (1958). Smallpox in Tottenham; 1957. *Lancet*, *1*, 1061-1064.

Hopkins, D. R. (1980). Ramses V: earliest known victim. *World Health*, *5*, 22-26.

Hopkins, D. R. (2002). *The Greatest Killer: Smallpox In History*. University of Chicago Press.

Hounsome, R. (2007). *The Very Nearly Man: An Autobiography*. Matador.

Hughes, A. L., Irausquin, S., & Friedman, R. (2010). The evolutionary biology of poxviruses. *Infect Genet Evol*, *10*, 50-59.

Hughes, E. B. C. (1978). *Smallpox outbreak—Medical School August*

1978. Diary of events by the Dean Professor Brodie Hughes. University of Birmingham special collection. Ref. pZ1-pZ675 H7 N.
"Husband may miss smallpox wife's funeral" (1978, September 13). *Birmingham Evening Mail*, p. 4.
"Husband tells of life without Janet" (1979, January 4). *Daily Express_g*, p. 4.
Hussain, I. (2013). The story of the first MERS patient. *Nature Middle East*. Retrieved from https://www.natureasia.com/en/nmiddleeast/article/10.1038/nmiddleeast.2014.134
"I'm still amazed more weren't infected" (2011, June 11). *Birmingham Mail*. Retrieved from https://www.thefreelibrary.com/'I'm+still+amazed+more+weren't+infected'.-a0259359829
Irons, J. V., Sullivan, T. D., Cook, E. B., Cox, G. W., & Hale, R. A. (1953). Outbreak of smallpox in the lower Rio Grande Valley of Texas in 1949. *Am J Public Health Nations Health*, *43*, 25-29.
Iyer, L. M., Balaji, S., Koonin, E. V., & Aravind, L. (2006). Evolutionary genomics of nucleo-cytoplasmic large DNA viruses. *Virus Res*, *117*, 156-184.
Jahrling, P. B., Hensley, L. E., Martinez, M. J., Leduc, J. W., Rubins, K. H., Relman, D. A. *et al.* (2004). Exploring the potential of variola virus infection of cynomolgus macaques as a model for human smallpox. *Proc Natl Acad Sci U S A*, *101*, 15196-15200.
"Janet Parker" (1978). *University of Birmingham Bulletin*, *333*, 3.
Jefferson, T. (1806). From Thomas Jefferson to George C. Jenner, 14 May 1806. *Founders Online, National Archives* http://founders.archives.gov/documents/Jefferson/99-01-02-3718
Jenner, E. (1798). An Inquiry Into the Causes and Effects of the Variolae Vaccinae. London: Sampson Low. Retrieved from http://www.gutenberg.org/ebooks/29414
Joarder, A. K., Tarantola, D., & Tulloch, J. (1980). *The eradication of smallpox from Bangladesh*. World Health Organization, South-East Asia Regional Office. New Delhi: World Health Organization South-East Asia Regional Office. (South-East Asia Series No 8).
Jones, L., Ristow, S., Yilma, T., & Moss, B. (1986). Accidental human vaccination with vaccinia virus expressing nucleoprotein gene. *Nature*, *319*, 543.
Kaiser, J., & Malakoff, D. (2014). U.S. halts funding for new risky virus studies, calls for voluntary moratorium. *Science*.

http://www.sciencemag.org/news/2014/10/us-halts-funding-new-risky-virus-studies-calls-voluntary-moratorium

Kemp, G. E. (1975). Viruses other than arenaviruses from West African wild mammals. Factors affecting transmission to man and domestic animals. *Bull World Health Organ*, *52*, 615-620.

Kemp, G. E., Causey, O. R., Setzer, H. W., & Moore, D. L. (1974). Isolation of viruses from wild mammals in West Africa, 1966-1970. *J Wildl Dis*, *10*, 279-293.

Kendall, M. (2009). Owen Lyndon Wade: clinical pharmacologist, 1921-2008. *Br J Clin Pharmacol*, *68*, 468-469.

Khalakdina, A., Costa, A., & Briand, S. (2016). Smallpox in the post eradication era. *Wkly Epidemiol Rec*, *91*, 257-264.

Kotar, S. L., & Gessler, J. E. (2013). *Smallpox*. Jefferson, North Carolina: McFarland.

Kupferschmidt, K. (2018). Critics see only risks, no benefits in horsepox paper. *Science*, *359*, 375-376.

La Scola, B., Audic, S., Robert, C., Jungang, L., de Lamballerie, X., Drancourt, M. *et al.* (2003). A giant virus in amoebae. *Science*, *299*, 2033.

Lane, J. M., & Poland, G. A. (2011). Why not destroy the remaining smallpox virus stocks. *Vaccine*, *29*, 2823-2824.

Laws, R. (2017, February 14). The day Bob Marley walked through Birmingham *The Birmingham Mail*. Retrieved from http://www.birminghammail.co.uk/whats-on/theatre-news/day-bob-marley-walked-through-12592119

Lewis, F. M., Chernak, E., Goldman, E., Li, Y., Karem, K., Damon, I. K. *et al.* (2006). Ocular vaccinia infection in laboratory worker, Philadelphia, 2004. *Emerg Infect Dis*, *12*, 134-137.

Li, Y., Carroll, D. S., Gardner, S. N., Walsh, M. C., Vitalis, E. A., & Damon, I. K. (2007). On the origin of smallpox: correlating variola phylogenics with historical smallpox records. *Proc Natl Acad Sci U S A*, *104*, 15787-15792.

Lidén, C., & Brehmer-Andersson, E. (1988). Occupational dermatoses from colour developing agents. Clinical and histopathological observations. *Acta Derm Venereol*, *68*, 514-522.

Ligon, B. L. (2004). Monkeypox: a review of the history and emergence in the Western hemisphere. *Semin Pediatr Infect Dis*, *15*, 280-287.

Lim, P. L., Kurup, A., Gopalakrishna, G., Chan, K. P., Wong, C. W., Ng, L. C. *et al.* (2004). Laboratory-acquired severe acute respiratory syndrome. *N Engl J Med*, *350*, 1740-1745.

Lock, S. (2012). Obituary: Christopher Booth. *Br Med J*, *345*, e5768.

Lodge, D. (1975). *Changing Places*. Harvill Secker.
Loman, N. J. (2016) Behind the paper: Real time, portable sequencing for Ebola surveillance. http://lab.loman.net/2016/02/03/behind-the-paper-real-time-portable-sequencing-for-ebola-surveillance/
"Lonely vigil of prisoner at No. 9" (1978, August 26). *Daily Express*, p. 2.
Lourie, B., Nakano, J., Kemp, G., & Setzer, H. (1975). Isolation of poxvirus from an African Rodent. *J Infect Dis*, *132*, 677-681.
MacAskill, W. (2015). *Doing good better: effective altruism and a radical new way to make a difference*. Guardian Faber Publishing.
Mack, T. M. (1972). Smallpox in Europe, 1950-1971. *J Infect Dis*, *125*, 161-169.
MacNeil, A., Reynolds, M. G., & Damon, I. K. (2009). Risks associated with vaccinia virus in the laboratory. *Virology*, *385*, 1-4.
Manela, E. (2010). A pox on your narrative: writing disease control into Cold War history. *Diplomatic History*, *34*, 299-323.
Mansworth, S. (2002). DEADLY DISEASE; Analysis: Survivors of the 1962 South Wales smallpox outbreak have helped to paint a terrifying portrait of how the UK would cope with a bio-terrorist attack. https://www.thefreelibrary.com/DEADLY+DISEASE%3b+Analysis%3a+Survivors+of+the+1962+South+Wales+smallpox.-a082591810
Marconi, P. M., Campagna, G., Fabri, G., & Schiavino, D. (1999). Allergic contact dermatitis from colour developers used in automated photographic processing. *Contact Dermatitis*, *40*, 109.
Massung, R. F., Liu, L. I., Qi, J., Knight, J. C., Yuran, T. E., Kerlavage, A. R. *et al.* (1994). Analysis of the complete genome of smallpox variola major virus strain Bangladesh-1975. *Virology*, *201*, 215-240.
Mauldin, M. R., Antwerpen, M., Emerson, G. L., Li, Y., Zoeller, G., Carroll, D. S. *et al.* (2017). Cowpox virus: What's in a Name. *Viruses*, *9*, pii: E101
McCarthy, K. (n.d.). *The Smallpox Episode Birmingham August 1978, the last episode of smallpox in human history*. University of Birmingham special collection. Ref. pZ1-pZ675 H7 N.
McCollum, A. M., Austin, C., Nawrocki, J., Howland, J., Pryde, J., Vaid, A. *et al.* (2012). Investigation of the first laboratory-acquired human cowpox virus infection in the United States. *J*

Infect Dis, *206*, 63-68.
McCollum, A. M., & Damon, I. K. (2014). Human monkeypox. *Clin Infect Dis*, *58*, 260-267.
McCollum, A. M., Li, Y., Wilkins, K., Karem, K. L., Davidson, W. B., Paddock, C. D. *et al.* (2014). Poxvirus viability and signatures in historical relics. *Emerg Infect Dis*, *20*, 177-184.
McGinty, L. (1979). Smallpox Laboratories, What Are the Risks? *New Scientist*, *81*, 8-14.
"Medical officer halts work on smallpox laboratory project" (1978, September 13). *The Times*, p. 2.
Mempel, M., Isa, G., Klugbauer, N., Meyer, H., Wildi, G., Ring, J. *et al.* (2003). Laboratory acquired infection with recombinant vaccinia virus containing an immunomodulating construct. *J Invest Dermatol*, *120*, 356-358.
Mervyn, H. G. (1925). Studies of the Viruses of Vaccinia and Variola.
Meselson, M., Guillemin, J., Hugh-Jones, M., Langmuir, A., Popova, I., Shelokov, A. *et al.* (1994). The Sverdlovsk anthrax outbreak of 1979. *Science*, *266*, 1202-1208.
Mezencev, R., & Mereish, K. (2005). How similar are poxviruses? *Science (New York, NY)*, *308*, 1259-1260.
"Midnight knock starts parents' ordeal" (1978, August 25). *Birmingham Evening Mail*, p. 5.
Miele, F. (1995). Darwin's Dangerous Disciple: An Interview with Richard Dawkins. *Skeptic magazine*, *3*.
Millard, C. K. (1943). Outbreak of Small-pox in Glasgow. *Br Med J*, *1*, 288-289.
Millard, C. K. (1945). Edinburgh Outbreak of Smallpox, 1942. *Br Med J*, *1*, 304-305.
Monthly Weather Report of the Meteorological Office (1950). December 1950. *67*.
"Mother of dead woman has smallpox" (1978, September 15). *The Times*, p. 2.
Motolinía, T. (1914). *Historia de los indios de la Nueva España: escrita a mediados del siglo XVI. Herederos de J. Gili.* Retieved from https://archive.org/details/historiadelosind00moto
Muzny, C. A., King, H., Byers, P., Currier, M., Nolan, R., & Mena, L. (2009). Vulvar vaccinia infection after sexual contact with a smallpox vaccinee. *Am J Med Sci*, *337*, 289-291.
Nagler, F. P., & Rake, G. (1948). The Use of the Electron Microscope in Diagnosis of Variola, Vaccinia, and Varicella. *J Bacteriol*, *55*, 45-51.
Negri, A. (1906). Über Filtration des Vaccinevirus. *Zeitschrift für*

Hygiene und Infektionskrankheiten, *54*, 327-346.
Nelson, J. B. (1943). The stability of variola virus propagated in embryonated eggs. *J Exp Med*, *78*, 231-239.
Nicol, W. (1980). Exotic infectious diseases: smallpox. *R Soc Health J*, *100*, 41-47.
Noble, J. (1970). A study of New and Old World monkeys to determine the likelihood of a simian reservoir of smallpox. *Bull World Health Organ*, *42*, 509-514.
Nolen, L. D., Osadebe, L., Katomba, J., Likofata, J., Mukadi, D., Monroe, B. *et al.* (2016). Extended Human-to-Human Transmission during a Monkeypox Outbreak in the Democratic Republic of the Congo. *Emerg Infect Dis*, *22*, 1014-1021.
Normile, D. (2004). Infectious diseases. Second lab accident fuels fears about SARS. *Science*, *303*, 26.
Noyce, R. S., Lederman, S., & Evans, D. H. (2018). Construction of an infectious horsepox virus vaccine from chemically synthesized DNA fragments. *PLoS One*, *13*, e0188453.
"Obituary A. B. Christie." (1992). *Br Med J*, *304*, 443.
"Obituary Brodie Hughes. Neurosurgeon in sight and sound" (1989, April 26). *The Guardian*, p. 47.
"Obituary E. B. C. Hughes." (1989). *Br Med J*, *298*, 1245.
"Obituary G. E. Breen." (1981). *Br Med J*, *283*, 1747.
"Obituary: Henry Samuel Bedson." (1978). *The Lancet*, *312*, 641.
Oliveira, J. S., Figueiredo, P. O., Costa, G. B., Assis, F. L., Drumond, B. P., da Fonseca, F. G. *et al.* (2017). Vaccinia Virus Natural Infections in Brazil: The Good, the Bad, and the Ugly. *Viruses*, *9*, pii: E340
Olson, V. A., & Shchelkunov, S. N. (2017). Are We Prepared in Case of a Possible Smallpox-Like Disease Emergence? *Viruses*, *9*, 242.
Openshaw, P. J., Alwan, W. H., Cherrie, A. H., & Record, F. M. (1991). Accidental infection of laboratory worker with recombinant vaccinia virus. *Lancet*, *338*, 459.
Orellana, C. (2004). Laboratory-acquired SARS raises worries on biosafety. *Lancet Infect Dis*, *4*, 64.
Osman, A. (1978, September 9). Coroner and press men clash over hounding and telephoning of smallpox chief and his family *The Times*, p. 2.
"Pakistanis' windows broken. "Smallpox" insults at Bradford." (1962, January 20). *The Guardian*, p. 3.
Paschen, E. (1906). Was wissen wir über den Vakzineerreger. *Münchner medizinische Wochenschrift*, *53*, 2391-2393.

Patterson, K. B., & Runge, T. (2002). Smallpox and the Native American. *Am J Med Sci*, *323*, 216-222.

Pattinson, T. "Obituary: Clive Jenkins." (1999, September 22). Obituary: Clive Jenkins. *The Independent*.

Peck, J., & Tickell, A. (2002). Neoliberalizing space. *Antipode*, *34*, 380-404.

Peiris, J. S., Yuen, K. Y., Osterhaus, A. D., & Stöhr, K. (2003). The severe acute respiratory syndrome. *N Engl J Med*, *349*, 2431-2441.

Pennington, H. (2002). Smallpox scares. *London Review of Books*, *24*, 32-33.

"Philip Cox, radar operator – obituary." (2015, March 15). *The Telegraph*. Retrieved from http://www.telegraph.co.uk/news/obituaries/11473278/Philip-Cox-radar-operator-obituary.html

Pidd, H. (2013, May 28). Lucy Meadows coroner tells press: 'shame on you' *The Guardian*. Retrieved from https://www.theguardian.com/uk/2013/may/28/lucy-meadows-coroner-press-shame

Pike, R. M. (1976). Laboratory-associated infections: summary and analysis of 3921 cases. *Health Lab Sci*, *13*, 105-114.

Pinker, S. (2018). *Enlightenment Now: The Case for Reason, Science, Humanism, and Progress*. Penguin UK.

Piskurek, O., & Okada, N. (2007). Poxviruses as possible vectors for horizontal transfer of retroposons from reptiles to mammals. *Proc Natl Acad Sci U S A*, *104*, 12046-12051.

"PO engineers hold out for 35-hour week." (1978, August 8). *The Guardian*, p. 24.

"Press harried smallpox professor, says coroner" (1978, September 9). *The Guardian*, p. 3.

Preston, R. (2002). *The Demon in the Freezer*. Headline.

Price, J. (2003). Smallpox cases in Brighton. *The Round Hill Reporter* http://www.roundhill.org.uk/main.php?sec=history&p=Smallpox_cases_in_Brighton

Qin, L., Favis, N., Famulski, J., & Evans, D. H. (2015). Evolution of and evolutionary relationships between extant vaccinia virus strains. *J Virol*, *89*, 1809-1824.

Quammen, D. (2012). *Spillover: animal infections and the next human pandemic*. London: Bodley Head.

Quick, J., Loman, N. J., Duraffour, S., Simpson, J. T., Severi, E., Cowley, L. *et al.* (2016). Real-time, portable genome sequencing for Ebola surveillance. *Nature*, *530*, 228-232.

Raoult, D., Audic, S., Robert, C., Abergel, C., Renesto, P., Ogata, H.

et al. (2004). The 1.2-megabase genome sequence of Mimivirus. *Science*, *306*, 1344-1350.

Razi, A. B. M. I. Z. (1848). *A Treatise on the Small-Pox and Measles*. London: The Sydenham Society. Retrieved from https://archive.org/details/39002086344042.med.yale.edu

Reardon, S. (2014a). Infectious diseases: Smallpox watch. *Nature*, *509*, 22-24.

Reardon, S. (2014b). 'Forgotten' NIH smallpox virus languishes on death row. *Nature*, *514*, 544.

Reed, D. L., Light, J. E., Allen, J. M., & Kirchman, J. J. (2007). Pair of lice lost or parasites regained: the evolutionary history of anthropoid primate lice. *BMC Biol*, *5*, 7.

Relman, D. A., Schmidt, T. M., MacDermott, R. P., & Falkow, S. (1992). Identification of the uncultured bacillus of Whipple's disease. *N Engl J Med*, *327*, 293-301.

Ricketts, T. F. (1908). *The diagnosis of smallpox*. Cassell. Retrieved from https://archive.org/details/diagnosisofsmall01rick

Riyesh, T., Karuppusamy, S., Bera, B. C., Barua, S., Virmani, N., Yadav, S. *et al.* (2014). Laboratory-acquired buffalopox virus infection, India. *Emerg Infect Dis*, *20*, 324-326.

Roe, A., & Roe, M. (2013). Obituaries: Reginald Arthur Shooter. *Br Med J*, *348*, g1241.

Ronson, J. (2016). *So you've been publicly shamed*. Riverhead Books.

Roy, J. (2010). *Smallpox Zero: An Illustrated History of Smallpox and Its Eradication*. Atlanta: Emory Global Health Institute.

Rubin, B. A. (1980). A note on the development of the bifurcated needle for smallpox vaccination. *WHO Chron*, *34*, 180-181.

Rubins, K. H., Hensley, L. E., Jahrling, P. B., Whitney, A. R., Geisbert, T. W., Huggins, J. W. *et al.* (2004). The host response to smallpox: analysis of the gene expression program in peripheral blood cells in a nonhuman primate model. *Proc Natl Acad Sci U S A*, *101*, 15190-15195.

Rubins, K. H., Hensley, L. E., Relman, D. A., & Brown, P. O. (2011). Stunned silence: gene expression programs in human cells infected with monkeypox or vaccinia virus. *PLoS One*, *6*, e15615.

Ruffer, M. A., & Ferguson, A. R. (1911). Note on an eruption resembling that of variola in the skin of a mummy of the twentieth dynasty (1200–1100 B.C.). *J Pathol*, *15*, 1-3.

Rustemeyer, T., & Frosch, P. J. (1995). Allergic contact dermatitis from colour developers. *Contact Dermatitis*, *32*, 59-60.

Rybicki, E. (2015). *A Short History of the Discovery of Viruses*. Apple iBook. https://itunes.apple.com/us/book/a-short-history-of-the-discovery-of-viruses/id1001627125?mt=11

Sample, I. (2014, December 4). Revealed: 100 safety breaches at UK labs handling potentially deadly diseases. *The Guardian*. Retrieved from https://www.theguardian.com/science/2014/dec/04/-sp-100-safety-breaches-uk-labs-potentially-deadly-diseases

Sample, I. (2018, February 9). Safety blunders expose lab staff to potentially lethal diseases in UK *The Guardian*. Retrieved from https://www.theguardian.com/science/2018/feb/09/safety-blunders-expose-uk-lab-staff-to-potentially-lethal-diseases

Schrick, L., Tausch, S. H., Dabrowski, P. W., Damaso, C. R., Esparza, J., & Nitsche, A. (2017). An Early American Smallpox Vaccine Based on Horsepox. *N Engl J Med*, *377*, 1491-1492.

Sharp, P. M., & Hahn, B. H. (2011). Origins of HIV and the AIDS pandemic. *Cold Spring Harb Perspect Med*, *1*, a006841.

Shchelkunov, S. N. (2009). How long ago did smallpox virus emerge? *Arch Virol*, *154*, 1865-1871.

Shchelkunov, S. N., Massung, R. F., & Esposito, J. J. (1995). Comparison of the genome DNA sequences of Bangladesh-1975 and India-1967 variola viruses. *Virus Res*, *36*, 107-118.

Shchelkunov, S. N., Totmenin, A. V., Loparev, V. N., Safronov, P. F., Gutorov, V. V., Chizhikov, V. E. *et al.* (2000). Alastrim smallpox variola minor virus genome DNA sequences. *Virology*, *266*, 361-386.

Shchelkunova, G. A., & Shchelkunov, S. N. (2017). 40 Years without Smallpox. *Acta Naturae*, *9*, 4-12.

Shooter, R. A. (1980). *Report of the investigation into the cause of the 1978 Birmingham smallpox occurrence*. London: HMSO.

"Shops clear shelves of tinned salmon" (1978, August 1). *The Guardian*, p. 1.

Silver, S. (2015). Laboratory-acquired lethal infections by potential bioweapons pathogens including Ebola in 2014. *FEMS Microbiol Lett*, *362*, 1-6.

Singh, K. (2009). Laboratory-acquired infections. *Clin Infect Dis*, *49*, 142-147.

Singh, K. (2011). It's time for a centralized registry of laboratory-acquired infections. *Nat Med*, *17*, 919.

Singh, R. K., Hosamani, M., Balamurugan, V., Bhanuprakash, V., Rasool, T. J., & Yadav, M. P. (2007). Buffalopox: an emerging and re-emerging zoonosis. *Anim Health Res Rev*, *8*, 105-114.

"Sir Christopher Booth obituary" (2012, August 31). *The Guardian*. Retrieved from https://www.theguardian.com/society/2012/aug/31/sir-

christopher-booth
"Smallpox" *Hansard* HC Deb vol 652 col 32-37 (1962) Retrieved from http://hansard.millbanksystems.com/commons/1962/jan/23/smallpox
"Smallpox 'beaten' and 260 cleared" (1978, September 11). *The Guardian*, p. 26.
"Smallpox (Birmingham)" *Hansard* HC Deb vol 961 col 434-448 (1979) Retrieved from http://hansard.millbanksystems.com/commons/1979/jan/24/smallpox-birmingham
Smallpox 1961-2. (1963). London: HMSO.
"Smallpox and race relations." (1962, January 24). *The Guardian*, p. 10.
"Smallpox case death 'due to heart attack'" (1978). *The Times*, p. 5.
"Smallpox case inquiry" (1966, May 13). *The Guardian*, p. 1.
"Smallpox case is delayed" (1979, January 23). *The Guardian*, p. 3.
"Smallpox chief drama" (1978, September 2). *Daily Express*, p. 1.
"Smallpox expert is critical" (1978, September 2). *The Guardian*, p. 1.
"Smallpox family in new tragedy" (1978, September 15). *Daily Express*, p. 19.
"Smallpox father dies" (1978, September 6). *The Guardian*, p. 3.
"Smallpox Outbreak - Meschede, Federal Republic of Germany, 1970" (1970). *Wkly Epidem Rec*, *45*, 249-256.
"Smallpox warning from worried countries" (1978, September 2). *Daily Express*, p. 2.
"Smallpox: 2 new suspects" (1978, September 10). *Sunday Express*, p. 1.
Smith, M., & Sample, I. "Coronavirus victim's widow tells of grief as scientists scramble for treatment" (2013, March 15). *The Guardian*. Retrieved from https://www.theguardian.com/science/2013/mar/15/coronavirus-victim-widow-scientists-treatment
Smithson, C., Imbery, J., & Upton, C. (2017). Re-Assembly and Analysis of an Ancient Variola Virus Genome. *Viruses*, *9*. pii: E253
Steinhardt, E., Israeli, C., & Lambert, R. A. (1913). Studies on the cultivation of the virus of vaccinia. *J Infec Dis*, *13*, 294-300.
Steward, G. F., Culley, A. I., Mueller, J. A., Wood-Charlson, E. M., Belcaid, M., & Poisson, G. (2013). Are we missing half of the viruses in the ocean. *ISME J*, *7*, 672-679.
Stewart, J. (n.d.). Smallpox1962. An online archive of the

outbreaks in Wales and England. https://smallpox1962.wordpress.com
Stubbs, D. (2016, August 9). Eric Clapton & Enoch Powell To Morrissey: Race In British Music Since '76. Retrieved from http://thequietus.com/articles/20701-eric-clapton-racism-morrissey
"Suicide man 'not hounded'" (1980, February 25). *The Guardian*, p. 3.
"Suicide plea of smallpox chief" (1978, September 8). *Birmingham Evening Mail*, p. 1.
Tainsh, J. M. (1962). Eleven cases of smallpox. *Lancet*, *1*, 996-999.
Takemura, M. (2001). Poxviruses and the origin of the eukaryotic nucleus. *J Mol Evol*, *52*, 419-425.
"The Weather" (1978, September 1). *The Guardian*, p. 26.
Thiessen, M. A. (2014, October 20). A 'Dark Winter' of Ebola Terrorism? *Washington Post*. Retrieved from https://www.washingtonpost.com/opinions/marc-thiessen-a-dark-winter-of-ebola-terrorism/2014/10/20/4ebfb1d8-5865-11e4-8264-deed989ae9a2_story.html
"Tight security at smallpox inquest" (1978, September 13). *The Guardian*, p. 4.
Tolstoy, L. (1922). War and Peace (Translated Louise and Aylmer Maude). Retrieved from http://www.gutenberg.org/ebooks/2600
"Tories press for laboratory code" (1978, September 4). *The Guardian*, p. 2.
Tovey, D. (2004). The Bradford smallpox outbreak in 1962: a personal account. *J R Soc Med*, *97*, 244-247.
"Treacy, Rt Hon. Sir Colman Maurice (born 28 July 1949), a Lord Justice of Appeal, since 2012." (2018). *WHO'S WHO & WHO WAS WHO*. Retrived from http://www.ukwhoswho.com/view/10.1093/ww/9780199540884.001.0001/ww-9780199540884-e-37981
Tucker, J. B. (2002). *Scourge: The Once and Future Threat of Smallpox*. Grove Press.
Uglow, J. (2002). *The Lunar Men*.
"Union leader blames 'new' virus for smallpox death" (1978, October 19). *The Times*, p. 8.
"Union sues on smallpox" (1979, May 18). *The Guardian*, p. 4.
"UNSAFE!" (1979, January 4). *Daily Express*, p. 8.
Uryvaev, L. V. (2011). In memory of V. M. Zhdanov. *Epidemiology and Vaccinal Prevention*. http://www.epidemvac.ru/arhiv/2011/08/pamyati-vm-

zhdanova

Valdivia-Granda, W. A., Kann, M. G., & Malaga, J. (2007). Transcriptional interactions during smallpox infection and identification of early infection biomarkers. *Pac Symp Biocomput*, 100-111.

Varma, A. (2013, March 23). Birmingham grandad is UK's second Coronavirus victim *Birmingham Mail*. Retrieved from https://www.birminghammail.co.uk/news/health/birmingham-grandad-abid-hussain-uks-1877516

Voice of America (2009). Asia Marks 30 Years since World Declared Free of Smallpox. https://www.voanews.com/a/a-13-2009-07-31-voa16-68743717/410219.html

Vorou, R. M., Papavassiliou, V. G., & Pierroutsakos, I. N. (2008). Cowpox virus infection: an emerging health threat. *Curr Opin Infect Dis*, *21*, 153-156.

Wade, M. (1978a). *On the Sidelines*. University of Birmingham special collection. Ref. pZ1-pZ675 H7 N.

Wade, N. (1978b). New smallpox outbreak leads scientist to suicide. *Science*, *201*, 1108.

Wade, O. L. (1996). *When I Dropped the Knife: The Joys, Excitements, Frustrations and Conflicts of a Life in Academic Medicine*. Edinburgh: The Pentland Press.

Wade, O. L. (1978c). *Diary kept by Professor O. L. Wade concerning smallpox alert*. University of Birmingham special collection. Ref. pZ1-pZ675 H7 N.

Wahl-Jensen, V., Cann, J. A., Rubins, K. H., Huggins, J. W., Fisher, R. W., Johnson, A. J. *et al.* (2011). Progression of pathogenic events in cynomolgus macaques infected with variola virus. *PLoS One*, *6*, e24832.

Waller, J. (2002). *The Discovery of the Germ*. New York: Columbia University Press.

Wanklyn, W. M. (1913). *Administrative Control of Smallpox*. London.

"Was the Birmingham Outbreak Really Smallpox?" (1978). *New Scientist*, *80*, 155.

Wehrle, P. F., Posch, J., Richter, K. H., & Henderson, D. A. (1970). An airborne outbreak of smallpox in a German hospital and its significance with respect to other recent outbreaks in Europe. *Bull World Health Organ*, *43*, 669-679.

Weinstein, I. (1947). An Outbreak of Smallpox in New York City. *Am J Public Health Nations Health*, *37*, 1376-1384.

Wertheim, J. O., Smith, M. D., Smith, D. M., Scheffler, K., & Kosakovsky Pond, S. L. (2014). Evolutionary origins of human herpes simplex viruses 1 and 2. *Mol Biol Evol*, *31*, 2356-2364.

Williams, G. (2010). *Angel of Death: The Story of Smallpox*. Palgrave Macmillan.

Witcover, J. (2014). Lincoln's vice-presidential switch changed history *Chicago Tribune*. Retrieved from http://www.chicagotribune.com/news/columnists/sns-201411141300--tms--poltodayctnyq-a20141116-20141116-column.html

"Witton Isolation Hospital, Birmingham" *Hansard* HC Deb vol 746 col 1961-1974 (1967) Retrieved from http://hansard.millbanksystems.com/commons/1967/may/12/witton-isolation-hospital-birmingham

Wolfe, N. D., Dunavan, C. P., & Diamond, J. (2007). Origins of major human infectious diseases. *Nature*, *447*, 279-283.

World Health Organization. (1980). *Declaration of Global Eradication of Smallpox*. Proceedings from World Health Assembly Resolution WHA333. Retrieved from http://apps.who.int/iris/bitstream/10665/223060/1/WER5520_148-148.PDF

Wurtz, N., Papa, A., Hukic, M., Di Caro, A., Leparc-Goffart, I., Leroy, E. *et al.* (2016). Survey of laboratory-acquired infections around the world in biosafety level 3 and 4 laboratories. *Eur J Clin Microbiol Infect Dis*, *35*, 1247-1258.

Young, A. (2014, August 17). Hundreds of bioterror lab mishaps cloaked in secrecy *USA TODAY*. Retrieved from https://www.usatoday.com/story/news/nation/2014/08/17/reports-of-incidents-at-bioterror-select-agent-labs/14140483/

Yutin, N., Wolf, Y. I., & Koonin, E. V. (2014). Origin of giant viruses from smaller DNA viruses not from a fourth domain of cellular life. *Virology*, *466-467*, 38-52.

Zaki, A. M., van Boheemen, S., Bestebroer, T. M., Osterhaus, A. D., & Fouchier, R. A. (2012). Isolation of a novel coronavirus from a man with pneumonia in Saudi Arabia. *N Engl J Med*, *367*, 1814-1820.

Zimmer, C. (2015). A Planet of Viruses. Second Edition. University of Chicago Press.

INDEX

Printed in Great Britain
by Amazon

51418227R00201